A Colour Atlas of

Geriatric Medicine

Asif Kamal
MBBS, MRCP
Consultant Physician in Geriatric Medicine, St George's Hospital, Lincoln

J C Brocklehurst
MD, MSc, FRCP (Glasgow & Edin.)
Professor of Geriatric Medicine, University of Manchester

Wolfe Medical Publications Ltd

Published by Wolfe Medical Publications Ltd, 1983
Printed by Royal Smeets Offset b.v.,
Weert, Netherlands
ISBN 0 7234 0812 2

This book is one of the titles in the series of Wolfe Medical Atlases, a series which brings together probably the world's largest systematic published collection of diagnostic colour photographs.
For a full list of Atlases in the series, plus forthcoming titles and details of our surgical, dental and veterinary Atlases, please write to Wolfe Medical Publications Ltd, Wolfe House, 3 Conway Street, London W1P 6HE.

General Editor, Wolfe Medical Atlases:
G. Barry Carruthers, MD(London)

Contents

Acknowledgements

We wish to express our most grateful thanks to all those who helped us in the preparation of this Atlas, especially our numerous sources and colleagues listed below who loaned us illustrations. Dr D. Prangell (**6 to 8, 11, 44, 189, 190**), Dr Ian Burton (**9**), Dr C. D. G. Beardwell (**19**), Mr E. N. Gleve (**20**), Dr J. P. Miller (**27, 231**), Dr P. J. August (**28, 51 to 53**), Dr Allen (**33**), Professor Stanley L. Robins and W. B. Saunders (**43, 92, 93, 97, 98, 101, 116**), Dr Tony Clark (**129a and b**), Dept. of Pathology, County Hospital, Lincoln (**46, 47**), Churchill Livingstone and Dr D. A. Leighton (**67**), Janssen Pharmaceutical Ltd (**77**), Churchill Livingstone and Professor M. S. Pathy (**82, 124, 125**), Saskatoon University (**85, 86**), Update Publications (**87, 89 to 91, 283**), Update Publications and Dr Michael Maisey (**94, 100**), Churchill Livingstone and Dr A. D. Dayan (**114, 117, 120**), Churchill Livingstone and Dr D. M. Bowen & Dr A. M. Davidson (**118**), Churchill Livingstone and Dr H. M. Wisniewski (**119, 121**), Dr John Carty (**128, 228, 252**), Dr B. Ottridge (**137**), Dr A. Pomerance (**151**), Dr Ian Paterson (**155**), Dr Brian Scott (**159, 161, 192 to 195, 197**), University Hospital of South Manchester, Xray Dept. (**173, 202, 203, 251**), Duphur Laboratories (**201, 205, 206**), Dr P. S. Haselton (**203a**), Churchill Livingstone (**213**), Churchill Livingstone and Dr R. Grahame (**260**), Churchill Livingstone and Professor A. N. Exton-Smith (**276**), Professor Douglas Gardner (**278, 279, 281**), London Foot Hospital and *Geriatric Medicine* (**306, 321**), Professor Stanley L. Robins and W. B. Saunders (**313**), Professor R. Marks and *Geriatric Medicine* (**333, 338**), Dr J. T. Leeming (**342**), Dr I. H. Taylor (**346**), Dr S. Mejzner (**351**), Dr R. H. MacDonald (**354, 358, 359, 361**).

Our sincere thanks are also due to Dr Michael Lye for his helpful advice on the manuscript, to Gus de Cozar and Peter Wilson of the Medical Illustrations Department of St. George's Hospital, Lincoln, to the Medical Illustration Department of University Hospital of South Manchester and to our secretaries. Our special thanks to Maureen Coffey for helping to collect the transparencies and typing the manuscript.

A. Kamal
J. C. Brocklehurst

Preface

Clinical presentation of disease in old age is often different from that in younger patients. This and the fact that old people also show the changes of ageing and of multiple pathology, makes clinical assessment, treatment, and rehabilitation all the more challenging.

Interpretation of these subtleties of disease in older patients demands a knowledge of the normal and abnormal phenomena associated with ageing. This Atlas shows some of the more important and interesting clinical features of geriatric medicine. The range of illustrations is as broad as possible; inevitably there is overlap with other specialities of medicine. This reflects the breadth of clinical practice in old age and bears out the often heard statement that geriatrics is the last remaining generalist area among the medical specialists.

This Atlas is a comprehensive introduction to geriatric medicine and complements standard reference textbooks on the subject. The emphasis throughout is on clinical features and presentation. Details of treatment, management, and rehabilitation are not included because of their complex and extensive nature.

The Atlas begins with **three** introductory chapters:

1 **Geriatric medicine**
2 **Special features of illness in old age**
3 **Assessment of an elderly patient**

These are followed by illustrated sections divided on an anatomical basis (i.e. head, face and neck, upper limbs, and so on).

Where relevant, some pictures or groups of pictures are supported by a somewhat longer textual description of the condition illustrated – its aetiology and importance in the elderly. In some cases differential diagnosis is also considered in table form.

We hope that this Atlas will be a valuable aid for all who care for ill and frail old people, especially doctors, nurses, physiotherapists, occupational therapists, and medical students. It should also be of considerable use to postgraduate students who are preparing for higher professional examinations.

1 Geriatric medicine

Industrialised countries of the world have experienced dramatic population changes in the 20th century. There has, for example, been a considerable increase in the proportion of elderly persons. At the beginning of this century, 4.7 per cent of the population of Britain was 65 years of age and over. By 1980 the figure had risen to 14.5 per cent. By the early part of the 21st century it seems likely that this steep rise in the 65-plus group will end, but the proportion of those who are 75 years of age and over will continue to rise. Indeed, a 20 per cent increase in the number of people in Britain who are 75 years of age and over may be expected within the next 20 years; this in the face of almost zero total population growth.

These changes are the result of radical improvements in public health – nutrition, environment, elimination of infectious disease by inoculations and vaccinations, and the spectacular reduction in infant mortality. Almost everyone may now expect to live to be old. While this marks a stage of great success in human development, it also brings its own problems.

As long as ageing is associated with frailty and an increasing likelihood of disabling illness, so the demands on health and welfare services by an ageing population will increase. These include demands on personal social services, on special housing and residential homes as well as on the hospital and community medical services.

By the year 2001, on current trends, elderly males could occupy 75 per cent and elderly females 90 per cent of all acute general hospital beds.

Definition of geriatric medicine

Geriatric medicine is a branch of general medicine concerned with the clinical, preventative, remedial and social aspects of health and disease in the elderly.

Modern geriatrics and new patterns of care

A well organised geriatric medicine service has a major role to play in dealing with the consequences of these demographic trends. Most people over 65 years of age live independently in the community. It is the prime function of the geriatric services to help to maintain this independence. The services should be able to prevent breakdown or to deal with it quickly enough to enable the elderly to continue caring for themselves and to help them to enjoy life.

The role of the newly retired

Retirement used to be the gateway to old age. This is no longer true. Today, people live longer but retire earlier. Retirement has become the 'third age' – a time of great opportunity but, to some, a time of bewilderment and boredom. The way in which a person copes with retirement may have a profound effect on his health in old age.

The role of the young

The young also have a considerable contribution to make towards the welfare of the elderly. Grandchildren and grandparents often have a special relationship which benefits both. Young people, through youth and voluntary groups, school and university schemes, and on an individual basis, can help old people in many ways. This can range from giving old people help with their shopping, house cleaning, gardening, laundry and painting. Young people could also be a source of companionship.

Attitudes towards the aged

Society has ambivalent attitudes towards the aged. There is a sizeable gap between the expressed concern for the needs of older people and the action taken to meet such needs. Generally, people feel hostile towards the aged, but at the same time they enjoy good relationships with the elderly within their own circle. Resentment and antagonism may arise from the lack of a clearly defined role for old people in modern industrialised society and also as a result of their economic dependency. Such negative attitudes are gradually being eroded by education and the development of geriatric medical units, as well as by special organisations which pinpoint the numerous problems.

Families, generally care for their aged – a fact which is not always acknowledged publicly. However, today over one-third of people who are 75 years of age and over have no surviving children and caring neighbours as well as back-up services are very important.

Inevitably some negative attitudes rub off on medical workers. Hostility or indifference towards the development of geriatric services has been a common phenomenon in many parts of the world. Fortunately, this changes as the geriatric service is able to demonstrate its achievements, and as medical and other students learn about the complexities of medicine and old age and how the service copes.

Deprivation of the aged

The most deprived members of the community are often old people. More than any other social group they live in low-standard housing – badly insulated, damp, draughty, and difficult to heat and sometimes with outside lavatories. Complications of such deprivation include accidental hypothermia, accidents, impairment of mobility, susceptibility to illness, depression, impaired nutrition and, in some cases, a resistance to discharge from hospital.

The complexity of financial benefits available to the old is such that many old people have no idea of their rights and entitlements. The key role of social workers and special organisations is thus apparent.

Nevertheless, the complications of poor nutrition are still commonplace among old people. These include scurvy, osteomalacia, hypokalemia and anaemia.

Breakdown in old age

Ageing is distinguished from disease by the fact that it is universal. From a practical point of view, however, its major quality is that it decreases function of cells, organs and so of the organism. Ageing thus predisposes to breakdown although ageing itself does not produce breakdown. Few old people escape the accumulation of chronic pathologies as they grow older, and the cumulative effect of this is another ingredient in the breakdown.

Multiple pathologies leading to multiple symptoms are often matched by the prescription of many drugs. Unfortunately these in themselves not infrequently predispose to breakdown in independent living, because either singly or in combination they may lead to significant loss of independence. Problems include mistakes in compliance caused by poor memory or poor vision; the changes in pharmacodynamics and pharmacokinetics which occur in ageing people and which many prescribers are still unaware of; and the tendency of some physicians to use drugs with profound side-effects in old age (such as the benzodiazepines) almost as placebos.

All these factors tend to cause breakdown in independent living in the elderly unless counterbalanced by such social and neighbourhood support systems as are available, and by the extent of physical and mental health which the old person maintains, and above all by the desire to retain independence. However, this uneasy equilibrium is easily destroyed by the addition of acute medical illness on the one side and the loss of social or other support on the other.

It is in responding to this breakdown, either that which occurs suddenly and acutely as an emergency or gradually over days or weeks, that the geriatric service has its most unique and important role.

Who is a geriatric patient?

Most patients under the care of geriatricians are in their late seventies and eighties and, apart from acute medical illness, they also have multiple chronic disabilities and/or complex social problems. Most geriatricians in the United Kingdom would see their work in the following terms:

1 Immediate admission from the community of elderly patients presenting with problems of extreme medical urgency.

2 Assessment of patients with similar but less urgent problems, either in their own homes, or at the hospital outpatient clinic.
3 The continuing management of physically disabling disease in old age through stages of rehabilitation, both in hospital and in the day hospital, and perhaps indefinite support in the community after that.
4 The long-term care of old people who are so physically disabled as to be unable to maintain independence in the community.
5 The short-term admission of elderly patients for holiday purposes, which is basically for the relief of relatives and family.
6 The transfer of patients from other hospital departments, either for rehabilitation or long-term care.
7 Participation in co-operative medical care with one or more of the following departments: psychiatry, orthopaedics, young disabled, stroke rehabilitation, and rheumatology and physical medicine.

The aims of geriatric medicine

1 Maintenance of health in old age by continuing social engagement and avoidance of disease.
2 Early detection and appropriate treatment of disease.
3 Maintenance of maximum independence consistent with irreversible disease and disability.
4 Sympathetic care and support during terminal illness.

Geriatric medicine is a dynamic process in which the patient's needs are assessed in detail by a multidisciplinary team. An appropriate plan of medical treatment, rehabilitation and social work is drawn up so as to restore the elderly patient to as normal a life as possible.

Structure of geriatric services

Geriatric medicine is a relatively young specialty and practice varies a great deal. In many parts of the world it is still at an early stage of development. While much of the success of a geriatric service depends on the resources and facilities available, the most important factor is the personality, drive and clinical ability of the geriatrician.

Most geriatric services in the UK are based on the principle of progressive patient care and consist of:

1 Acute admissions/assessment ward
2 Rehabilitation ward
3 Long-term care ward
4 Minimal care ward
5 Day hospital

and facilities such as outpatient department, domiciliary assessment visiting, combined clinics with orthopaedic surgeons and psychogeriatricians. Back-up hospital services include laboratory facilities, xrays and other imaging techniques, physiotherapy, occupational therapy, speech therapy, chiropody, and a social services department.

Acute assessment ward

Most admissions to a geriatric department are to an acute assessment ward. The basic function and management on this ward is similar to that of general medical wards. Elderly patients are admitted as emergencies or planned admissions for medical diagnosis, functional and social assessment and for treatment.

The ward must be properly equipped for the elderly with low beds and beds of variable height. There should be easy access to lavatories and the ward should be easily accessible to all other hospital services. The nurses should have special understanding and training in geriatric medicine, and the medical staff should include young doctors undergoing general medical training.

All discharges need careful planning with the involvement of the therapists, social workers and community support groups. Rehabilitation of the geriatric patient starts right from the beginning, but if this is likely to continue for several weeks after the initial assessment and treatment, then the patient is generally transferred to the rehabilitation ward.

Rehabilitation ward

It is in the rehabilitation ward that geriatric team work is most to the fore. The underlying physical problems are varied and include conditions such as cerebrovascular disease, cardiovascular disease, fracture of the femur, amputation, Parkinson's disease, and musculoskeletal disorders. The restoration of optimal function may require treatment over several weeks or months. The patients may be transferred here from the acute geriatric ward or medical, orthopaedic, and surgical wards. Management is usually through case conferences and once again discharge needs to be meticulously planned.

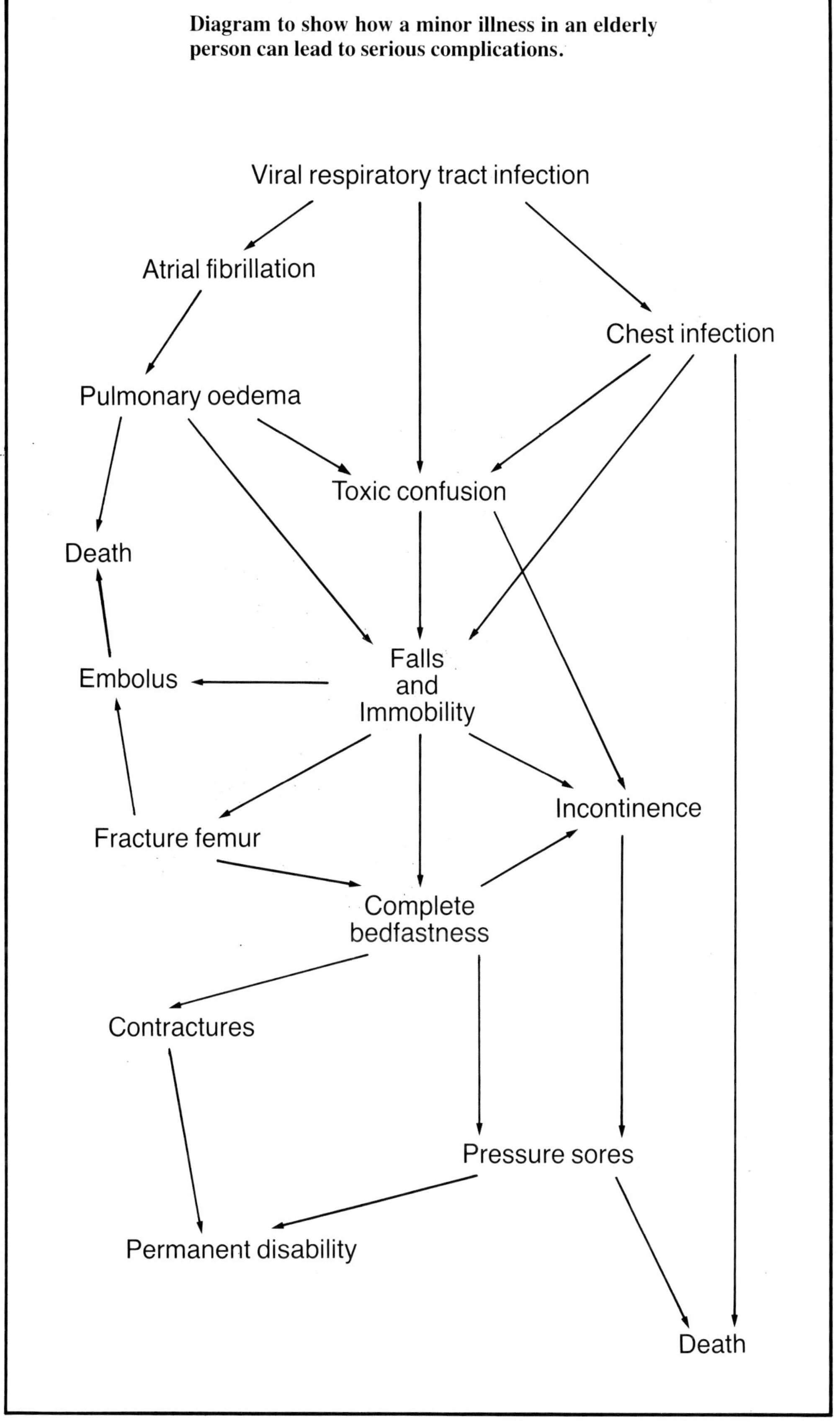
Diagram to show how a minor illness in an elderly person can lead to serious complications.
Viral respiratory tract infection
Atrial fibrillation
Chest infection
Pulmonary oedema
Toxic confusion
Death
Falls and Immobility
Embolus
Incontinence
Fracture femur
Complete bedfastness
Contractures
Pressure sores
Permanent disability
Death

Long-term care ward
If rehabilitation does not restore sufficient independence for discharge into the community, then long-term hospital care will be required. Wards providing this service have a very different function to those involved in assessment and rehabilitation. They become the patient's home and the most important person in the patient's life is the nurse.

Medical investigations and intensive remedial therapy play a small part. It is the quality of life which matters most, and this should stem from an appropriate blend of maximum privacy and maximum security. Single bedrooms are optimal if they can be provided. Areas for activities should include a quiet room where patients may escape from the noise and distractions which are so inseparably bound to most hospitals. Staff should include activities organisers and volunteers, relatives, and visitors should be encouraged at all times of the day.

In some geriatric departments the three types of ward described above are combined in one. This has some advantages inasmuch as the staff deal with patients with all kinds of problems. On the other hand, the homely atmosphere appropriate to the quality of life in a long-term care ward is inappropriate in the management of acutely ill patients, so that this compromise is more likely to be of benefit to the staff than to the patients.

Minimal care ward
If there is a shortage of residential accommodation and special housing, it may be convenient to develop a minimal care ward or convalescent ward, where patients may be transferred until suitable accommodation is found. Such wards usually have a lower ratio of nursing staff. Most patients on these wards tend to be fully ambulant and independent in self-care.

Geriatric day hospital
Geriatric day hospitals have shown considerable development over the last 20 years. They aim to provide some hospital facilities without the patients having to stay overnight and over the weekend. Patients may attend after inpatient assessment and rehabilitation, but about 50 per cent of the patients attending the day hospital come straight from the community, and so inpatient admission is avoided. The day hospital has four main objectives:

1 Rehabilitation.
2 Maintenance of treatment – to ensure that levels of independence achieved as a result of rehabilitation are kept at an optimal level.
3 Social care of the physically disabled – to provide social companionship for those who are housebound and isolated and so to prevent depression, or else relieve relatives and help them to cope for a longer period.
4 For medical and nursing assessment, investigations and treatment.

2 Special features of illness in old age

Presenting symptoms

Some of the features distinguishing medicine in old age from medicine in younger age groups are the four cardinal presenting symptoms of illness in old age. These are *mental confusion, incontinence, instability,* and *immobility.* Each is a symptom and the common underlying factor is the effect of ageing on the central nervous system. Because of the diminished reserve of cortical neurones many acute illnesses producing anoxaemia and toxaemia overcome the limited reserve of cerebral function and present as confusion. Similarly, the cerebral control of micturition is precarious because of ageing and thus many pathologies, both systemic and local, may precipitate incontinence. Similarly, balance is less certain and postural instability or falling is the third common presenting symptom. Finally, there is a tendency towards immobility, not only as a result of ageing in the central nervous system but also its effects on muscles and joints, together with chronic pathological changes such as osteoarthrosis and foot disorders. Therefore, much illness in old people presents with one of these four symptoms – each requires as careful a differential diagnosis as other symptoms such as pain, fever, vomiting, and dyspnea.

Acute illness in the elderly

Acute brain failure or acute confusional disorders are thus compounded of underlying age change of the brain, and an acute pathology which may further impair blood or oxygen supply to the brain, affect it by toxins or by direct involvement by vascular disorder.

Thus:

1 Acute anoxic brain failure may result from bronchopneumonia, congestive cardiac failure, acute bronchitis, pulmonary collapse or an acute impairment of cardiac output, associated with sudden onset of a rapid dysrhythmia or a myocardial infarct.
2 Acute infections such as pyelitis, pneumonia, sub-acute bacterial endocarditis, and influenza may all present with toxic acute brain failure. Metabolic toxaemia such as hepatic failure, uraemia, hyperglycaemia may all present with a toxic confusional state.
3 Acute poisoning with drugs and alcohol and hypoglycaemia may all present similarly.

Sometimes the confusion masks other common presenting symptoms such as pain in myocardial infarction and in acute appendicitis. An elderly person may of course present acutely with any of the wide range of medical illnesses found in other age groups; for example, acute abdomen, subarachnoid haemorrhage, urinary retention, acute pulmonary oedema, pulmonary embolism, etc.

Chronic illness in the elderly

The longer people live the more likely they are to contract chronic disabilities. Chronic airways obstructive disease probably affects about 20 per cent of elderly people today. Congestive cardiac failure may be insidious in its onset as may diabetes.

In the central nervous system cerebrovascular disease causing stroke is probably the commonest disability. Parkinsonism is also common in old people.

In the musculoskeletal system a major cause of disability is osteoarthrosis, particularly in the hip, knee and spine.

Peripheral vascular disease leading to intermittent claudication, leg ulceration and amputation is another common cause of disability.

Multiple pathologies

Having these aspects of acute and chronic illness in mind it is clear that the range of clinical presentation in old people is tremendous. For instance, a myocardial infarct presenting with mental confusion may precipitate incontinence, and the outcome may be affected also by underlying chronic obstructive airways disease and diabetes.

A small acute stroke may present with urinary incontinence, to which also partial immobility due to osteoarthrosis of the hip may contribute.

Anaemia, perhaps a symptom of diverticular disease of the colon or chronic blood loss from hiatus hernia, may present as a series of falls and a developing chairfast state.

Atherosclerosis

Probably the most important single pathological process underlying disability in old age is atherosclerosis. Unhappily, the cause of atherosclerosis still eludes us, although there is now a good deal of evidence about related factors. The most important association is that with high levels of total low-density lipoproteins. This occurs both in geographical areas where atherosclerosis is common and also in a series of pathological conditions associated with atherosclerosis; for example, the nephrotic syndrome, hyperthyroidsim, uncontrolled diabetes mellitus, and chronic biliary cirrhosis. Other important factors are hypertension, obesity, smoking, diet, and stress.

While atherosclerosis may appear anywhere throughout the vascular tree, its consequences in old age are mainly limited to the brain (cerebrovascular disease and multi-infarct dementia), the myocardium (ischaemia and infarction), and the peripheral arteries (leg ulcer and gangrene).

Stroke

While little progress has been made in treating the acute phase of stroke, in recent years there have been considerable advances in its prevention on the one hand and in rehabilitation on the other. The increasingly widespread control of hypertension in the middle-aged and the treatment of carotid transient ischaemic attacks by aspirin, other antiplatelet drugs, and anticoagulants have both contributed to the decline in the incidence of stroke. At the same time an increasing interest in rehabilitation has led to a realisation of the importance of perceptual disorders and disorders of body image, particularly in non-dominant hemisphere strokes.

The development of stroke rehabilitation units has led to a renewed interest among medical and paramedical staff in the management of stroke patients. Future trends are likely to see more domiciliary treatment with better advice to the patient and his relatives at home, so that they may have a clearer understanding of its very complex problems.

Musculoskeletal disease

Myopathies and arthropathies may all present as postural instability or as increasing immobility. The eminently treatable proximal myopathy of osteomalacia is being recognised in the elderly with much greater frequency. The operative treatment of osteoarthrosis has opened new horizons for many painfully disabled old people. The development of combined orthopaedic geriatric units is improving the outcome for the more difficult fractures of the femur.

Instability and falls

Recognition of the many possible causes of falls in old people is leading to a more rational approach in treatment, although some of the most common causes (drop-attacks) still defy explanation and prevention.

Incontinence

It is only in recent years that the widespread prevalence of incontinence among people of all age groups is becoming realised. Urodynamic assessment units have provided much information but drug therapy of the unstable bladder is still unsatisfactory. On the other hand, the management of stress incontinence and the realisation of the frequency of iatrogenic causes (chronic retention and overflow incontinence as a side-effect of antidepressant and anticholenergic drugs) is far more clearly understood. A better assessment of the place of indwelling catheters and of different types of body-worn protection is stemming from the development of specialist nurse advisors in this very difficult problem.

Constipation

This remains the great scourge of immobile old people, particularly those in long-term care and faecal incontinence is its symptom. The management of such a simple and unpleasant condition requires a great deal of investigation.

Hypothermia

One of the greatest successes in health education, in relation to old age, has been in spreading knowledge about hypothermia. As a result it is far more commonly recognised now than ten years ago. Nevertheless, sub-optimal housing conditions and a need (or perceived need) to save fuel, still affects thousands of old people during winter.

Disorders of the senses

A recent study has shown that a considerable number of people over 70 years of age suffer from hearing disorders which, if diagnosed by an audiologist, would certainly lead him to prescribe a hearing aid. The same study showed a significant correlation between depression and hearing impairment in old age. Amplification is not the whole answer to this problem although a small, behind-the-ear hearing aid is much more acceptable. The complexity of presbyacusis is now being recognised and the need for counselling, not just of the patient but of also those who come in contact, as how to speak to elderly deaf people is now being understood.

Much visual disorder is well dealt with by ophthalmologists although in many cases underlying senile macular degeneration, presently an incurable condition, limits the outcome of treatment.

Psychogeriatric problems

The pathological process which stands alongside atheroma, being the other most common cause of disability in old age, is senile dementia of the Alzheimer type. The pathological changes are similar to those occurring in Alzheimer's presenile dementia and some of these (for example, the senile plaque and neurofibrillary tangles) are found although to an extremely limited degree in the brains of very old normal people. The cause of this pathology is at present unknown, although theories include a slow virus infection, disorder of aluminium metabolism, and an inherited defect. Senile dementia of Alzheimer type together with multi-infarct dementia are possibly the two most feared illnesses in the latter part of life. It is estimated that 6 per cent of the over-65s and 20 per cent of the over-80s have these diseases in moderate and severe form. The problems these conditions generate for families and for the community are well known.

The speciality of psychogeriatrics has developed to provide a special expertise among psychiatrists in the total management of mental illness in the aged. This includes depression, paraphrenia and other disorders as well as the dementias. In the diagnosis of dementia a close collaboration between psychiatrist and geriatrician is important, and is found in most of the developing psychogeriatric units. Perhaps one of the most important aspects of the diagnosis of dementia is to discover potentially treatable causes like Vitamin-B_{12} deficiency, subdural haematoma, normal pressure hydrocephalus, and meningioma.

Malignant disease

Malignant disease is the second commonest cause of death in old age (the first being heart disease), and the commonest site in both sexes is the gastrointestinal system, particularly the colon and rectum. In some ways it is the most important site because the outcome of the surgical management of colorectal malignancy, if diagnosed at an early stage, is very good. Overall, carcinoma of the prostate is the most common malignancy in aged males. Carcinoma of the breast is runner-up in aged females. Both of these diseases are compatible with many years of life in old age.

Special hospices providing expert terminal care have developed in most of the cities in the United Kingdom and are being developed throughout the world. However, these are more likely to be centres of excellence and trend-setters than the place for the management of all terminal stages of cancer. They have been particularly successful in developing a rational policy of analgesia (ensuring a pain-free death), and in teaching doctors and nurses the importance of the psychological as well as the somatic approach to malignant disease.

Infection

An increasing realisation of the pleomorphic presentation of infection in old age is occurring. The need for blood cultures in patients presenting with acute brain failure for which other causes are not apparent – and particularly if they have a disease of the heart valves or infection of the bladder – is now well established.

Other common disorders

There are certain other diseases which have an inherent predilection for the elderly. Many of these disorders may present in a less dramatic way and in a considerable number of cases the mode of presentation may be altered too; for example, painless myocardial infarction presenting with acute brain failure, chronic constipation causing depression, etc. Conditions seen frequently in geriatric medical practice include Parkinsonism, motor-neuron disease, herpes zoster, polymyalgia rheumatica, giant-cell arteritis, pernicious anaemia, folate deficiency, leukaemias, hypothyroidism, tuberculosis, osteomalacia, osteoporosis, hyperosmolar non-ketotic diabetic crisis, scurvy, ischaemic colitis, hiatus hernia, and diverticular disease of the colon. This list is of course incomplete, but serves to indicate the range and diversity of geriatric medicine.

3 Assessment of an elderly patient

The general approach to history and clinical examination in old people is along the same lines as in younger patients. However, numbers of additional procedures should be undertaken in the elderly – this chapter is concerned with these procedures.

History

History is all important and with elderly patients more time is required because of deafness, poor memory, confusion, suspicion, and slow responses. Always ask simple, straightforward questions. If it cannot be reliably obtained from the patient then every effort must be made to interview someone who knows what has been the march of events; for example, neighbours, relatives, district nurse, home nurses, etc. The first thing to determine is when the patient was last perfectly normal. In the confused old person the history may be crucial in distinguishing between acute and chronic forms of brain failure. If there is reason to suspect that the history being obtained is unreliable, then some form of mental assessment must be carried out during the examination. Allowance must be made for the benign memory loss of normal ageing, in which recall of dates and names may be difficult but the story will be coherent and logical. On the other hand, the patient with mild to moderate dementia who is confabulating may present so plausible a story that it has every appearance of normality, until checked against that of the relatives or neighbours.

In the case of falls a good description is needed. It is usually best to get the patient to concentrate on one fall, probably the most recent, and describe it in detail.

Always ask about micturition habits – how often the patient has to get up at night to pass urine and whether there is any urgency by day. Ask specifically about bedwetting and wetting the clothes.

Dizziness is a difficult symptom to elucidate. It is very seldom that a history of rotational vertigo emerges and dizziness in most cases is probably a lightheadedness, which most elderly people experience in a transitory manner occasionally. It is not a sympton which requires treatment per se.

The social history is particularly relevant in old people having in mind bereavement, family contact, dietary habits, and the nature of housing and services that are used. It is also important to find out whether the patient's house is centrally heated, whether the toilet is situated a distance away from the main dwelling, the pattern of daily living, and the degree of independence within the house.

Mental testing may be introduced during or at the end of the history. It is useful to use a simple ten-question questionnaire such as that shown in Table 1. This will not only give an indication of normal cognitive function or moderate or severe abnormality; it will also record baseline data which may be used as points of reference on subsequent occasions. If the patient is sensible it is best to introduce the questionnaire as a test of memory, and it is usually accepted uncomplainingly as such.

Examination

There are certain points that must be remembered while examining an elderly patient. One must remember the prevalence of multiple pathology and also the normal age-related changes. The examination should be gentle at all times and one should try and avoid complicated manoeuvres.

First, get the patient to stand up and if possible, assess postural stability with the eyes open and closed, and the gait.

The general and systemic examination proceeds in the normal standard way. Common signs of ageing will be seen in the face – the wasting of orbital fat and of the muscles of the face, the arcus senilus, wrinkling of the skin, hair changes, and sometimes scars on the bridge of the nose indicating falls in the past. Other signs to look for are pigmentation, scratch marks, intertrigo, senile keratosis, bruises, and state of pressure areas. Breasts should be examined in every case. In the root of the neck beware pulsations from a kinked carotid artery. Senile purpura is occasionally seen in the neck and very commonly seen on the extensor aspect of the hands and forearms. Its significance is only that it is associated with transparent skin. In younger patients of course, it is associated with steroid medication and rheumatoid arthritis. Look out for Heberden's and Bouchard's nodes and the usual nail changes. In the legs and feet pay particular attention to foot deformities such as overgrown toenails, hallux valgus, and corns. Distinguish between pitting oedema and lymphoedema. See if erythema abigne suggests hypothyroidism.

Cardiovascular system

Systolic murmurs often present problems in old people. Ejection systolic murmurs, best heard at the base with or without radiation into the neck, may be caused by aortic sclerosis and not stenosis. The former is a benign increasing rigidity of the aortic ring and the aortic cusps but no actual obstruction to flow. A lower pitched pan-systolic murmur is also commonly present indicating mitral incompetence by its irradiation around the axilla and possibly into the back. This may be associated with mitral stenosis, secondary to enlargement of the left ventricle or caused by prolapsing leaflet of the mitral valve as a result of necrosis of the valve or of a papillary muscle.

Always listen for murmurs in the carotid artery.

Triple rhythms (third sound, fourth sound summation gallops) are a common harbinger of ventricular failure.

Always measure blood pressure with the patient supine and then repeat after the patient has stood erect for two minutes. This manoeuvre reveals the presence of postural hypotension. Palpation of the peripheral arteries in the lower limbs will probably have been carried out during the general examination.

Respiratory system

In the respiratory system the procedure is a little different from that in younger people. First, deviation of trachea is common as a result of dorsal scoliosis and chest expansion tends to be limited. Hypostatic basal crepitations are common in the elderly and will disappear after a few maximal respirations.

Central nervous system (CNS)

Examination of the central nervous system will depend in part upon the assumed diagnosis. If brain failure is thought to be present, then a record of the primitive reflexes should be included (grasp and groping reflex, snout and sucking reflex, and the palmomental and patellar tap reflexes). Their presence indicates widespread involvement of the frontal lobes.

Tremor has to be diagnosed carefully. A familial and a senile tremor are similar. They persist during activity or indeed may get worse, and they may or may not go away at rest. Choreoathetotic tremor is usually characteristic but Parkinsonian tremor is overdiagnosed. Its quality is very characteristic and it diminishes on activity. Orofacial movements and other dyskinesias should alert one to the toxic effect of phenothiazines or L-dopa. Some facial tics and plucking at the bedclothes are late signs of dementia. Age changes in neurotransmission in the long spinal tracts is thought to account for the diminution or absence of vibration sense of many old people in whom the sensation is retained in the upper limbs. For the same reason ankle jerks are quite often absent.

Gastrointestinal tract (GIT)

In the gastrointestinal tract always look at the tongue and examine the teeth or dentures. Monilial infections are not uncommon and in their absence a white, sodden tongue may be a nonspecific sign of illness, particularly in the gastrointestinal tract, or it may be one of the signs of Vitamin-B deficiency. In constipated patients faeces can be felt not only in the left iliac fossa but often in the transverse colon; the caecum, distended and doughy, is often palpable. Beware of tortuosity or aneurysm of the abdominal aorta – it is often misdiagnosed as an abdominal mass. Note also whether or not the bladder is distended. All women with urinary incontinence should have the perineum inspected, looking for leakage on coughing or for atrophy or redness of the genital epithelium, with or without superadded infection, indicating atrophic vaginitis. Vaginal examination is not always necessary, but it sometimes reveals a long-forgotten pessary, which is best removed.

In faecal incontinence and in any alimentary tract disorder, rectal examination is mandatory.

Tests

On any suspicion of hypothermia the temperature should be measured with a low-reading thermometer. If an ordinary clinical thermometer is the only one available it should be shaken right down. One should suspect the presence of hypothermia if there is no measurable rise. If the consultation and examination is the first that has been carried out for a year or more, then haematology and routine biochemistry should be performed, and a chest xray and an ECG carried out. These procedures will sometimes provide unexpected clues and in any case will provide baseline data for the future. The 48-hour Holter cardiac monitoring is now fairly generally available and may help to elucidate intermittent confusional episodes. However, remember that published series show as high an incidence of dysrhythmias in elderly control subjects as in symptomatic patients. Therefore, no causal relationship can be imputed unless the timing of the confusional episode is recorded at the same time: 48-hour monitoring will sometimes indicate ventricular arrhythmias or episodes of fast-flutter fibrillation which will respond to treatment.

The use of ultrasound or other imaging techniques and computerised axial tomography (CAT scan) are now becoming generally available and in many situations are as useful in the very old as in the young. However, the CAT scan is not yet regarded as an essential test in the differential diagnosis of dementia. Its place is where a focal lesion is strongly suspected – and particularly one that is remediable.

Further tests and investigations will of course be required depending upon the suspected diagnosis and for the monitoring of clinical progress.

The benefits of the investigations should be weighed carefully against the possible therapeutic benefits. However, it is absolutely wrong to deny an elderly patient any investigative manoeuvre just because he is old.

Table 1. Short mental status questionnaire for assessing the mental status in chronic brain failure (dementia).

(Score 1 for each correct response)

1 What is your name?
2 What is the name of this place? or Where are we now?
3 What year is this?
4 What month (or season) is this?
5 What day of the week is it today?
6 How old are you?
7 What is the name of the Prime Minister/the President of this country?
8 When did World War I start?
***Remember these three items. I will ask you to recall them in a few minutes. ***Standard items, bed, chair, window – have patient repeat before proceeding.
9 Count backwards from 20 to 1 (any uncorrected error – score 0).
10 Repeat the three items I asked you to remember. (Score ½ for any item remembered, or 1 for all three.)

Normal: 8 or above
Mild to moderate: 4–7
Moderate to severe: less than 4

4 Disorders of the head, face and neck

1

1 Healthy elderly face. This lady is over 100 years of age, but has a healthy, relatively young looking face, with only few signs of extreme old age.

2 Ageing face. This lady is also 100 years of age; the face shows signs of old age, with loss of periorbital fat and onset of baldness. Note the ectropion and evidence of recent fall.

3 Wasted face. A 60 year old man, looking older than his age. He has cachexia, secondary to carcinoma of stomach.

2

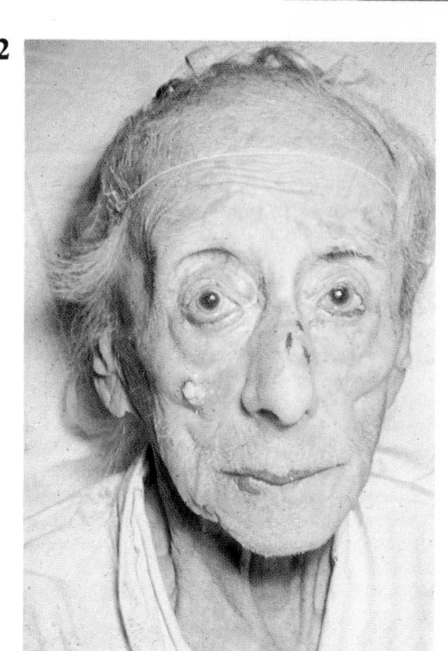

3

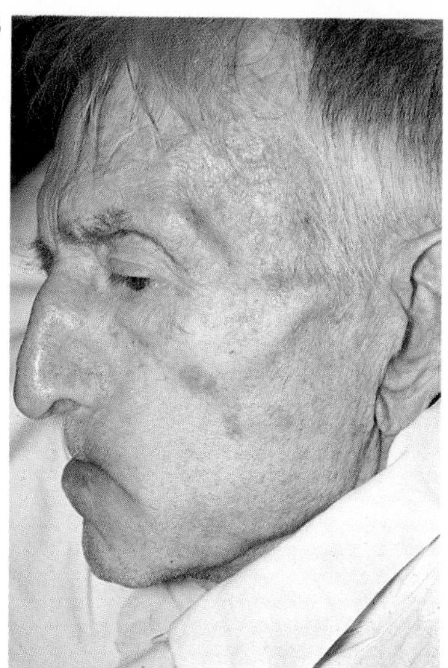

Anaemia in old age

Anaemia is said to be present when the haemoglobin is less than 13 grams in men and 12 grams in women.

Anaemia occurs in 5–20% of the elderly population. There are six main types:

1 Iron-deficency anaemia
2 Megaloblastic anaemia
3 Anaemia of chronic disease
4 Sideroblastic anaemia
5 Hypoplastic anaemia
6 Haemolytic anaemia

Iron-deficiency anaemia

Causes:
Poor nutrition, poverty, immobility, isolation.
Defective absorption – gastritis, post-gastrectomy malabsorption.
Excessive blood loss – peptic ulcer, hiatus hernia and oesophagitis, gastric carcinoma, colonic diverticular disease, carcinoma of large bowel, haemorrhoids, vaginal bleeding, haematuria.
Drugs – salicylates and some other analgesics, steroids.

Clinical features

Tend to be non-specific in early stages. Pallor, weakness, glossitis, confusion, falls, CCF, dysphagia (Plummer-Vinson syndrome), koilonychia and features of the condition causing the anaemia. Hypochromic microcytic RBCs.

4

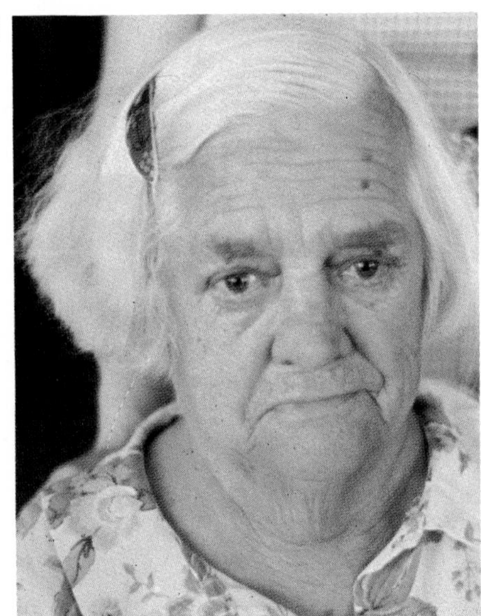

Megaloblastic anaemia

Vitamin-B_{12} deficiency:
Poor diet, pernicious anaemia, atrophic gastritis, gastrectomy, carcinoma of stomach, malabsorption, ileal resection.

Folate deficiency:
Poor diet and malabsorption, chronic diseases, neoplasm, liver disease, drugs, e.g. phenytoin.

Clinical features:
Non-specific signs of anaemia, yellow tinge to skin in pernicious anaemia, anorexia, glossitis, peripheral neuropathy, subacute combined degeneration, mild confusion, depression, dementia. Megaloblasts and macrocytes are typical haematological findings.

Sideroblastic anaemia

A type of hypochromic anaemia with ring sideroblasts in the bone marrow. Erythroblasts are loaded with iron (sideroblasts), but hypochromic anaemia results.

The primary aetiological factor is defective iron utilisation.

There are two main types:
1 Primary – acquired
2 Secondary – myeloproliferative disorders
Myeloma, carcinoma, collagen diseases, myxoedema, drugs, e.g. anti-TB, phenacetin, chloramphenicol.

Anaemia of chronic disease

Normochromic normocytic anaemia occurring in association with chronic diseases, e.g. TB, diverticulitis, rheumatoid arthritis, pressure sores, malignancy, hypothyroidism, renal failure.

Hypoplastic anaemia

Hypoplastic anaemia results from the failure of bone marrow and is not very common in old age. May be seen in association with myeloma, carcinomas, myeloproliferative disorders, and various drugs.

Haemolytic anaemia

Haemolytic anaemias are frequently seen in old age and some common causes are idiopathic autoimmune hemolytic anaemia, reticulosis, leukaemias, paroxysmal nocturnal hemoglobinuria, and drugs such as methyldopa and quinine.

5

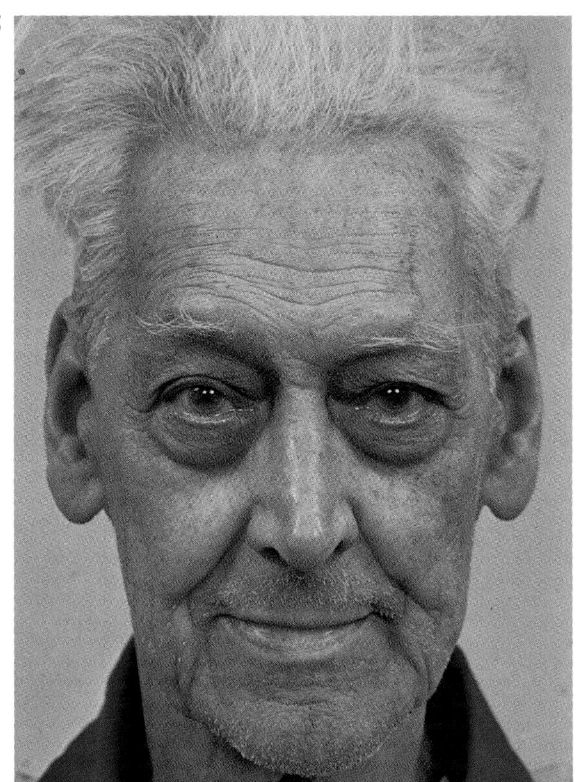

6

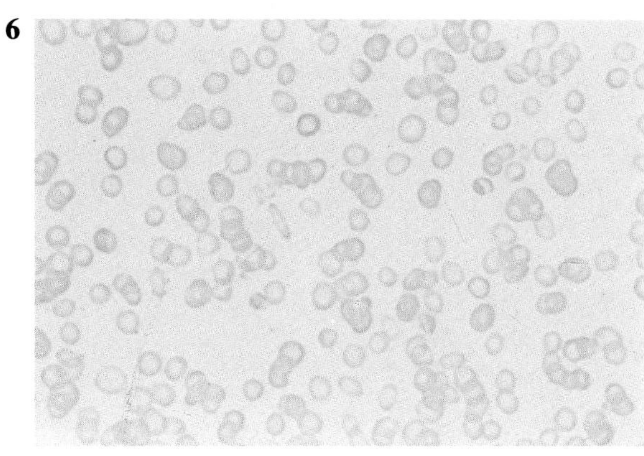

7

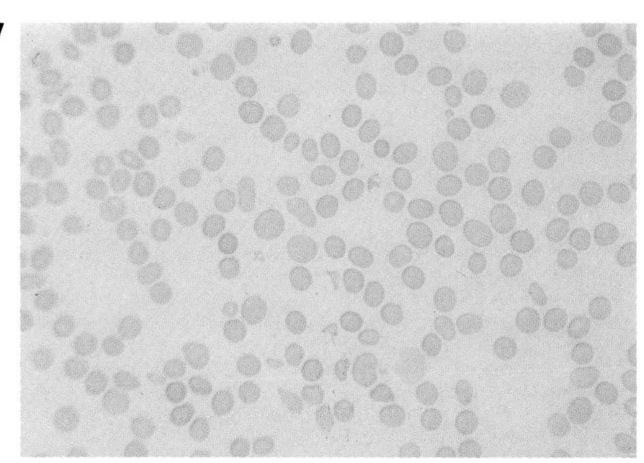

8

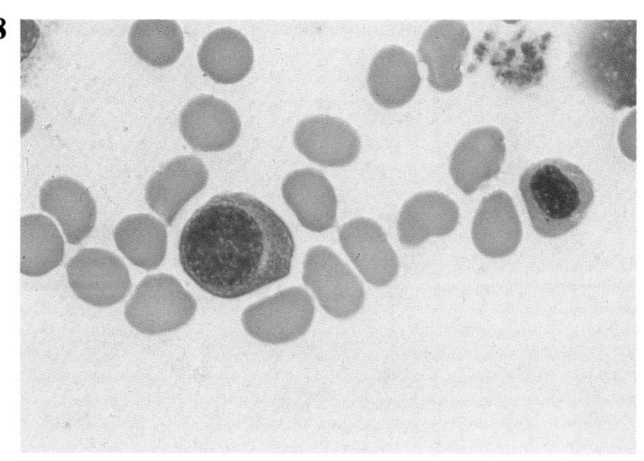

9

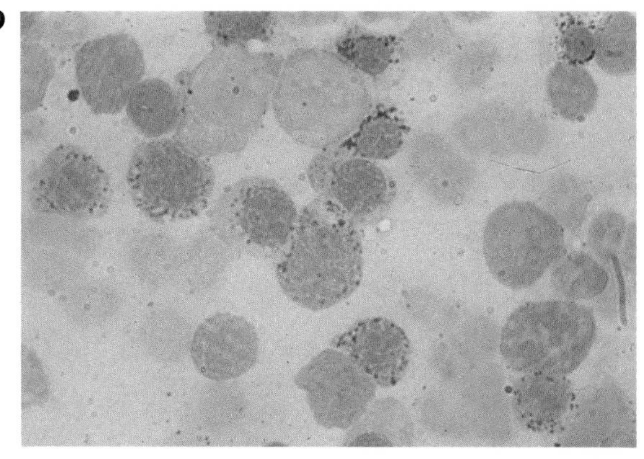

4 Facial pallor. Severe hypochromic anaemia with haemoglobin of 4.5 gm, secondary to chronic salicylate ingestion.

5 Pernicious anaemia. Pale face of a patient with pernicious anaemia. There is no significant weightloss.

6 Hypochromic RBCs. Blood film from a case of iron-deficiency anaemia. Note hypochromic red cells and pencil cells. (×*400*)

7 Megaloblastic anaemia. Blood film in megaloblastic anaemia showing oval macrocytes, marked anisocytosis and moderate poikilocytosis. (×*400*)

8 Megaloblastic anaemia. Bone marrow showing late (left) and intermediate (right) megaloblasts. (×*1000*)

9 Sideroblastic anaemia. Ring sideroblasts in bone marrow from a case of primary acquired sideroblastic anaemia.

10

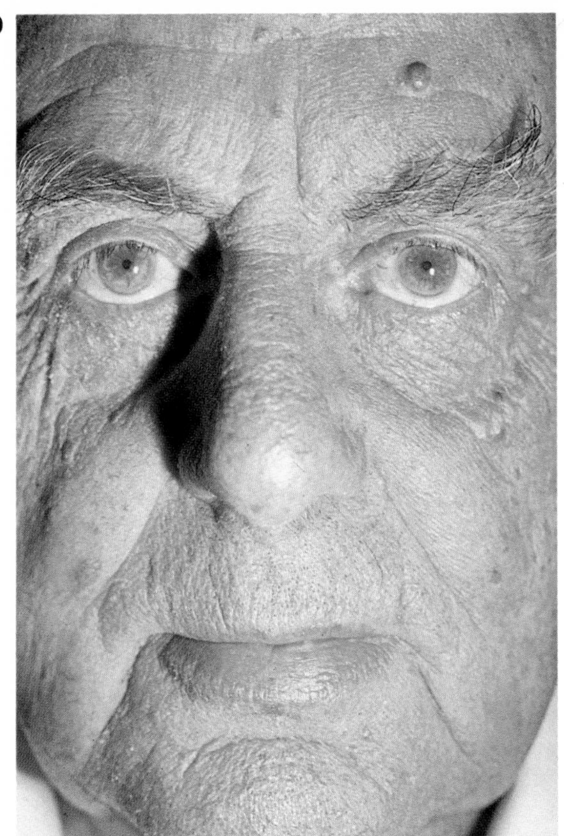

11

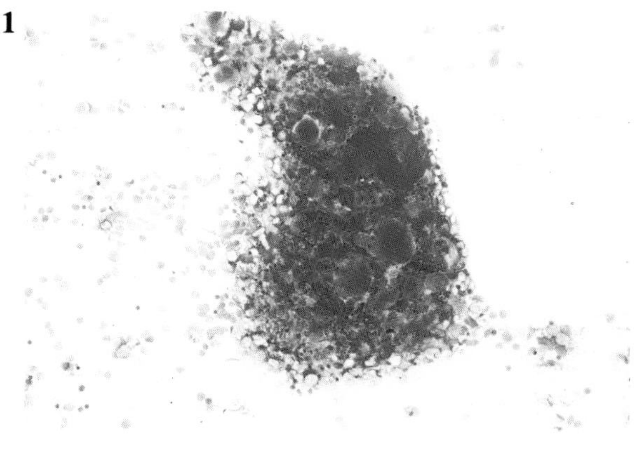

10 Polycythaemia. Plethoric face of an elderly man with polycythaemia rubra vera. The patient presented with features of cardiac failure.

11 Polycythaemia rubra vera. Fragment of bone marrow in a smear from a case of polycythaemia rubra vera. Note extreme hypercellularity, absence of fat spaces and great excess of megakaryocytes. (×*100*)

Causes of polycythaemia in the elderly

1 *Idiopathic* – polycythaemia rubra vera

2 *Secondary*
Chronic cardiac disease
Chronic pulmonary disease
High altitudes
Obesity
Meth. and sulphaemoglobinaemia
Carcinoma of the liver
Kidney disease
Uterine myomata
Phaeochromocytoma

3 *Relative*
Dehydration
'Stress' polycythaemia

Complications of polycythaemia

Venous thrombosis
Ecchymosis and bleeding
Hypertension
Coronary thrombosis and CHF
Cerebral thrombosis
Peptic ulcer
Gout
Chronic myelocytic leukaemia in polycythaemia rubra vera

12

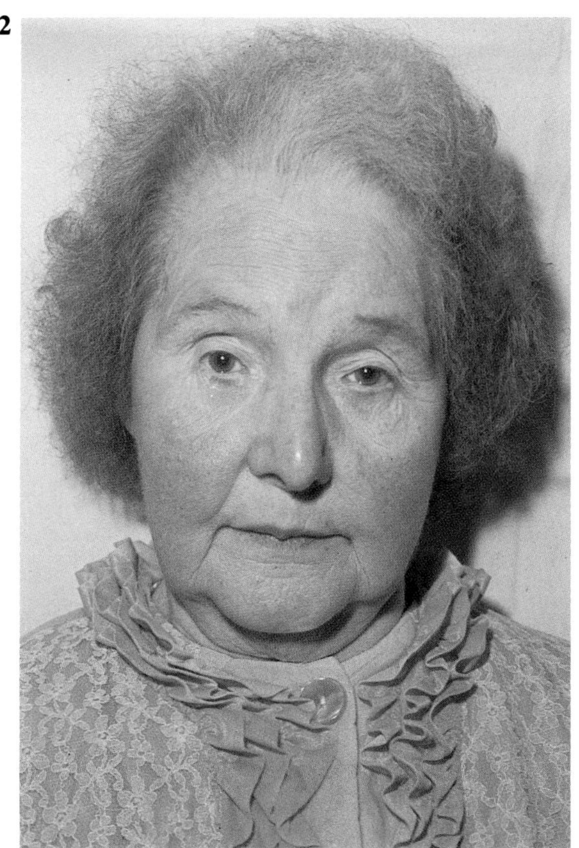

13

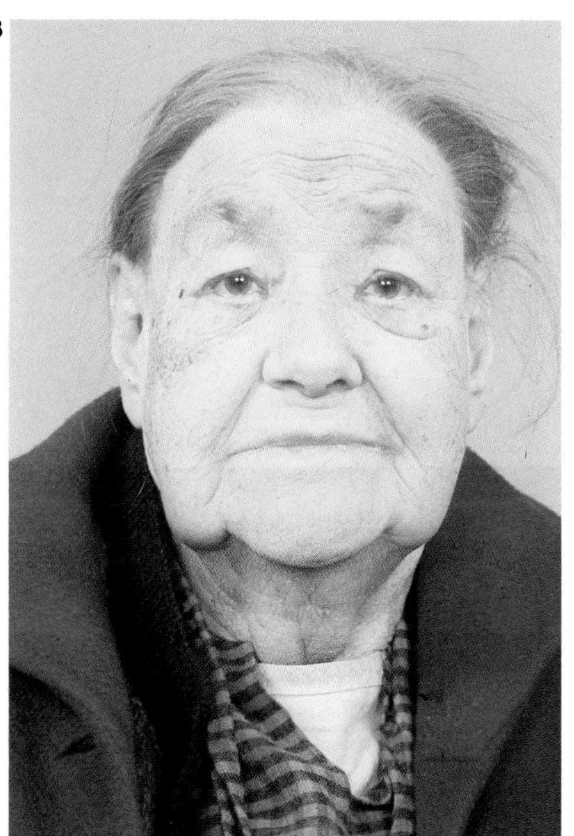

12 Myxoedema. Facial appearance of a case of mild hypothyroidism, whose main presenting complaint was longstanding depression.

13 Hypothyroidism. Facial appearance of a case of moderate hypothyrodism. The features are puffy and there is some coarsening of skin.

Hypothyroidism – myxoedema

Clinical features:

More common in elderly females. About 3–5% of admissions to geriatric units are found to be hypothyroid.
Insidious onset
Physical and mental deterioration
Depression
Constipation
Impaired mobility and falls
Increased sensitivity to cold
Loss of hair
Hoarseness of voice
Dry, coarse skin
Confusion leading to dementia
Slow relaxation of tendon jerks

Complications

Neuropathy
Hypothermia
Myxoedema coma
Carpal tunnel syndrome
Pericardial effusion
Ascites
Cerebellar ataxia

14a

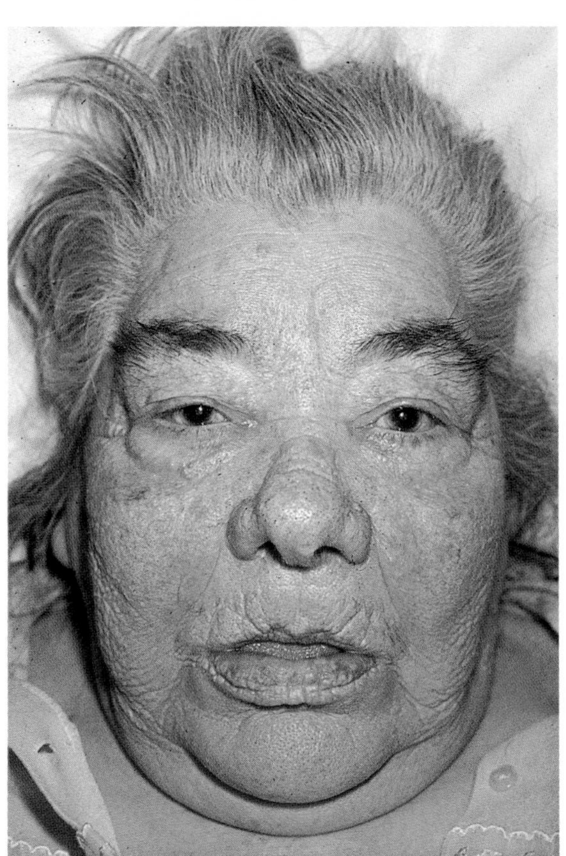

14a Myxoedema. This elderly lady was admitted suffering from hypothermia, with a rectal temperature of 31°C. Note the dry, puffy facial appearance with coarse hair. The skin is cold to touch and there is mental apathy. She was treated with gradual re-warming, antibiotics, intravenous fluids and tri-iodothyronine.

14b

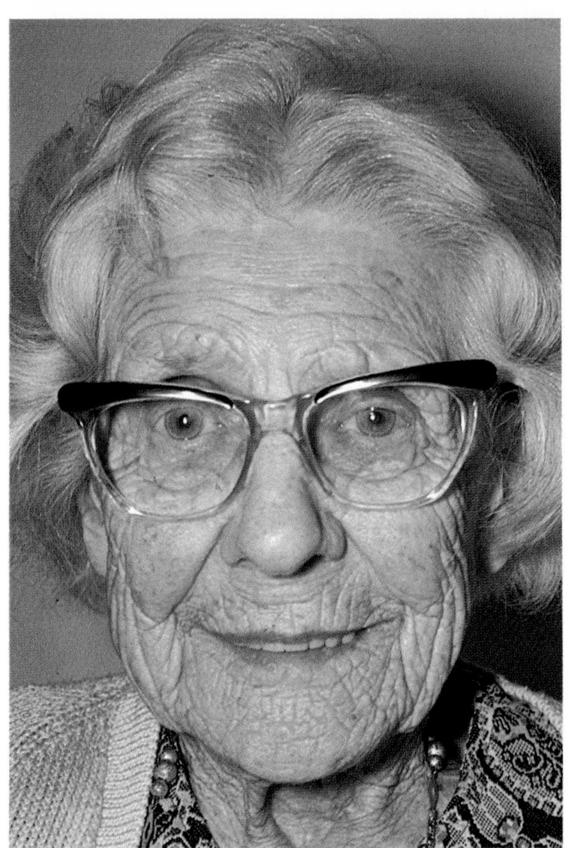

14b Myxoedema. This elderly lady was admitted to hospital with severe myxoedema. After five weeks treatment with thyroxine, she improved considerably. Her depression and lethargy disappeared. She is now active and more cheerful.

15

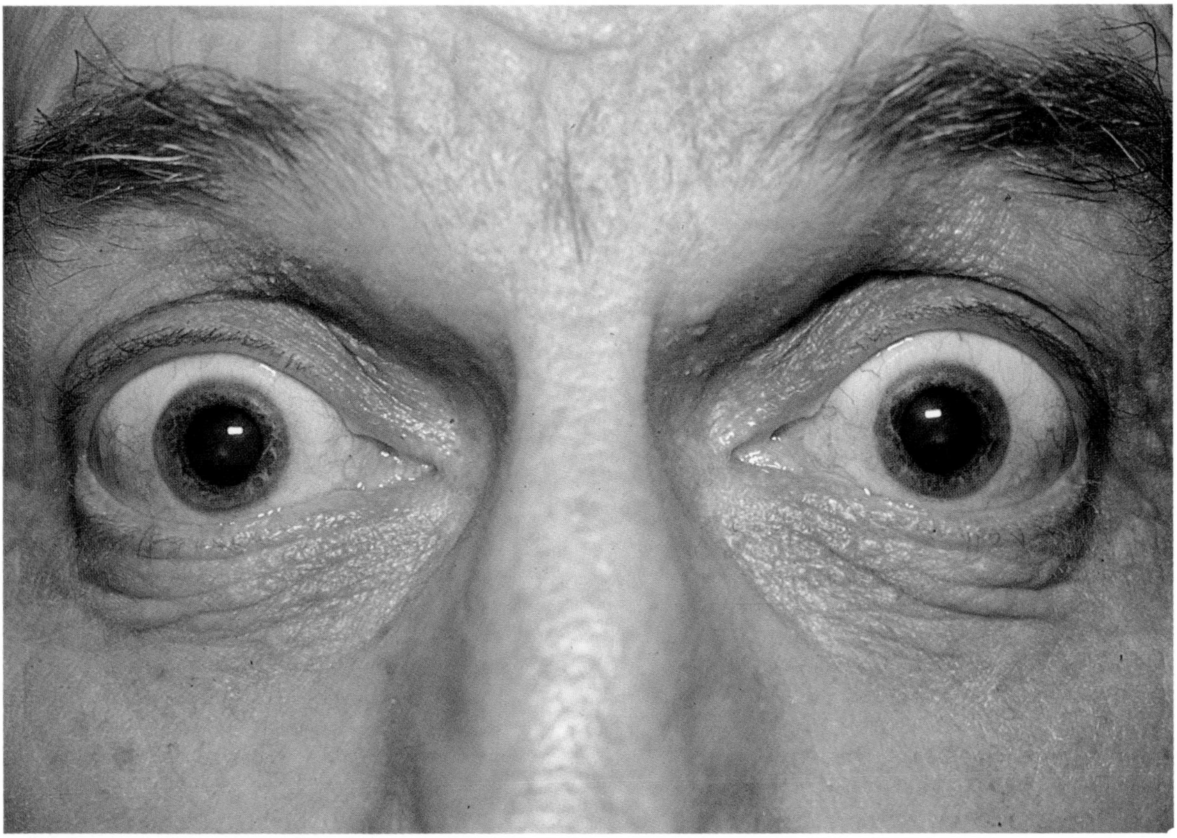

16

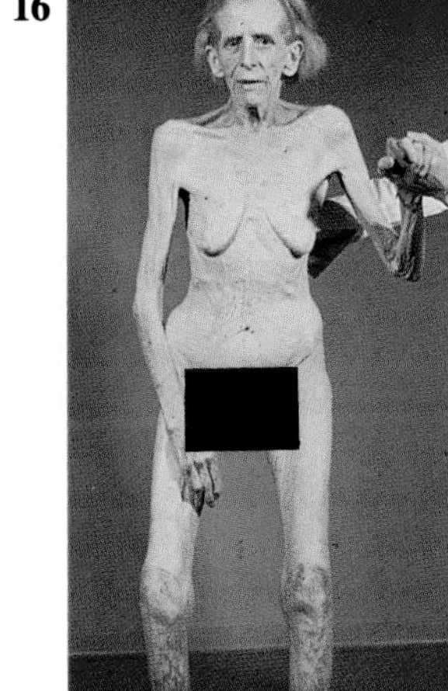

17

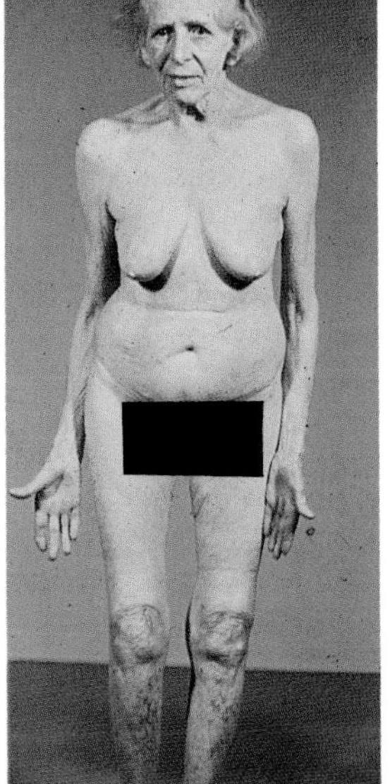

15 Thyrotoxicosis. Note the obvious exophthalmos with lid retraction. The patient also had atrial fibrillation.

16 Thyrotoxicosis. Elderly lady showing features of thyrotoxicosis. She is frail with considerable weightloss.

17 Treated thyrotoxicosis. Same patient as in **16**. The overactive thyroid has been treated. She has gained weight and feels well.

Thyrotoxicosis in the elderly

Clinical features

The classic features of thyrotoxicosis in younger age groups may be absent
Muscle weakness with cramps
Depression (apathetic thyrotoxicosis) and confusion
Weightloss
Diarrhoea
Atrial fibrillation which does not respond to Digoxin and CCF
Osteoporosis is fairly common

Signs that are usually absent in elderly

Exophthalmos and ophthalmoplegia
Warm, sweaty hands
Hyperkinesis
Thyroid bruit
Goitre

18

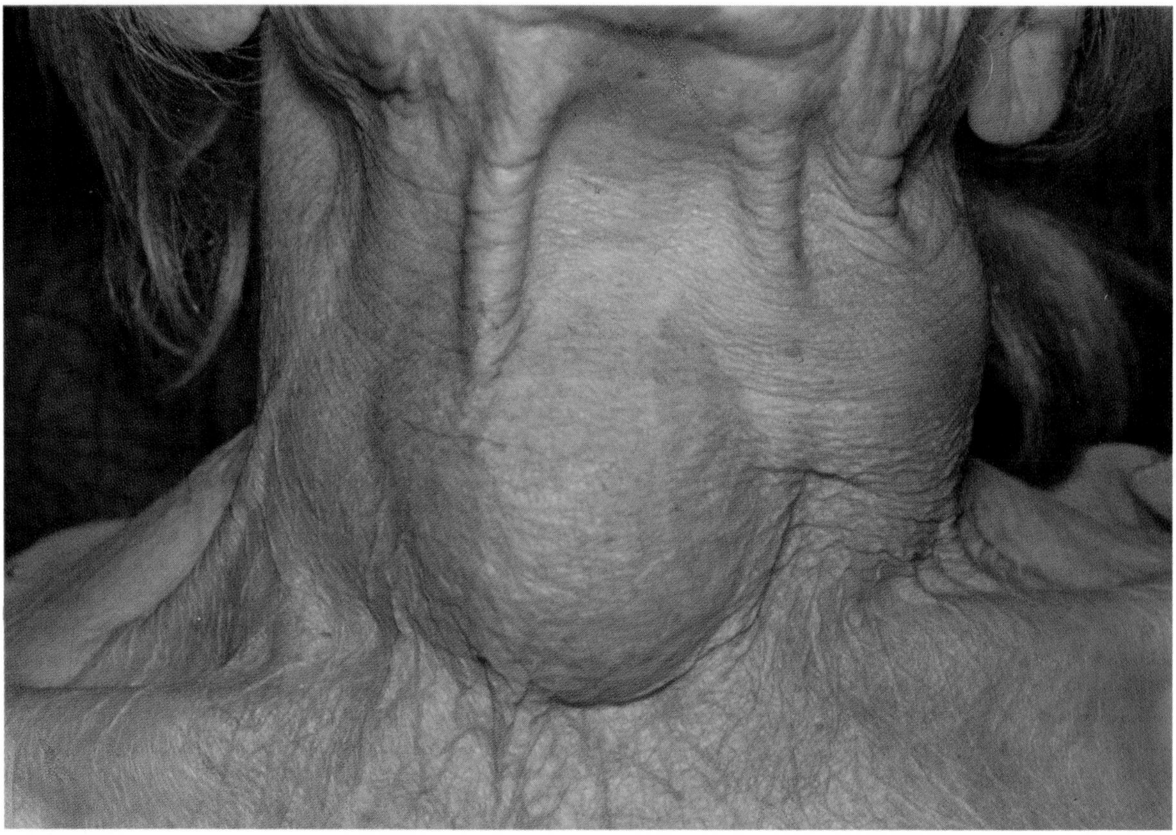

19a

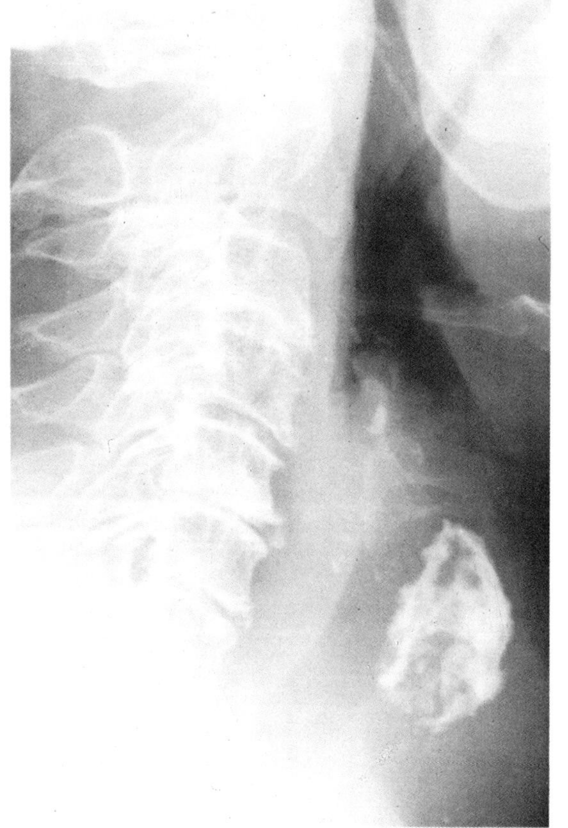

18 Goitre. Longstanding benign thyroid enlargement – a case of Derbyshire neck.*

19a A non-toxic goitre. A lateral Xray of the neck showing areas of calcification in a chronic non-toxic goitre.

19b Non-toxic goitre. An elderly lady with a large non-toxic goitre. It caused her only mild discomfort.

20 Thyroid carcinoma. This is an uncommon tumour in old age, but when it does occur it should be differentiated from simple goitre. The incidence is about 2.5 cases per 100,000 population per year. Hyperthyroidism or myxoedema is very rarely associated with this cancer.

*At one time benign goitre was common in the county of Derbyshire (England), because the drinking water supply lacked iodine.

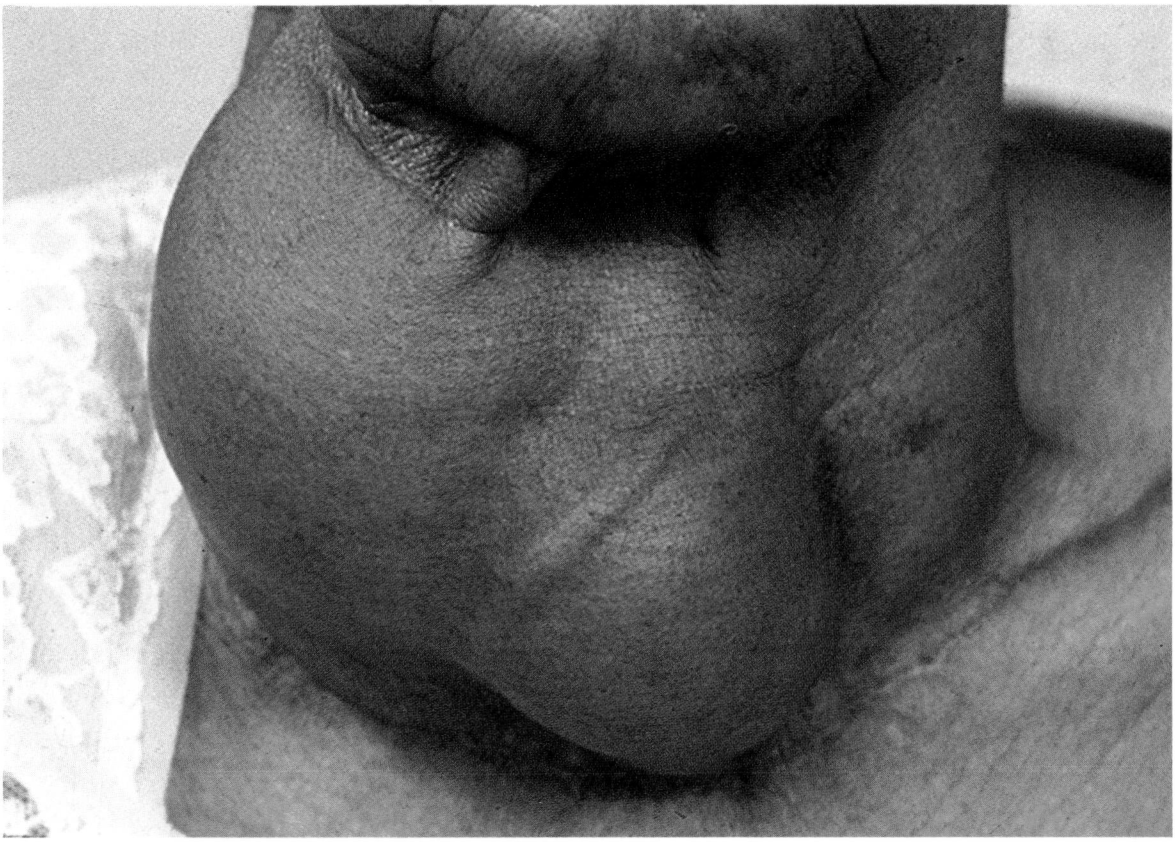

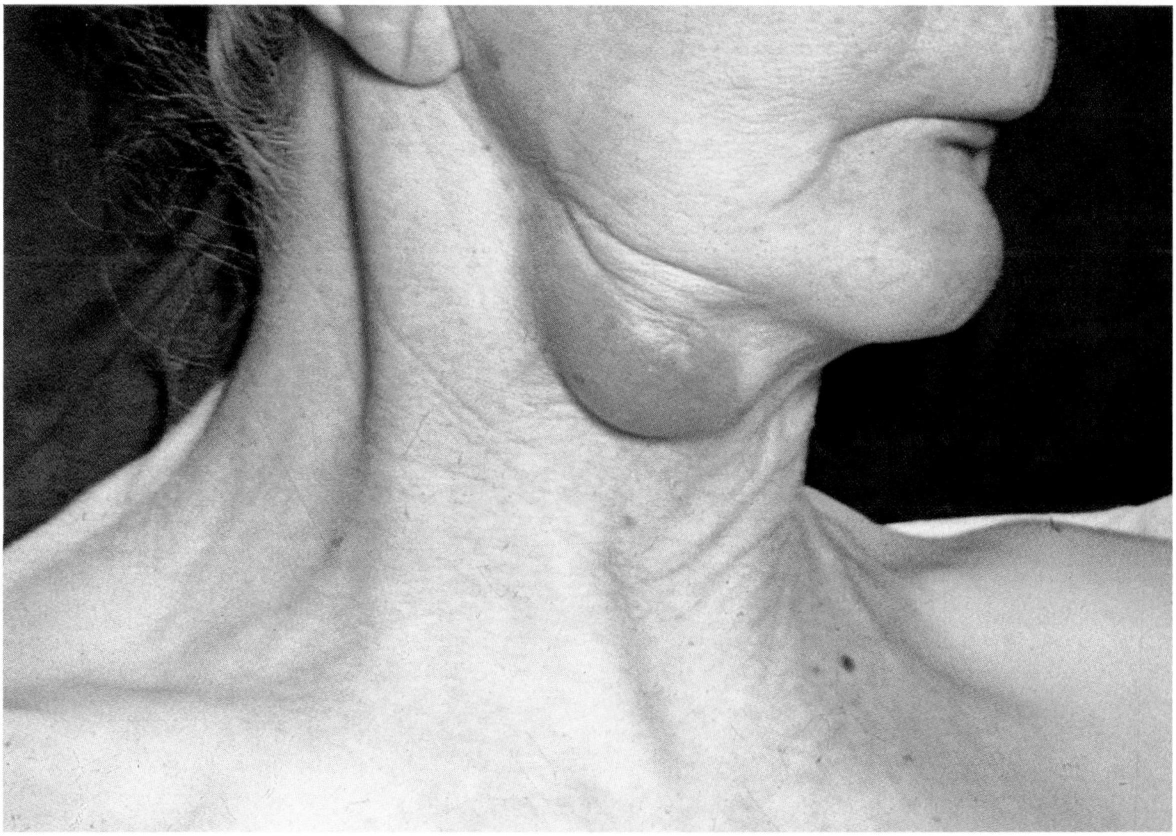

21

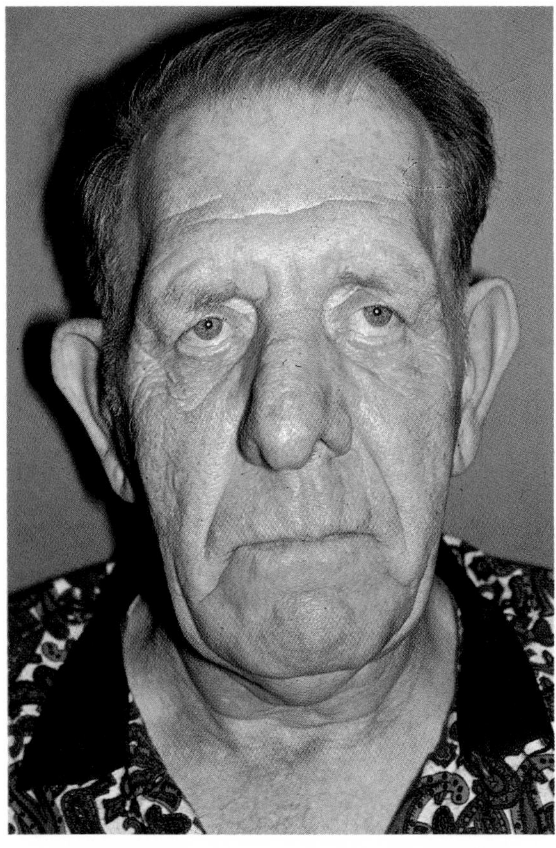

21 Acromegaly. The patient presented with lethargy, increased sweating and mild hypertension. Xray of the skull revealed an enlarged pituitary fossa.

22

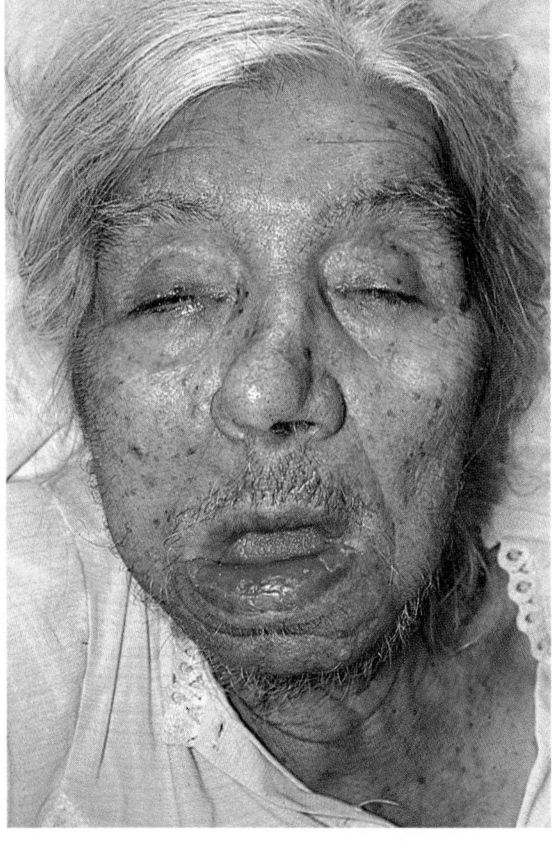

22 Acromegaly. This acromegalic female presented with extreme drowsiness. The facial features are enlarged and there is macroglossia. She also had visual disturbances, enlargement of the hands and feet, arthritic changes, mild cardiac failure, and glycosuria.

23 Pituitary tumour. Xray skull showing an enlarged pituitary fossa caused by a tumour. The patient, who was 80 years of age, had the classic features of acromegaly.

24 Acromegaly. Xray skull of another patient showing enlargement of pituitary fossa and also generalised thickening of bone.

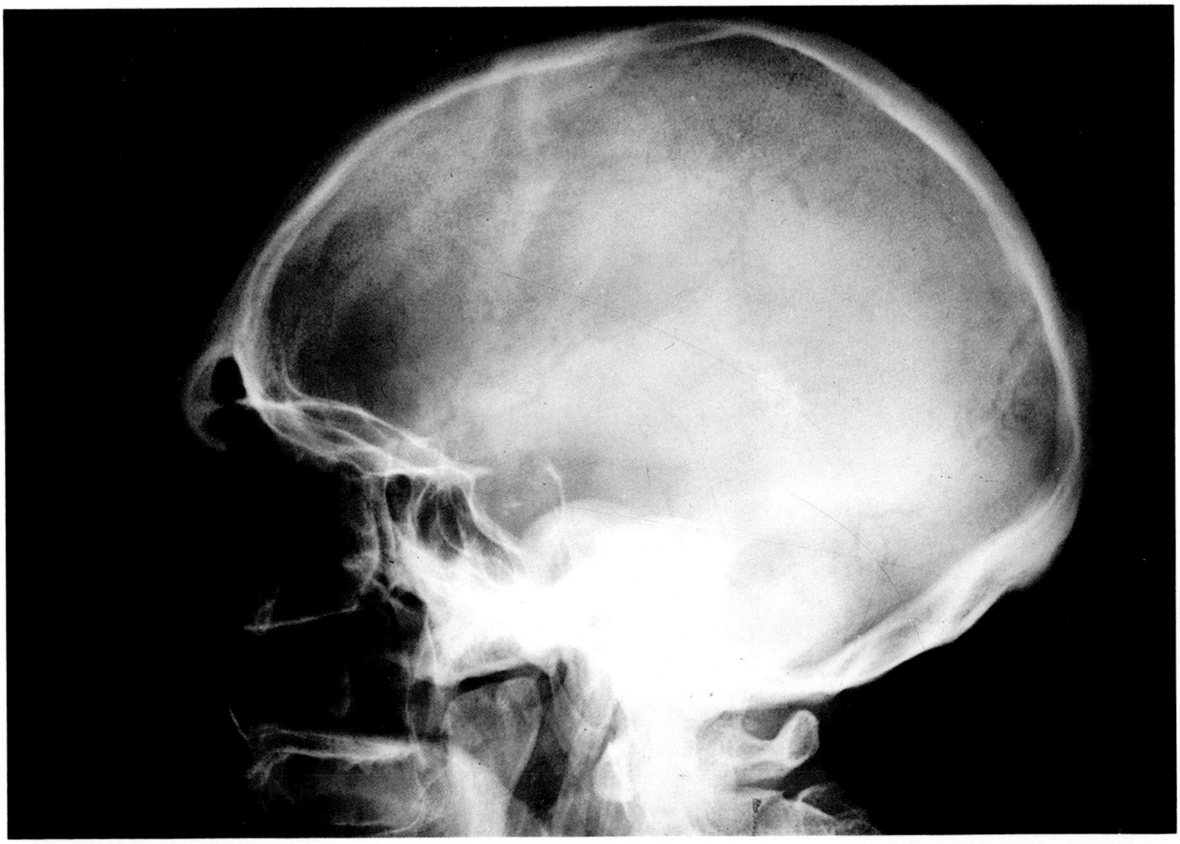

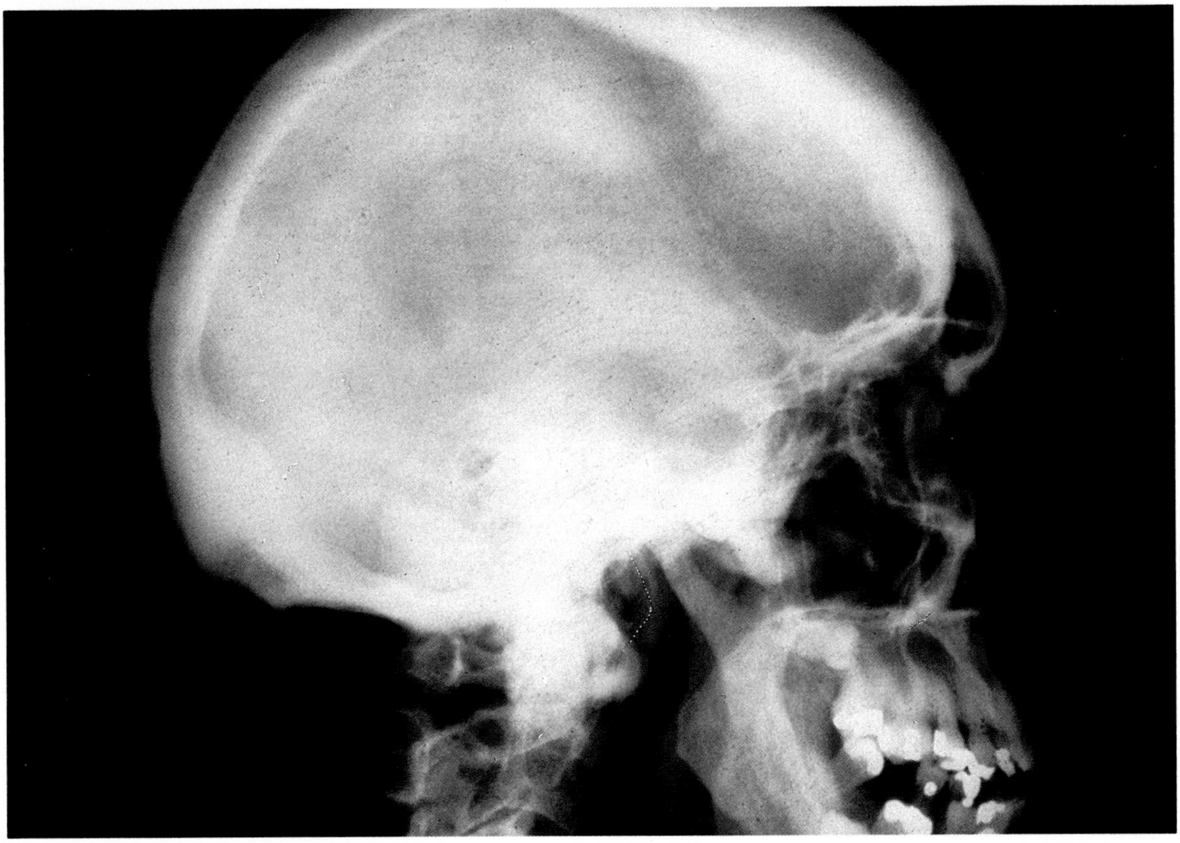

25a
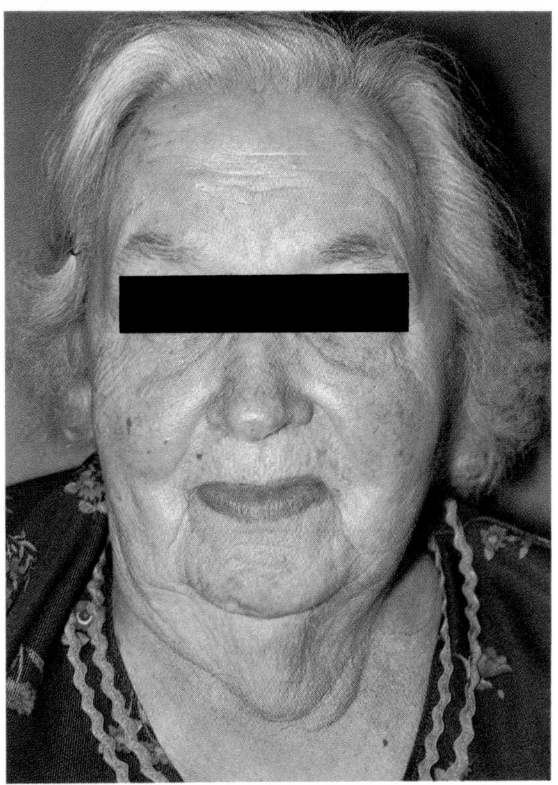

25a **Cushingoid face.** Flushed, puffy face of an elderly lady who was prescribed corticosteroids for rheumatoid arthritis.

Complications of systemic glucocorticosteroid therapy

1. Weight gain with water and sodium retention
2. Hypokalaemia
3. Hyperglycaemia
4. Cushingoid facies
5. Adrenal suppression and rebound of disease on stopping the drug
6. Hypertension
7. Hyperlipidemia
8. Osteoporosis, aseptic bone necrosis
9. GIT – dyspepsia, peptic ulceration, pancreatitis
10. CNS – euphoria, psychosis, increased intracranial pressure
11. Skin – Thinning of skin and easy bruising. Poor wound healing, acne, hypertrichosis
12. Myopathy
13. Cataracts
14. Hypothermia
15. Withdrawal phenomenon
16. Infections – viral, TB, fungal

25b **Cushingoid face.** Another case showing cushingoid features caused by chronic steriod ingestion for asthmatic bronchitis.

25b
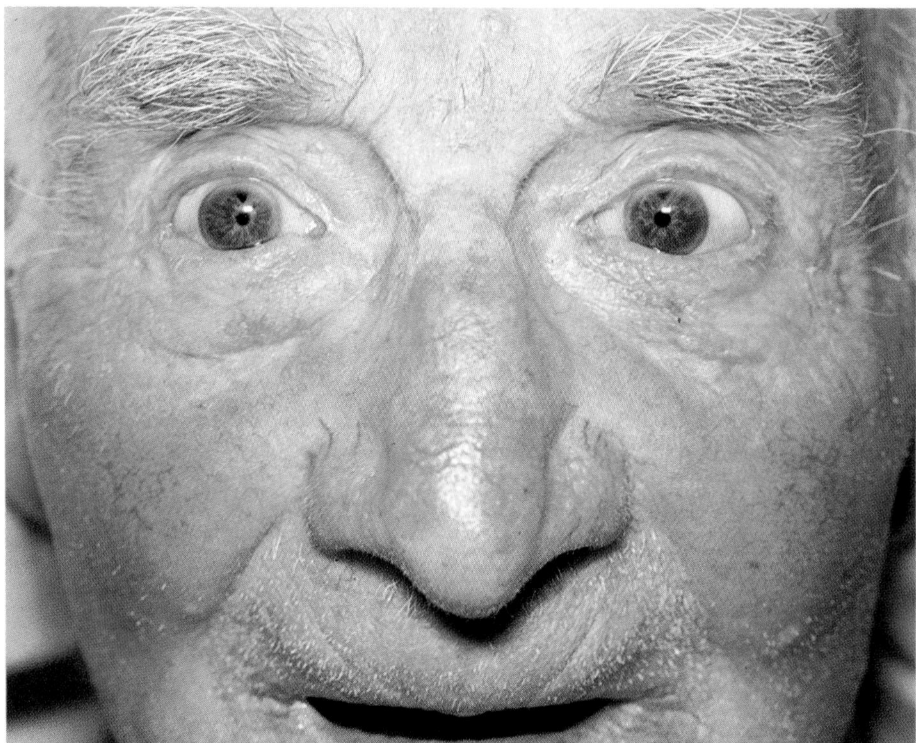

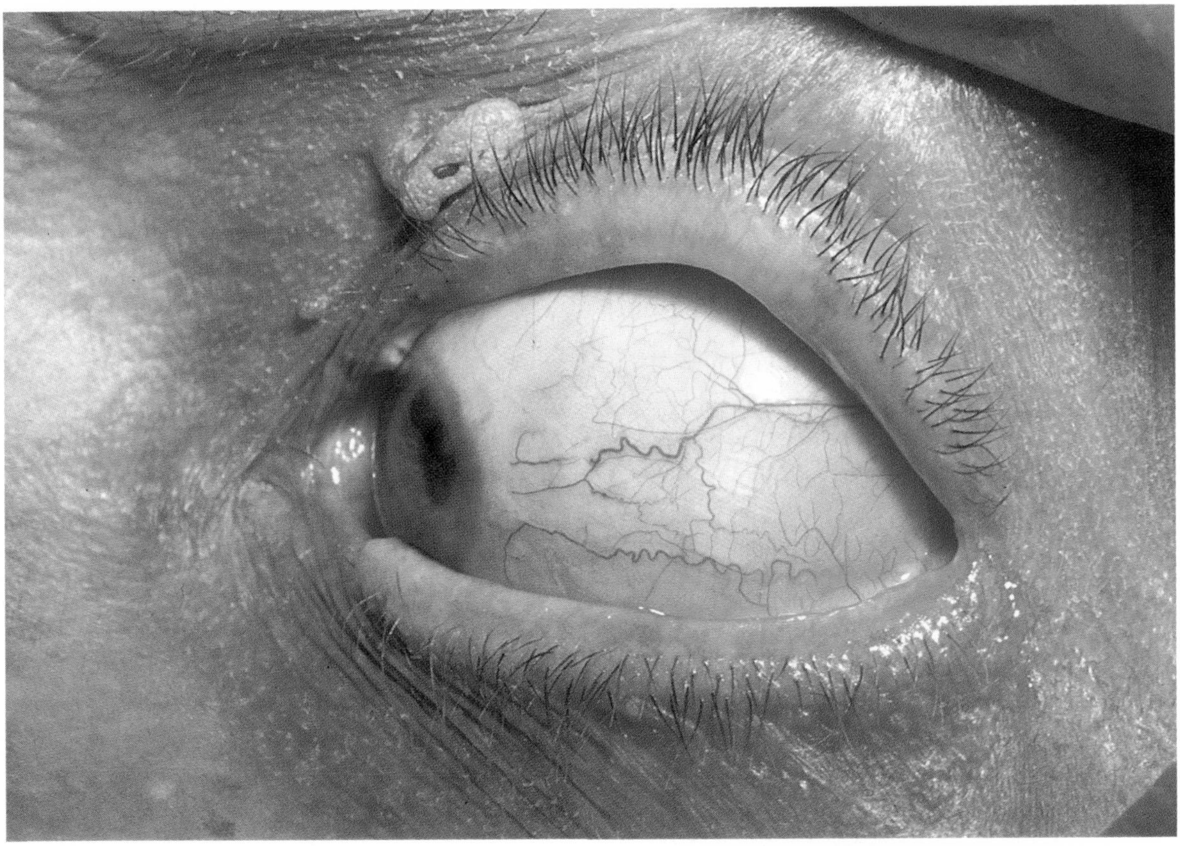

26 Jaundice. Icteric sclera in a case of obstructive jaundice caused by carcinoma in the porta hepatus.

27 Primary biliary cirrhosis. Note the deep jaundice and marked pigmentation.

27

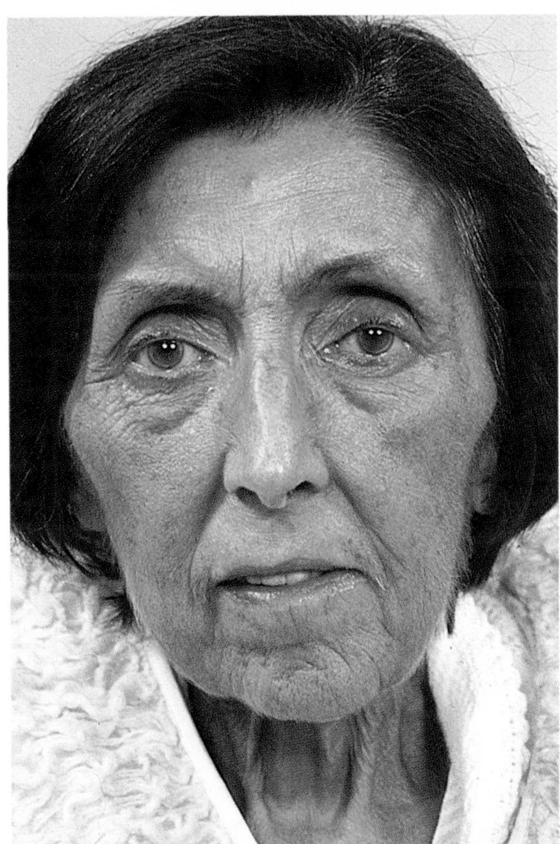

Jaundice

Some common causes of jaundice in old age are:

1 Biliary stone
2 Hepatic cancer, usually secondary
3 Carcinoma head of pancreas or ampulla
4 Liver cirrhosis
5 Porta hepatis lymph node enlargement
6 Viral hepatitis
7 Congestive heart failure
8 Pulmonary infarction
9 Drugs

28

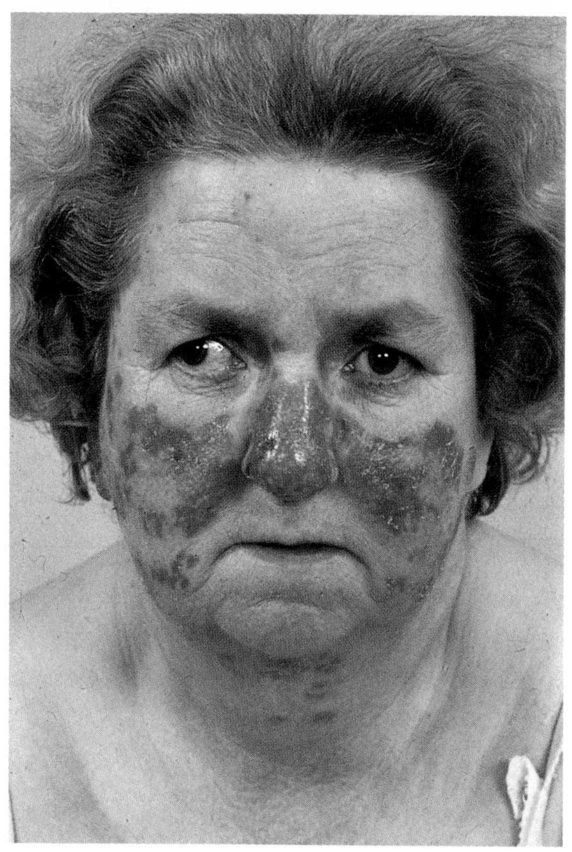

29

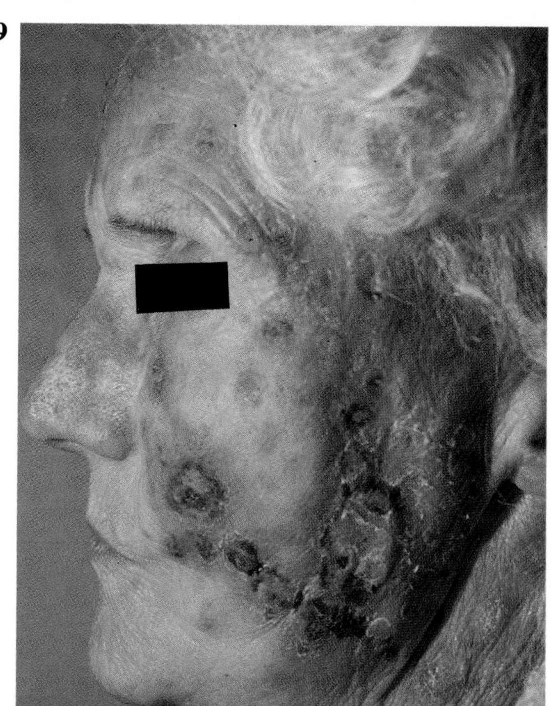

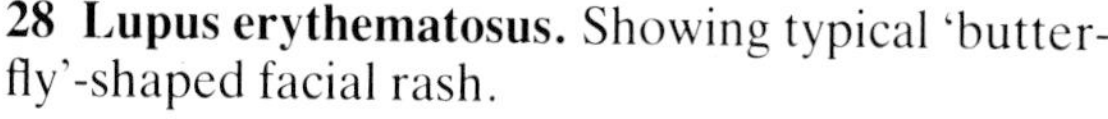

28 Lupus erythematosus. Showing typical 'butterfly'-shaped facial rash.

29 Lupus erythematosus. A more advanced case showing widespread rash with some necrotic lesions which are painless. This patient also had renal and pulmonary damage.

30a

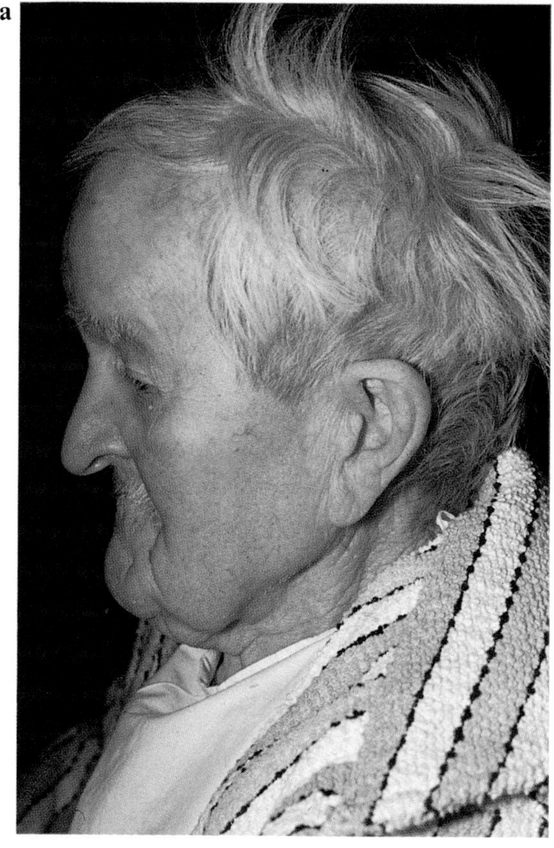

30a Paget's disease of the skull. Note the large skull and prominence of frontal bones. This patient was also deaf. In the elderly, Paget's disease is usually symptomless but can present with bone pain, deformities, cardiac failure, deafness, optic nerve involvement, and fractures. Osteogenic sarcoma is a rare complication.

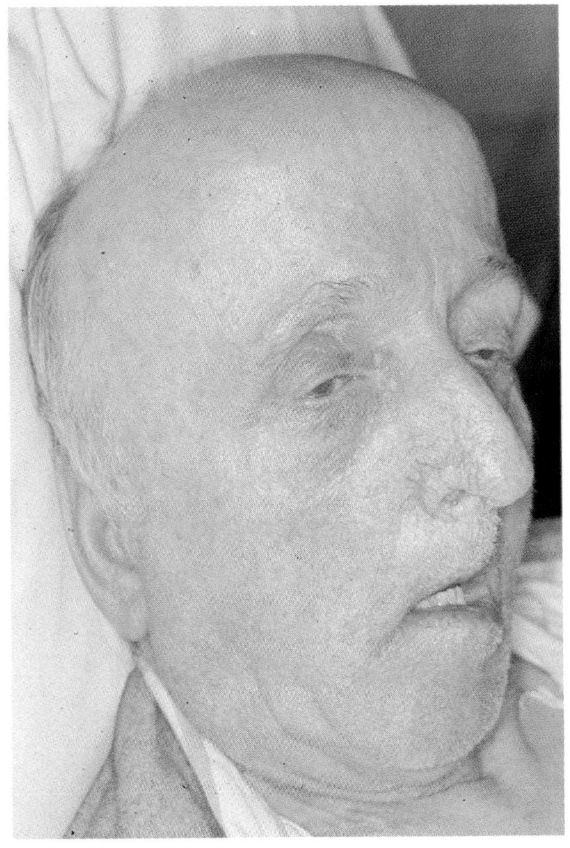

31

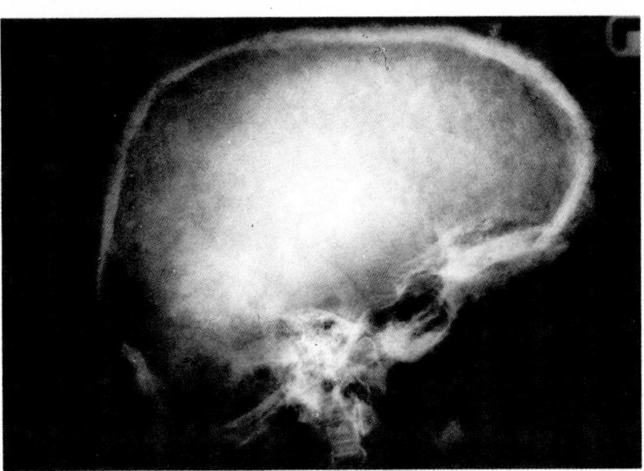

30b Paget's disease of skull. This elderely man has advanced Paget's disease and there is involvement of some cranial nerves. Note the right-sided facial palsy.

31 Paget's disease. Xray showing thickening of calvarium and the typical disorganised bony architecture.

32 Osteoporosis circumscripta. This condition occurs in association with Paget's disease. Note the rounded translucency in the skull.

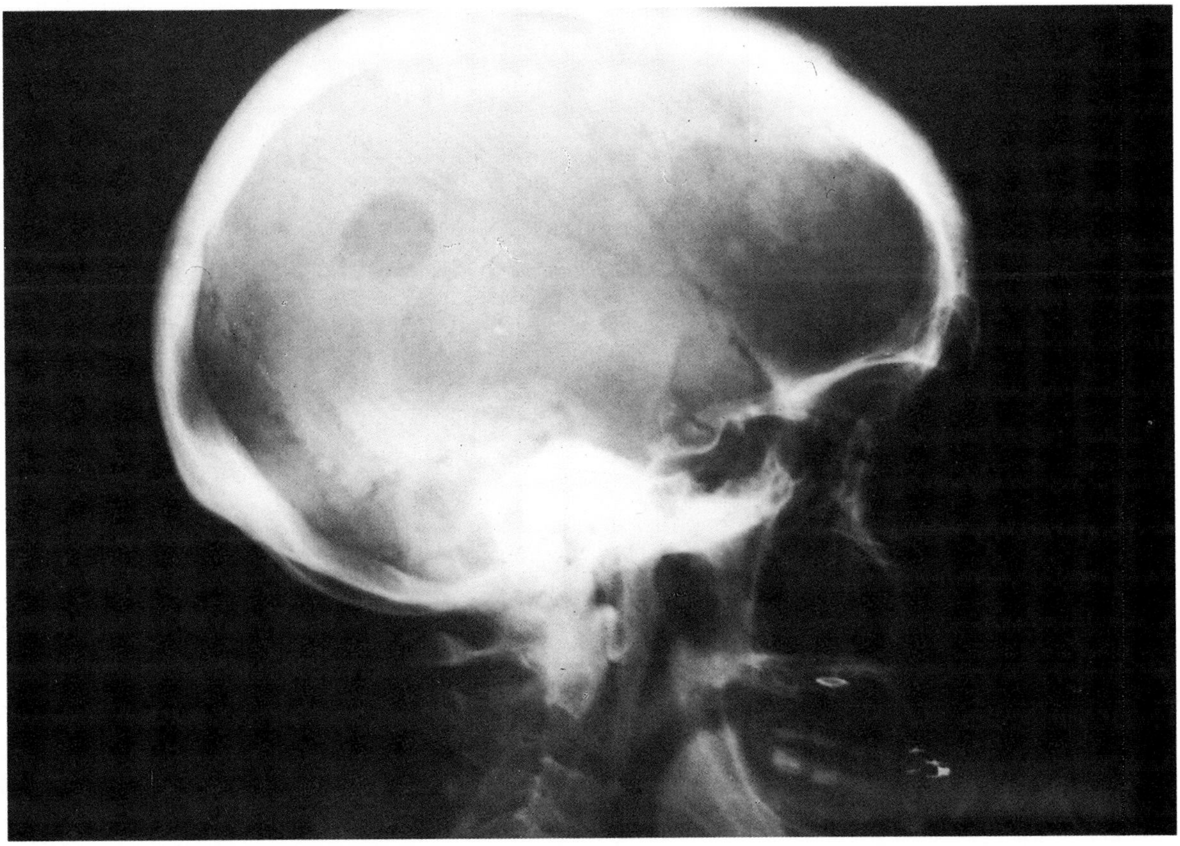

33a

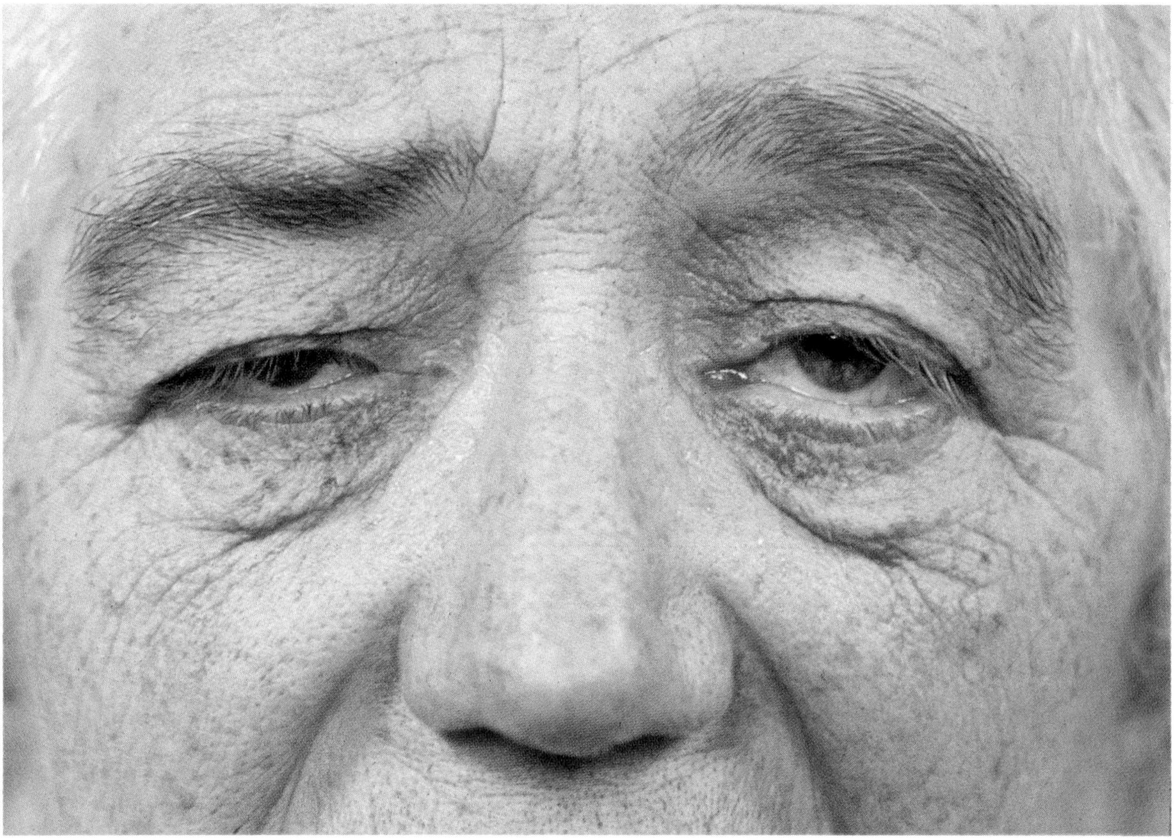

33b

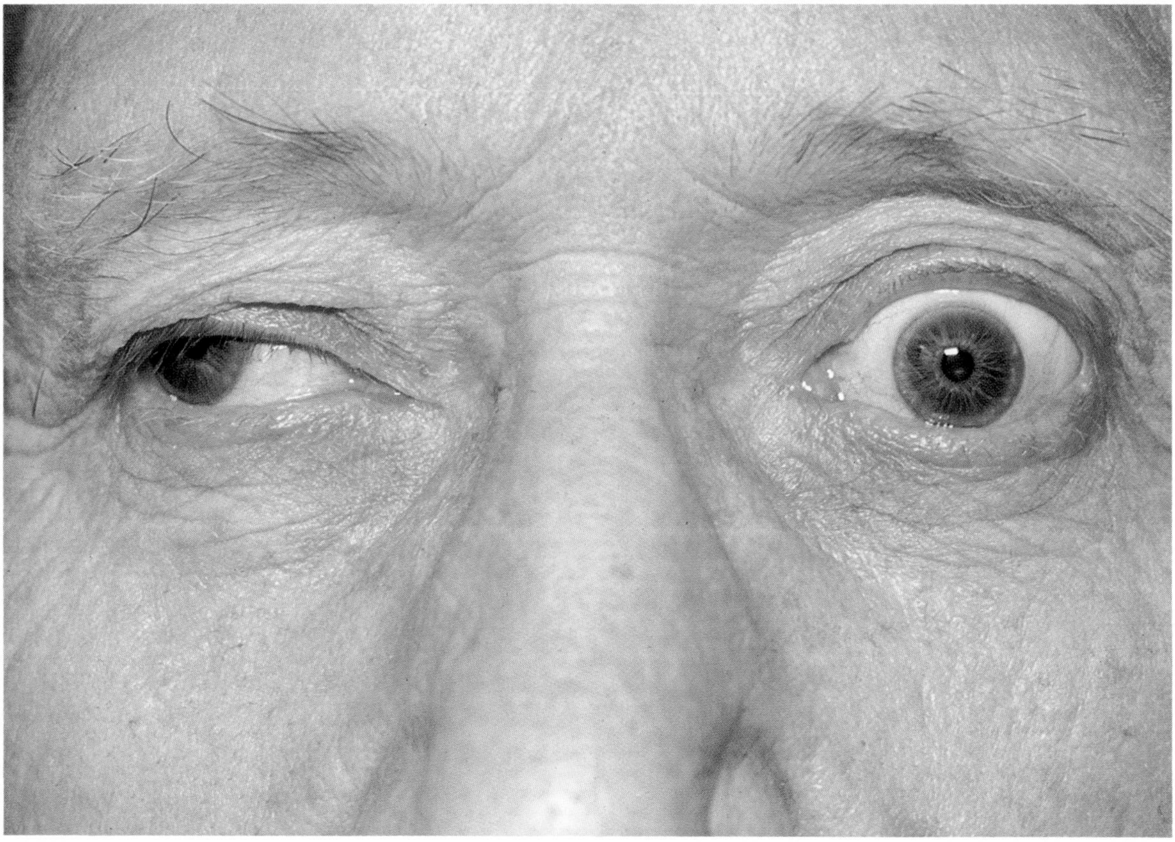

33a Myasthenia gravis. Face of an elderly lady showing bilateral ptosis and arching of the eyebrows. Older patients with myasthenia must be investigated for an occult tumour such as carcinoma of the lung.

33b Ophthalmoplegia. A case of third-nerve palsy showing right-sided ptosis and divergent strabismus. In the elderly the common causes are cerebrovascular disease, tumours, diabetes mellitus, and cranial arteritis.

34

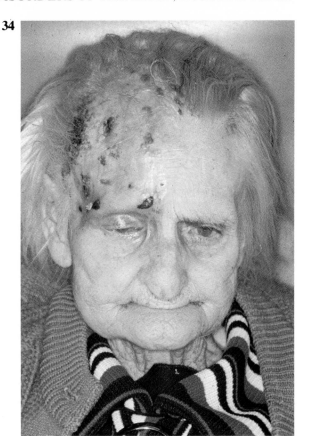

34 Ophthalmic herpes zoster. In this case there is involvement of the ophthalmic divisions of the fifth nerve; the main danger is permanent corneal scarring.

35

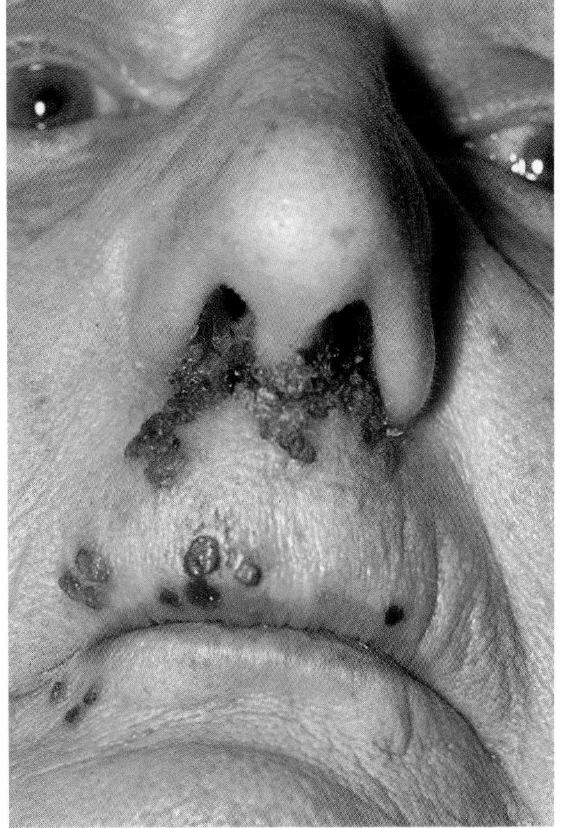

35 Herpes simplex. Painful eruption around the mouth and nostrils in a patient who had chest infection and toxic confusional state.

Herpes labialis results from activation of the herpes simplex virus by rise in temperature. It is common in bacterial infections of the respiratory system.

Complications of herpes zoster

1 Post-herpetic neuralgia and depression
2 Secondary bacterial infection
3 Ophthalmic herpes zoster
4 Ramsay-Hunt syndrome – herpes of geniculate ganglion resulting in severe facial palsy and vesicular eruption in external auditory canal
5 Encephalitis
6 Generalised herpes zoster

36

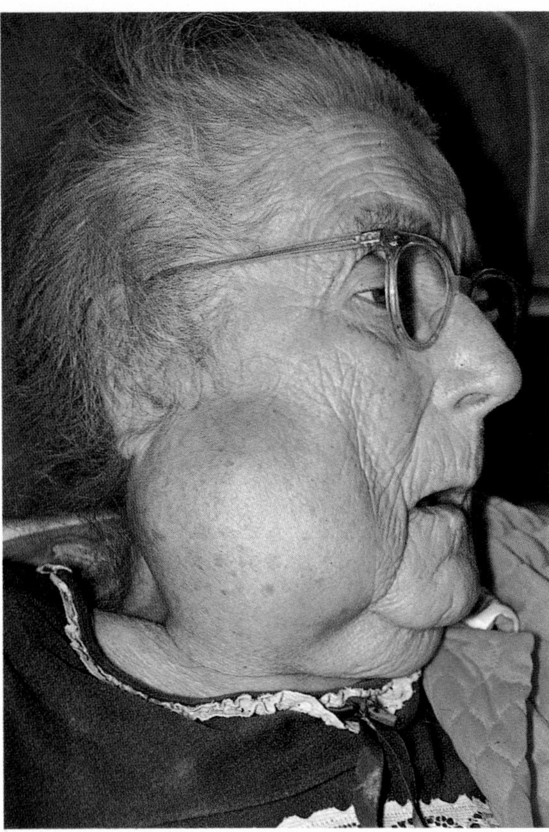

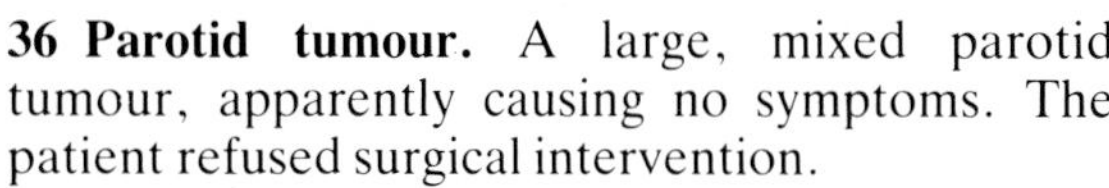

37

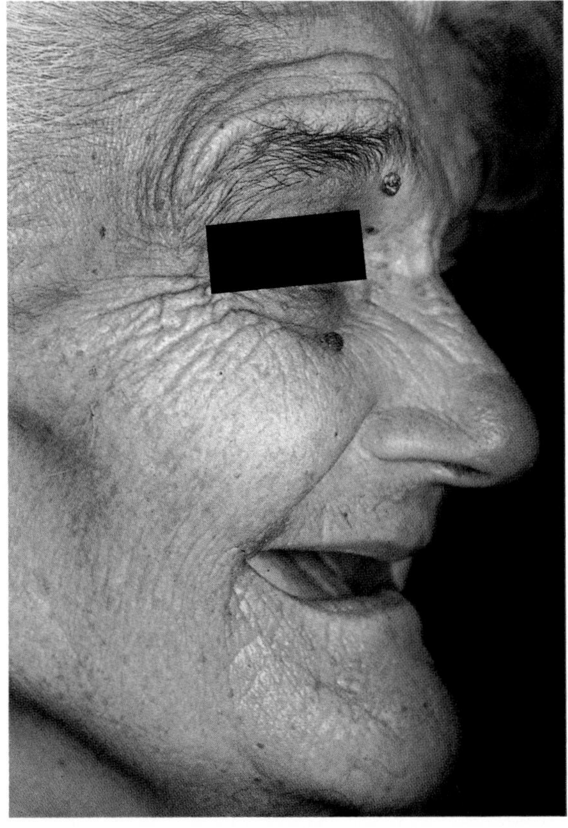

36 Parotid tumour. A large, mixed parotid tumour, apparently causing no symptoms. The patient refused surgical intervention.

37 Hyperpigmentation. Generalised facial hyperpigmentation in a Caucasian lady. She complained of weightloss and was found to have bronchogenic carcinoma. Further investigations revealed evidence of ectopic–ACTH syndrome and cerebral metastasis. Her symptoms were minimal and her general condition remained satisfactory for several months. She eventually developed a dementia-like picture.

Common causes of hyperpigmentation

- Racial or genetic
- Radiation, e.g. UVR
- 'Vagabond's itch' – chronic scratching
- Hypoadrenalism
- Acromegaly
- Phaeochromocytoma
- Ectopic ACTH from carcinomas
- Cachexia caused by malignancy
- Chronic infection, for example, endocarditis
- Malabsorption
- Pellagra
- Chronic hepatic disease
- Chronic renal failure
- Collagen diseases, for example, dermatomyositis
- Drugs, for example busulphan, ACTH, oestrogens, chlorpromazine, chloroquine
- Haemochromatosis

8

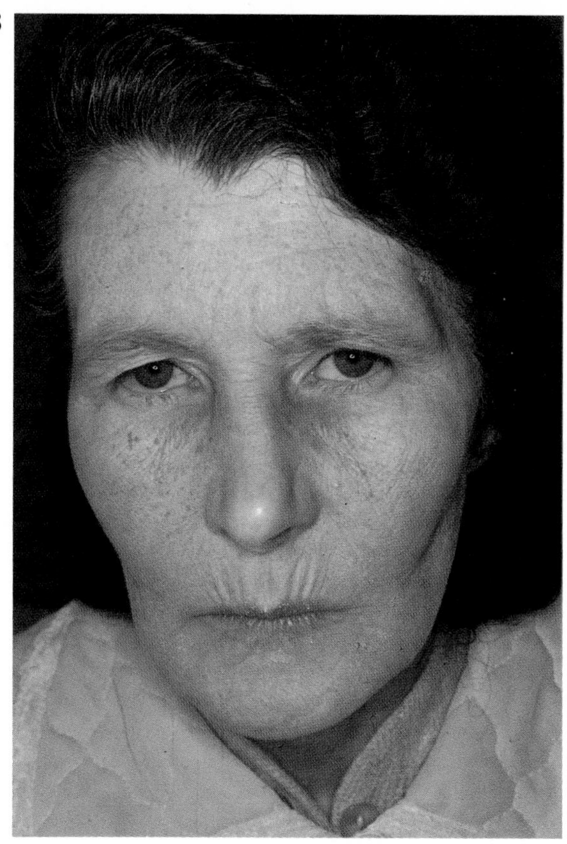

39

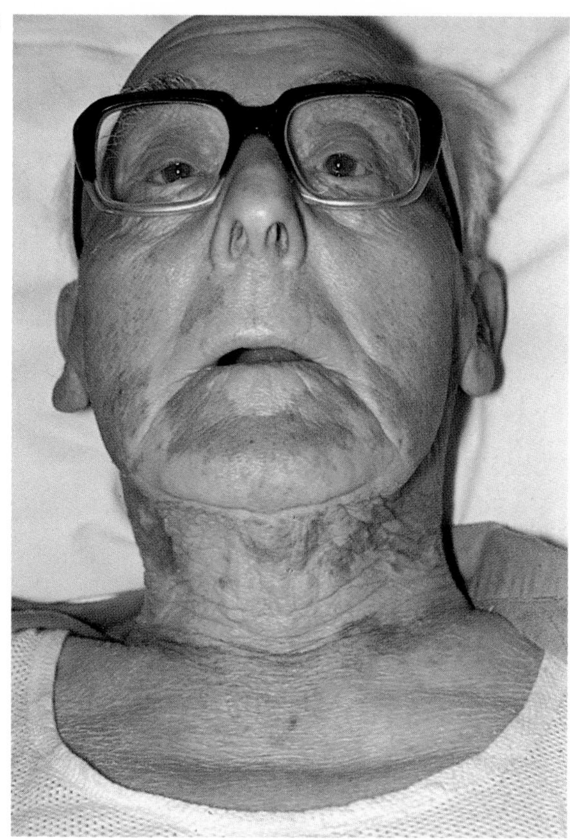

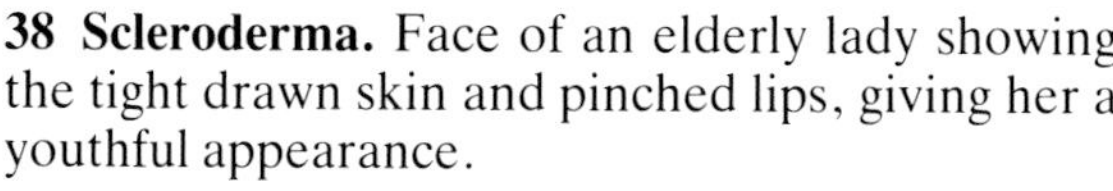

38 Scleroderma. Face of an elderly lady showing the tight drawn skin and pinched lips, giving her a youthful appearance.

39 Vitiligo. Typical patches of hypopigmentation in a patient with hypothyroidism. Chest Xray also revealed that he also had carcinoma of the bronchus, with recurrent laryngeal nerve paralysis.

Conditions associated with vitiligo

1 Autoimmune diseases
    Myxoedema
    Addison's disease
    Pernicious anaemia
    Diabetes mellitus
2 Alopecia areata
3 Malignant melanoma

Falls in the elderly

Occur in four per cent of elderly women and 24 per cent of elderly men

General features

1 Incidence increases linearly with age
2 More common in women
3 Most frequently indoors
4 Often happen when moving from bed, wheelchair or lavatory
5 Frequent in elderly people who are socially isolated, depressed or demented

Causes

1 Environmental causes – accidental falls
 - Tripping over objects, slips
 - Old, ill-fitting footwear
 - Slippery surfaces
 - Narrow steep stairs
 - Poor lighting
 - Pets, electrical flexes, etc

2 Musculoskeletal
 - Onychogryphosis (overgrown toenails)
 - Osteoarthritic feet, knees and hips
 - Corns, bunions, hammer toes
 - Hallux valgus
 - Oedema of the feet
 - Muscle weakness

3 Nervous system
 - Transient ischaemic attacks
 - CVAs in evolution
 - Epilepsy
 - Parkinsonism and other extrapyramidal disorders
 - Cerebellar disorders
 - Labyrinthine disorders
 - Visual impairment
 - Peripheral neuropathy

4 Cardiovascular
 - Silent myocardial infarction
 - Arrhythmias, heart block
 - Postural hypotension
 - Subclavian-steel
 - Anaemia

5 Drop attacks
 - Vertebrobasilar insufficiency with cervical spondylosis
 - Transient ischaemia of spinal cord
 - Myxoedema

6 Miscellaneous
 - Defaecation syncope
 - Micturation syncope
 - Hypoglycaemia
 - Vagovagal attacks
 - Carotid sinus hypersensitivity

Complications of falls in the elderly

Fractures, especially of long bones; e.g. fractured neck of femur
Hypothermia
Burns
Dehydration
Bronchopneumonia
Loss of confidence – immobility
Subdural haematoma

40 Torticollis. This occurred in an elderly schizophrenic who had been on long-term phenothiazine therapy. She also had orofacial dyskinesia.

41 Drug-induced rash. Erythematous skin rash; side-effect of an antibiotic. The whitish patches are caused by calamine application.

42a Head injury. This injury is the result of a minor fall. There was no fracture of the skull, but later the patient developed features of subdural haematoma.

42b Facial injury. This elderly lady suffered from recurrent drop-attacks. This particular fall had resulted in concussion and fracture of nasal bone. Recurrent falls are a common symptom of ill-health in the elderly and require thorough investigations.

40

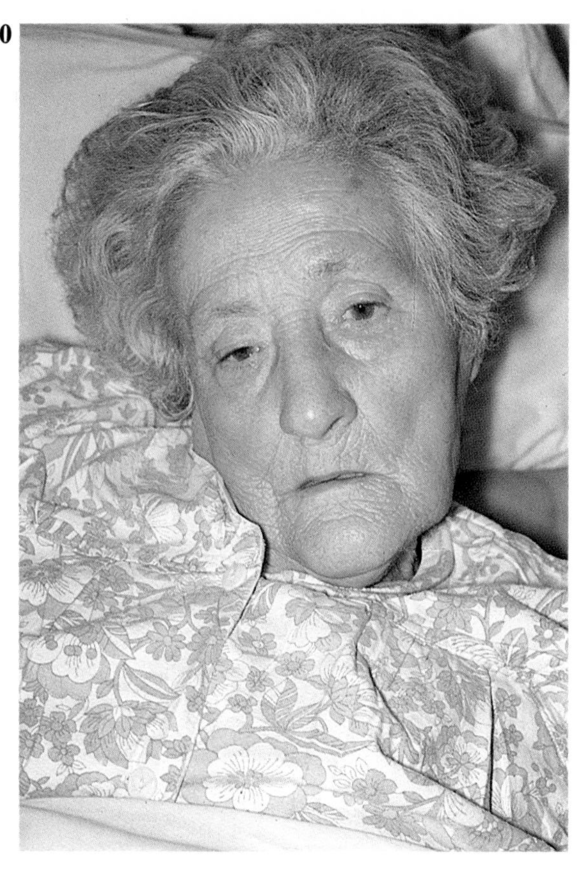

41

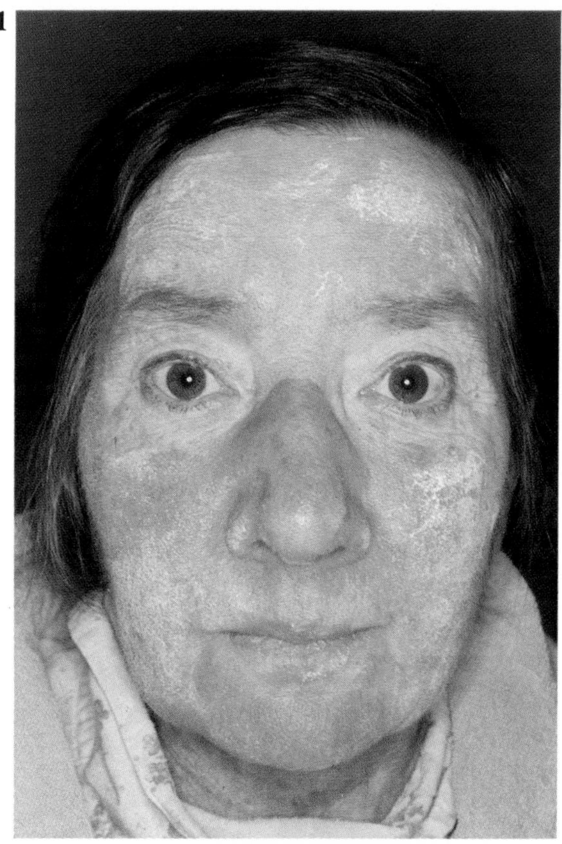

2a

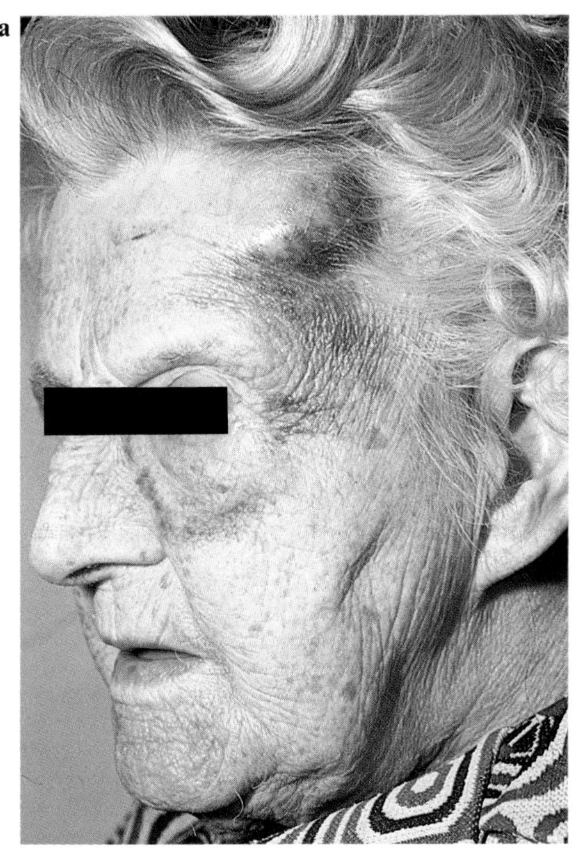

42b

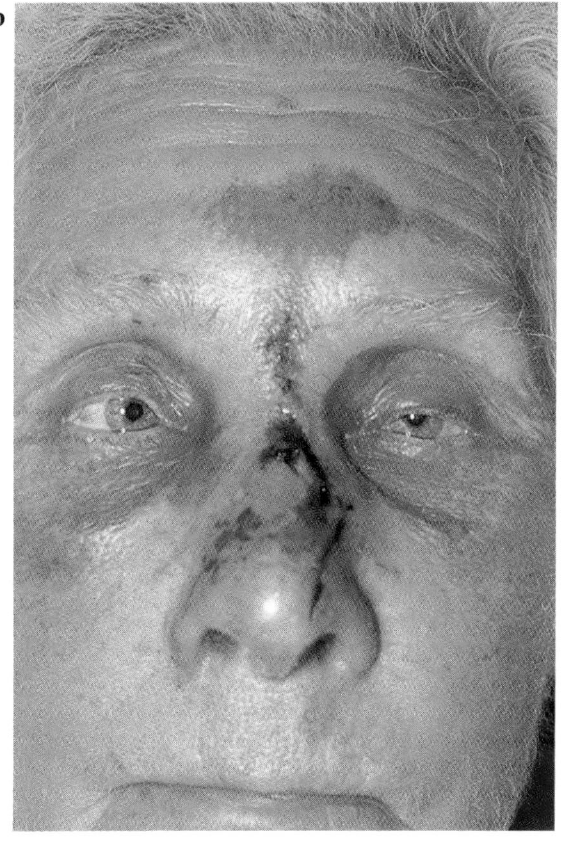

43

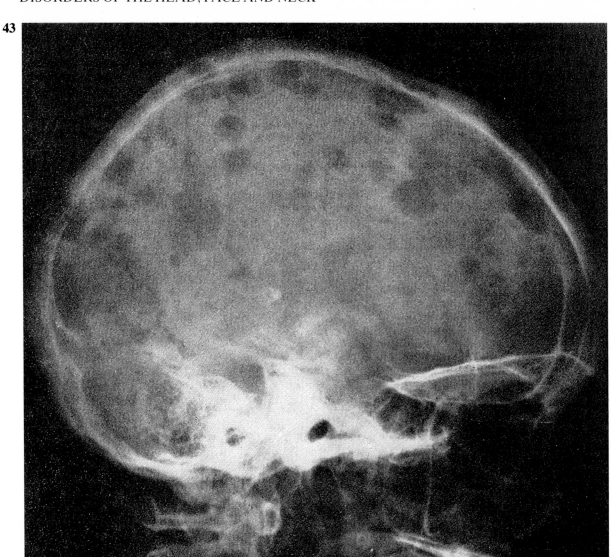

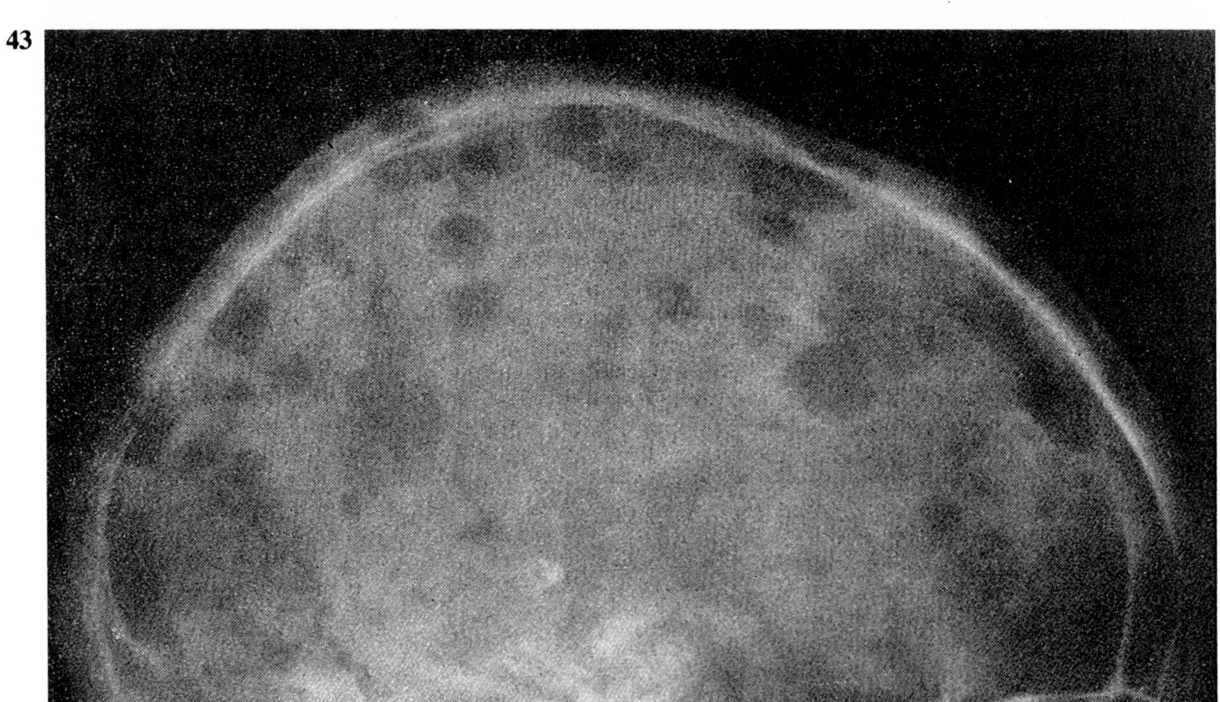

43 Plasma-cell myeloma. Xray skull showing classical appearance of multiple myeloma. Note the numerous 'punched out' translucencies.

44

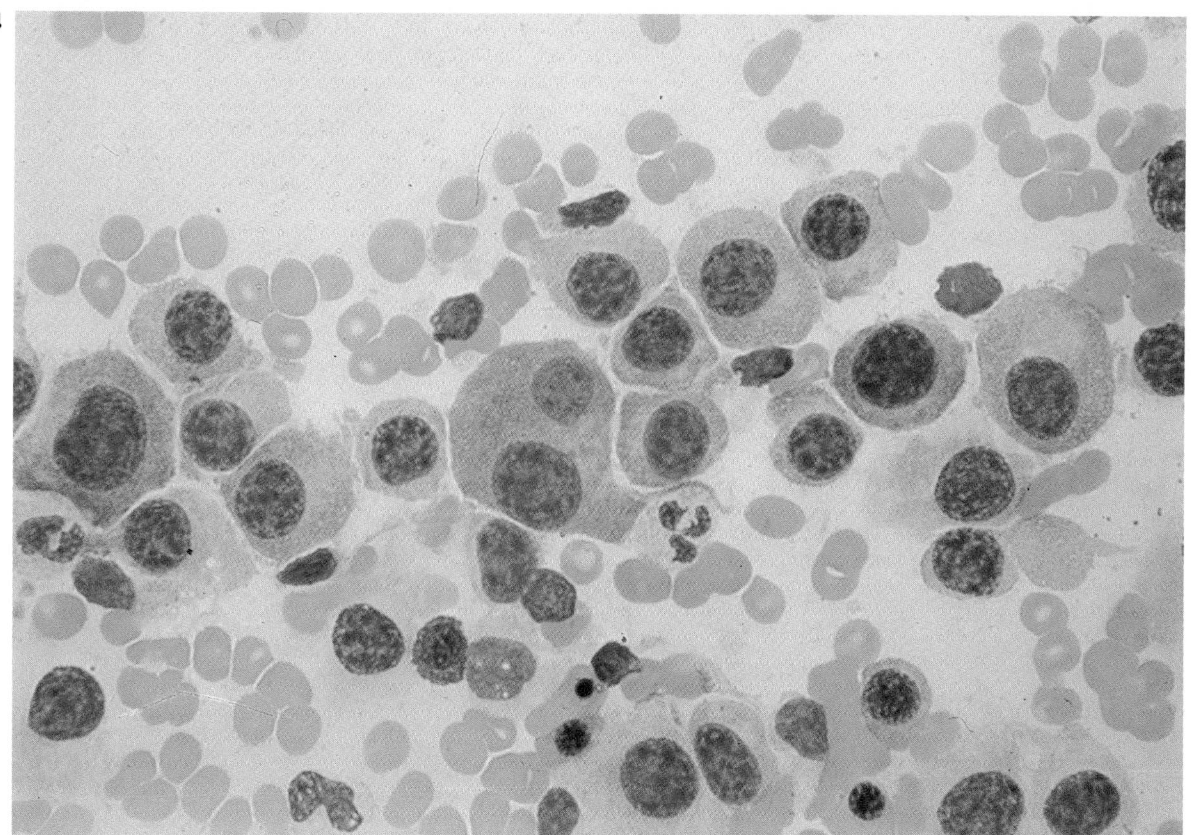

44 Multiple myeloma. Bone marrow showing excess of plasma cells. (×*500*)

Multiple myeloma

Malignant proliferation of plasma cells

Clinical features

General ill health and anorexia
Anaemias
Bone pains and pathological fractures
Hypercalcaemia and renal failure
Peripheral neuropathy
Amyloidosis
Reduced resistance to infection
Hyperviscosity syndrome
Vertebral collapse and cord compression

Investigations

Anaemia is common
ESR very high
Abnormal monoclonal band on plasma protein electrophoresis
Bence-Jones protein positive in 50 per cent
Increased number of abnormal plasma cells in bone marrow
Xray may show osteolytic lesions in skull

Temporal arteritis

This condition is a true panarteritis and affects vessels of all sizes.

The arterial wall is thickened by granulomatous tissue containing epithelioid and multinucleate giant cells, chronic inflammatory cell infiltration, necrotic foci and areas of fibrinoid change. Aneurysms may develop and sometimes there is segmental occlusion of affected vessels by thrombosis and intimal proliferation, leading to infarction of the tissues supplied by that blood vessel.

Most patients are over 70 years of age and female to male ratio is 3:1.

Clinical features Anorexia and weightloss, headaches and hyperalgesia of scalp. The temporal artery may be thickened, non-pulsating and tender.
Pain on chewing
Neck stiffness
Blurred vision, loss of vision
Fundi may show ischaemic papillopathy or central retinal artery occlusion. There may be coexistent polymyalgia rheumatica.

45

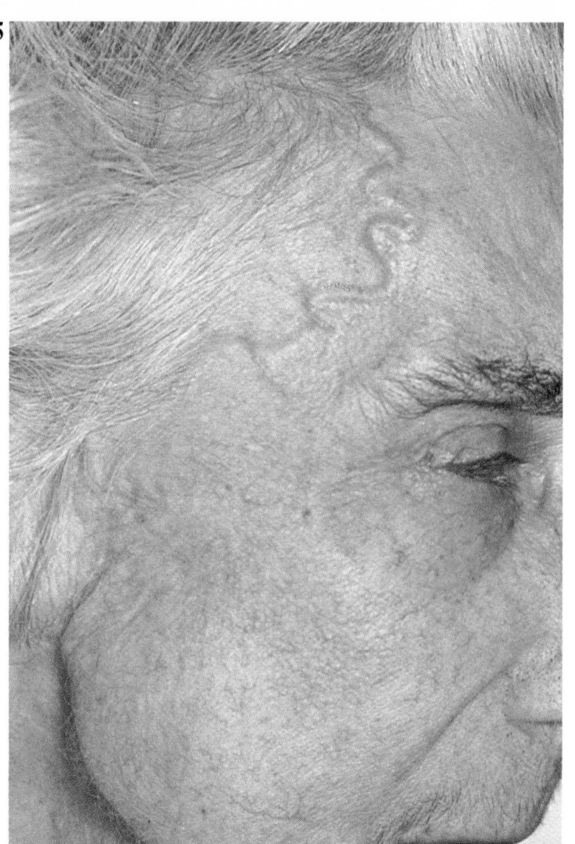

Polymyalgia rheumatica

A collagen disease related to temporal arteritis and occurring in old age.

Clinical features

General ill health and malaise
Anorexia
Aches and pains in the shoulders ('rheumatism')
Stiffness of arms and legs – difficulty in combing hair
Low-grade pyrexia
Headache and scalp tenderness
Normochromic normocytic anaemia
High ESR, usually over 50 mm/H
Increased serum immunoglobulins
Arterial biopsy will show giant-cell granulomata

45 Temporal arteritis. An elderly lady presenting with severe unilateral headaches. She had tenderness over temporal artery and ESR was significantly raised.

46 Temporal arteritis. Temporal artery biopsy showing inflammatory cell infiltration.

47 Temporal arteritis. Giant cells are visible among the inflammatory cell infiltration in the arterial wall.

46

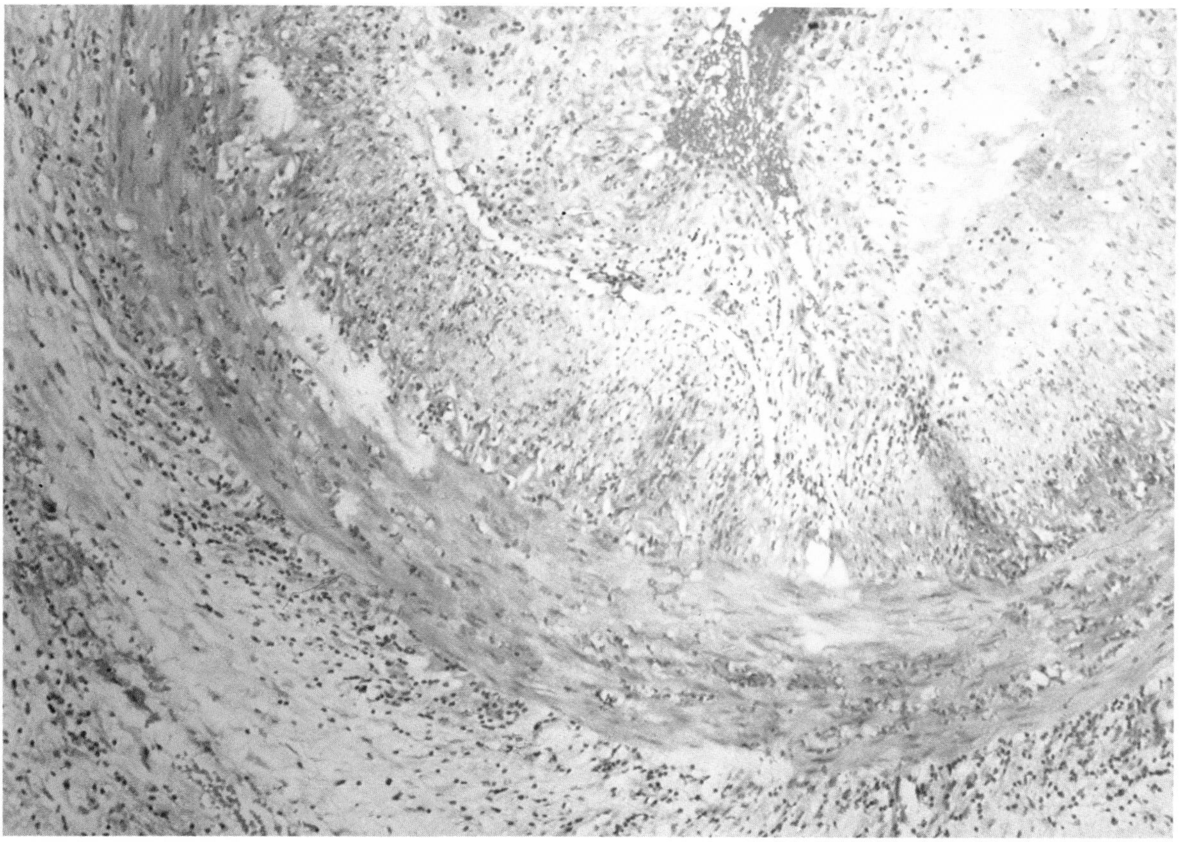

47

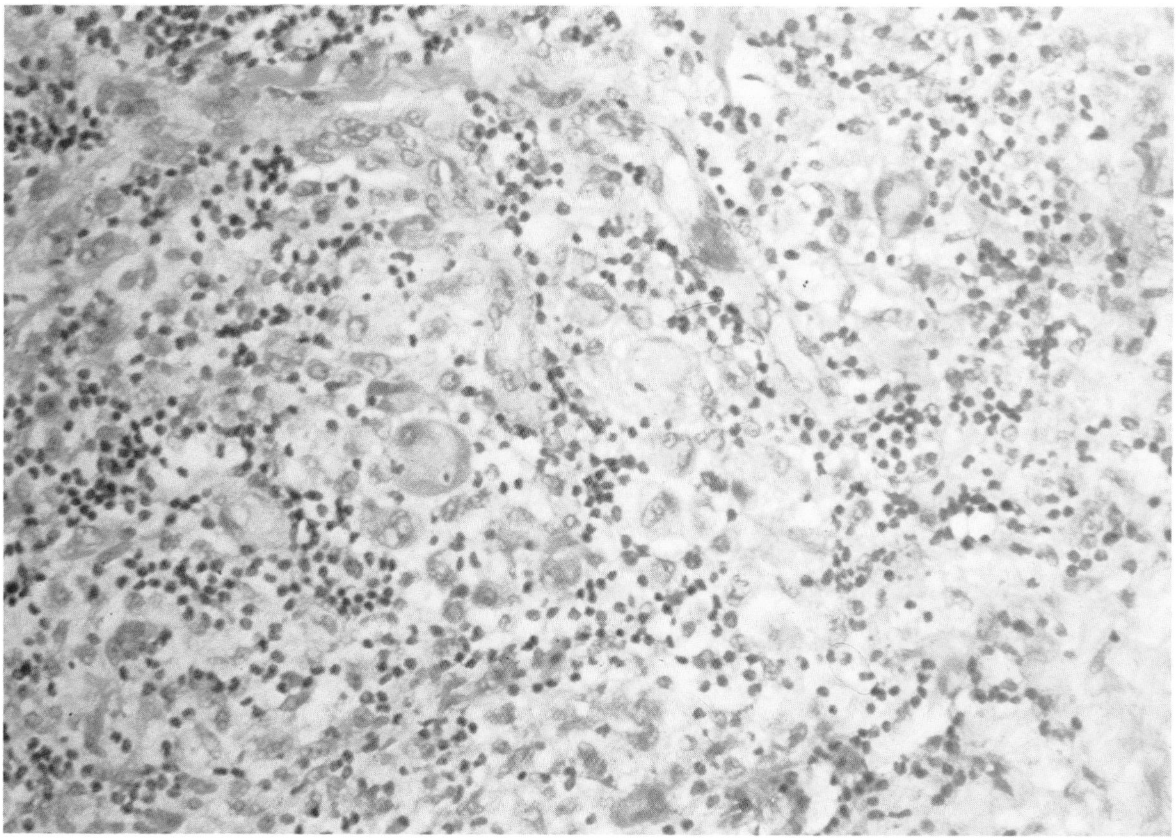

48

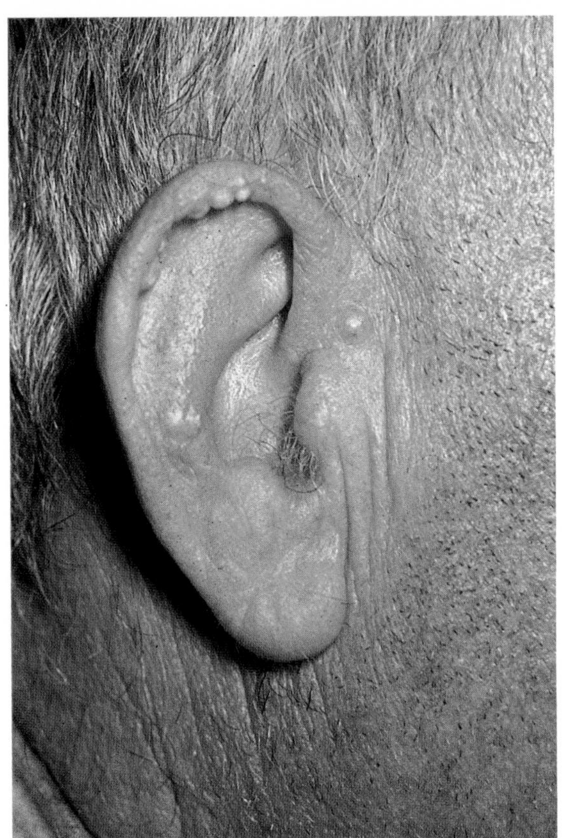

Common causes of hyperuricaemia in the elderly

Primary gout
Lymphomas
Multiproliferative disease
Chronic haemolytic disorders
Chronic renal failure
Starvation, vomiting
Diabetic ketoacidosis
Diuretics

48 Gout. The pinna of the ear shows tophaceous gouty deposits. The patient had chronic gout but the serum uric-acid level was normal.

49 Hyperostosis frontalis interna (arrowed). A benign radiological appearance seen in the elderly. It used to be thought that this was associated with cerebral atrophy, but the evidence does not bear this out.

49

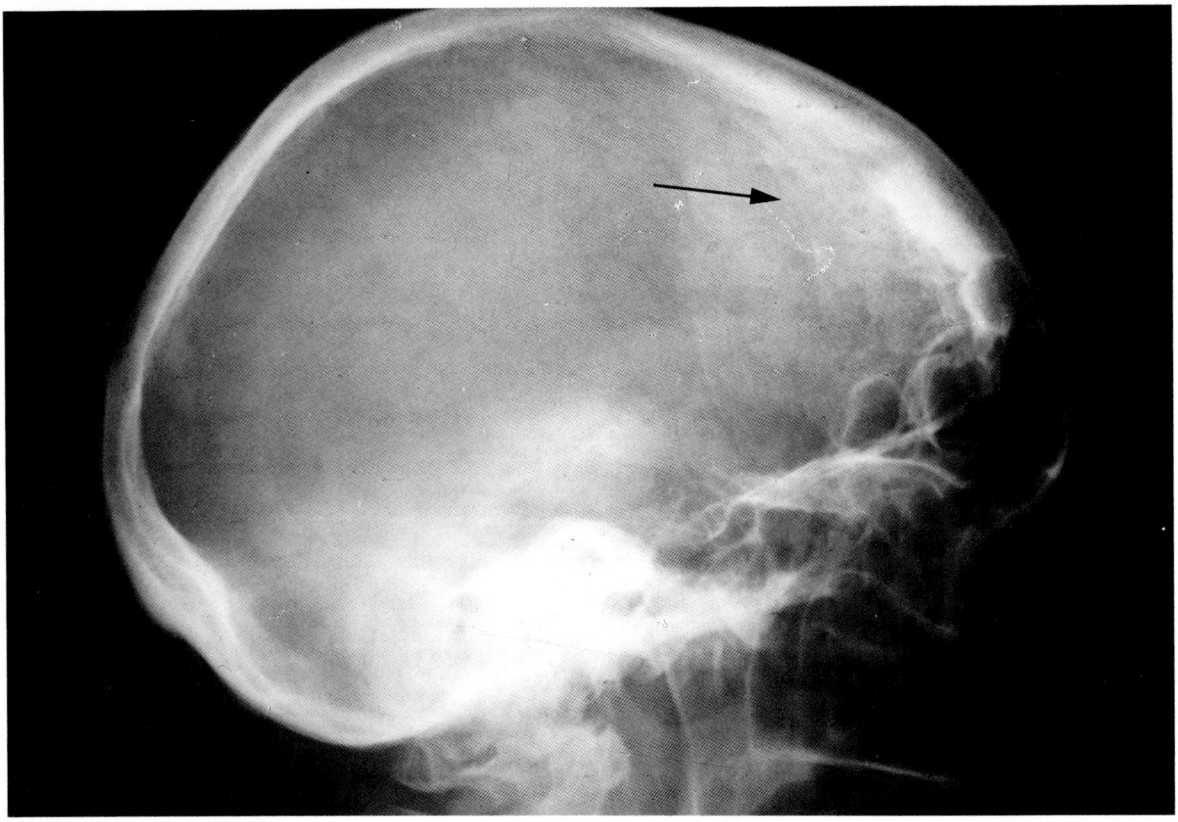

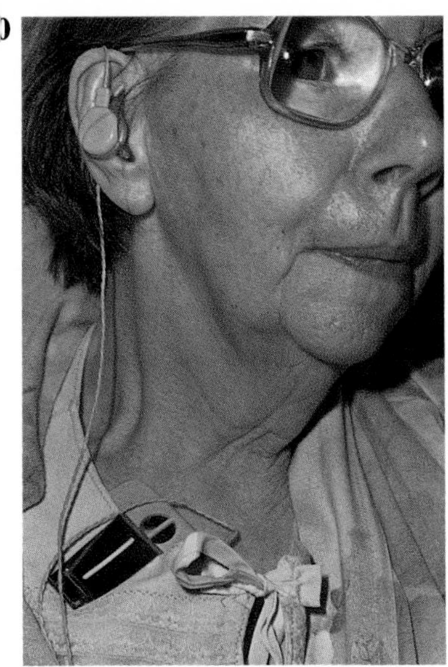

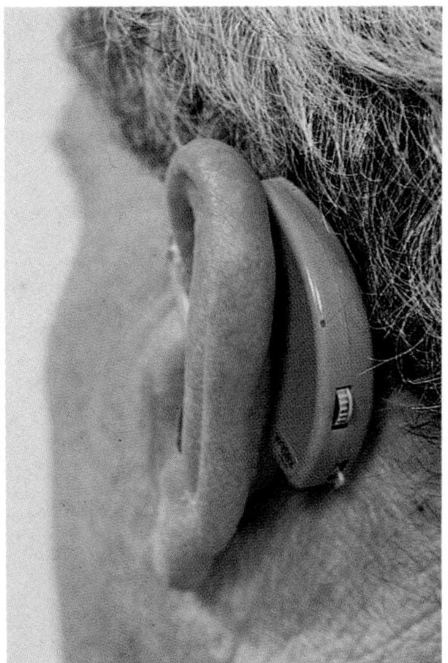

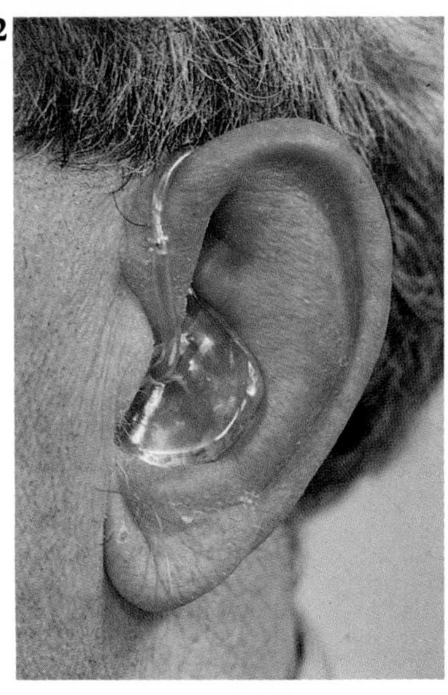

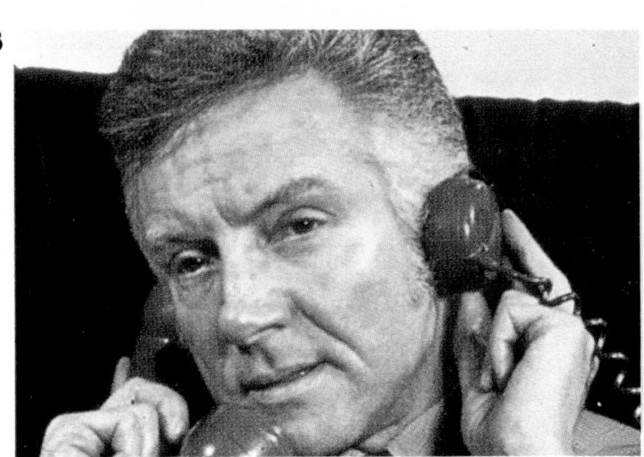

50 Hearing aid. This is a traditional form of hearing aid which is basically an electronic amplifier. This instrument has limitations and requires good maintenance and advisory facilities. Most elderly patients do not use the hearing aid properly.

51 and 52 Hearing aid. A more modern form of hearing aid which because of its small size and compactness has some advantages.

53 Deaf-aid telephone. Note the additional earpiece which improves the stereophonic hearing.

Deafness associated problems

Sensory deprivation
Social deprivation
Withdrawal
Depression
Slow responses
Agitation
Dementia

Deafness: common causes in the elderly

Presbyacusis – sensory neural hearing loss of between 10–60 dB
Wax in external auditory canal
Perforation of tympanic membrane
Otosclerosis
Meniere's disease
Herpes zoster infection
Acoustic neuroma
High-dosage or long lasting drugs
– quinine (for cramps)
kanomycin
neomycin
ethacrynic acid
frusemide

54

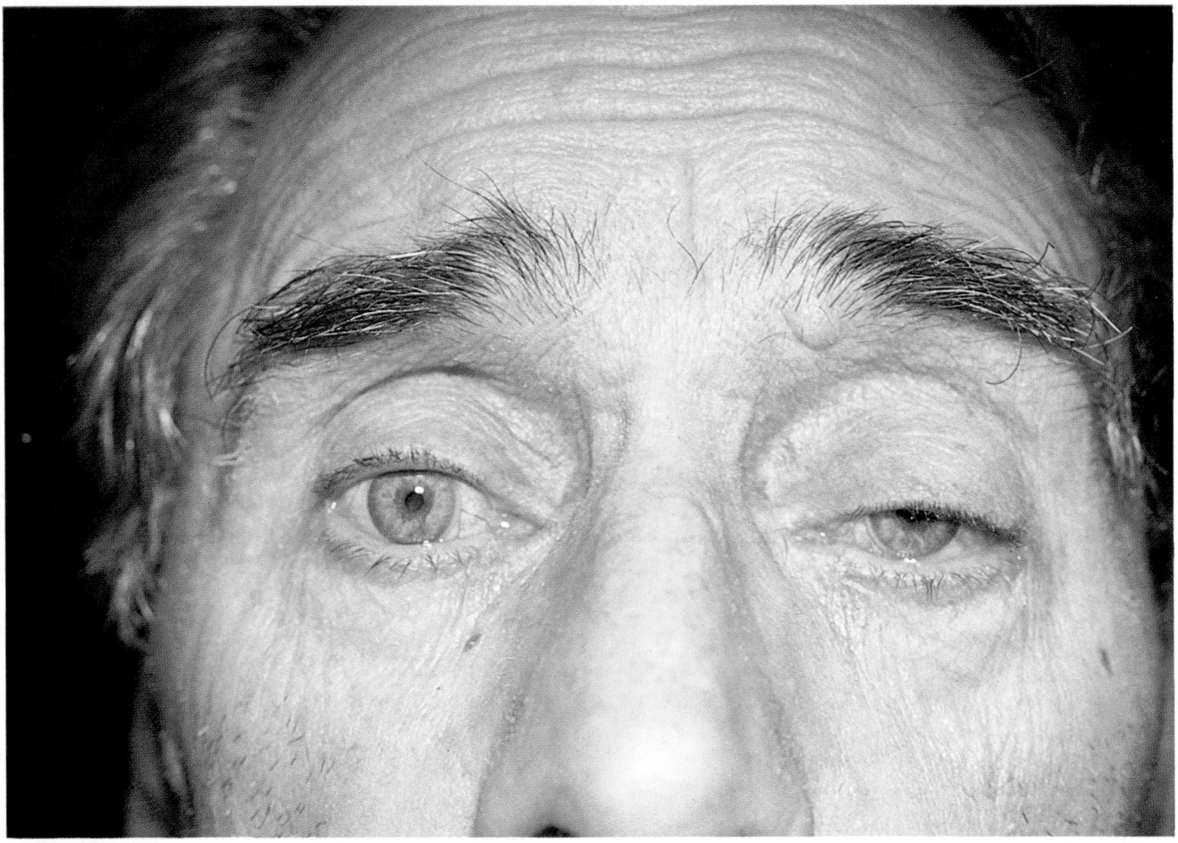

55

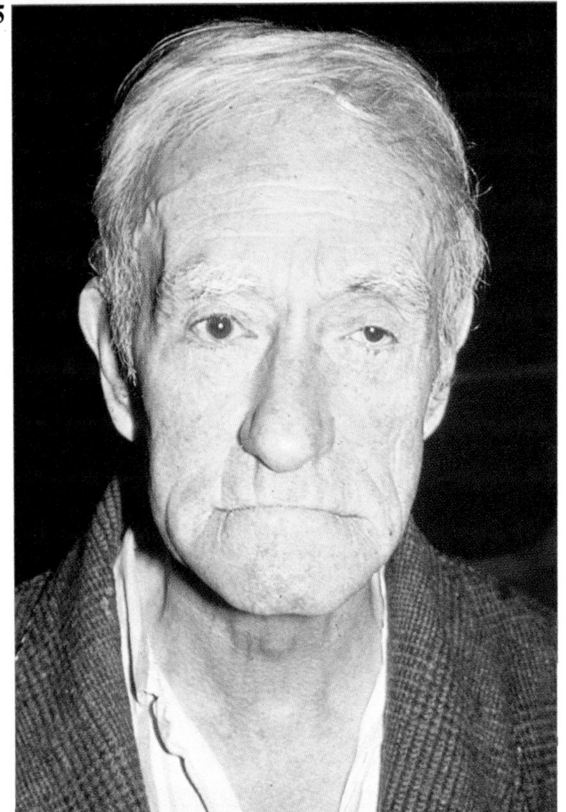

54 Ptosis. Left-sided ptosis caused by a lesion involving the cervical sympathetic chain.

55 Horner's syndrome. An elderly man with Horner's syndrome showing ptosis on the left side.

Causes of ptosis

A Congenital – simple ptosis
B Acquired
  1 *Neurogenic*
    Traumatic ophthalmoplegia
    Congenital 3rd nerve palsy
    Vascular lesions
    Tumors
    Ophthalmoplegic migraine
    Horner's syndrome
    Multiple sclerosis
  2 *Myogenic*
    Senile ptosis
    Myasthenia gravis
    Late acquired hereditary ptosis
    Corticosteroid-induced ptosis
  3 *Traumatic*
    Surgical and accidental

56 Nasolabial seborrhoea in facial palsy. This condition is associated with Vitamin-B complex deficiency (in association with cheilosis and angular stomatitis).

57 Facial palsy. Right-sided facial palsy which gradually improved over a period of months. It was associated with a CVA causing hemiplegia.

58 Xanthelasmas. The patient had a family history of ischaemic heart disease and presented with myocardial infarction. The blood lipids were only marginally raised.

57

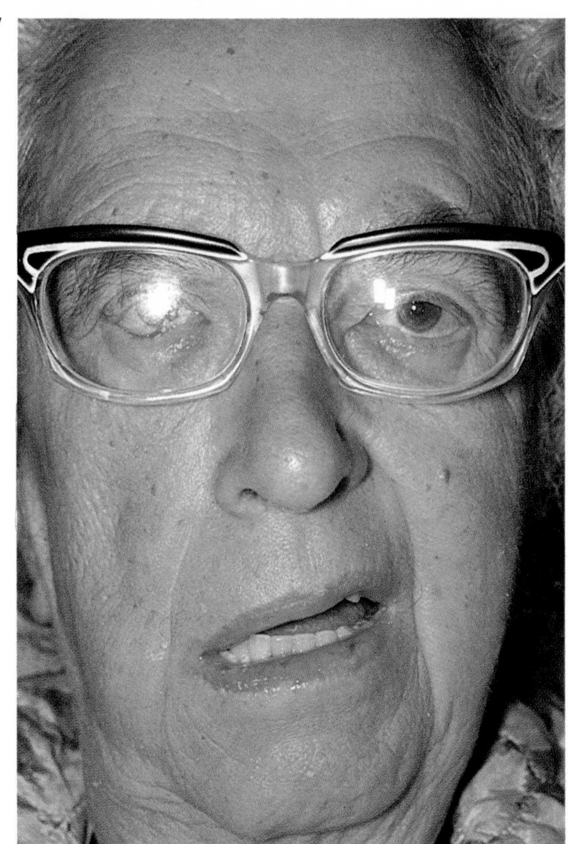

56

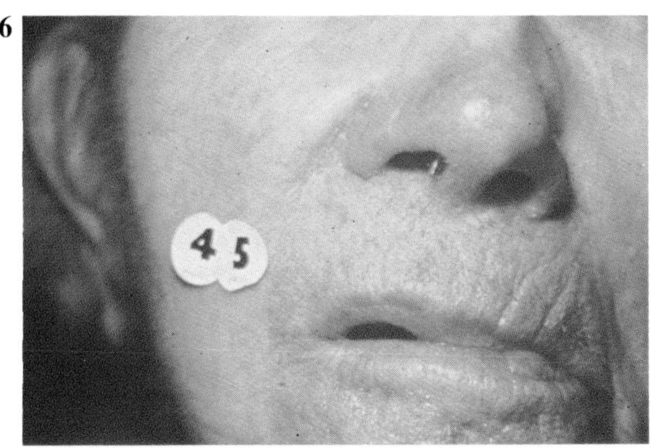

58

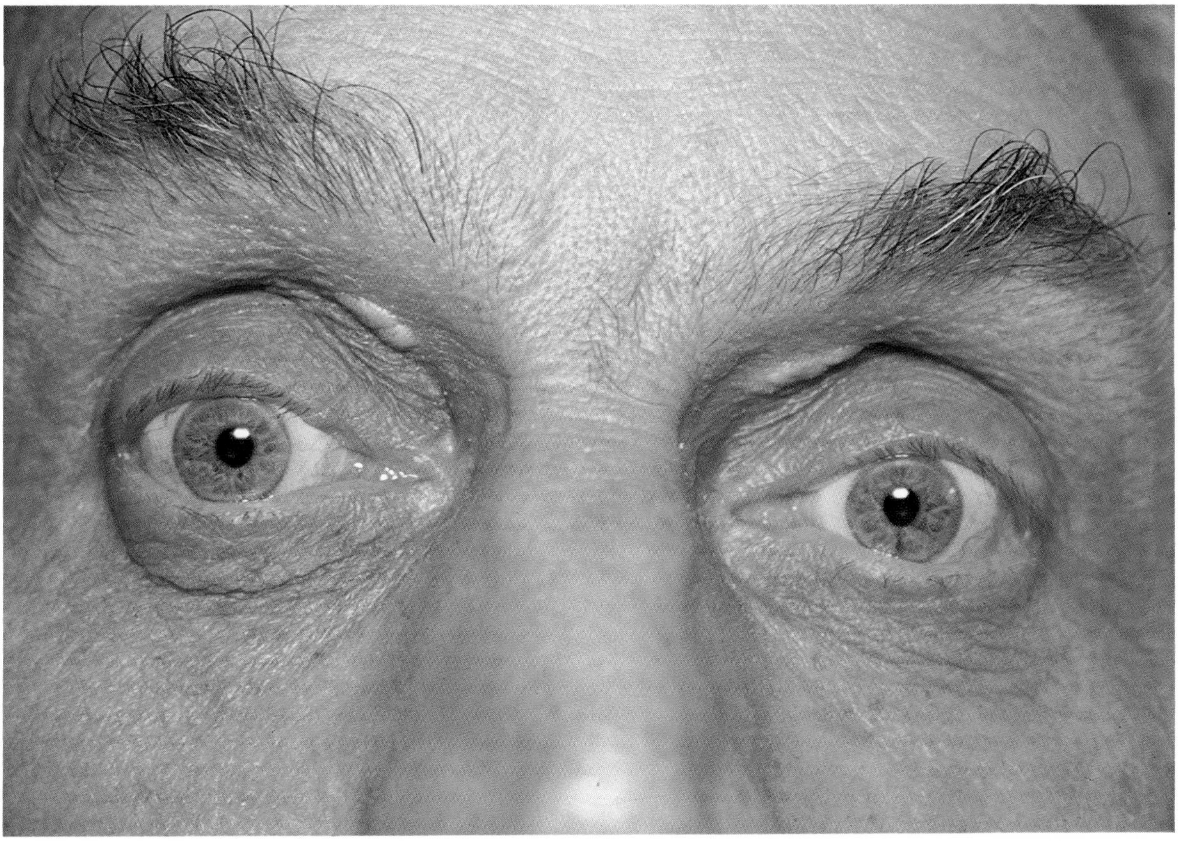

59

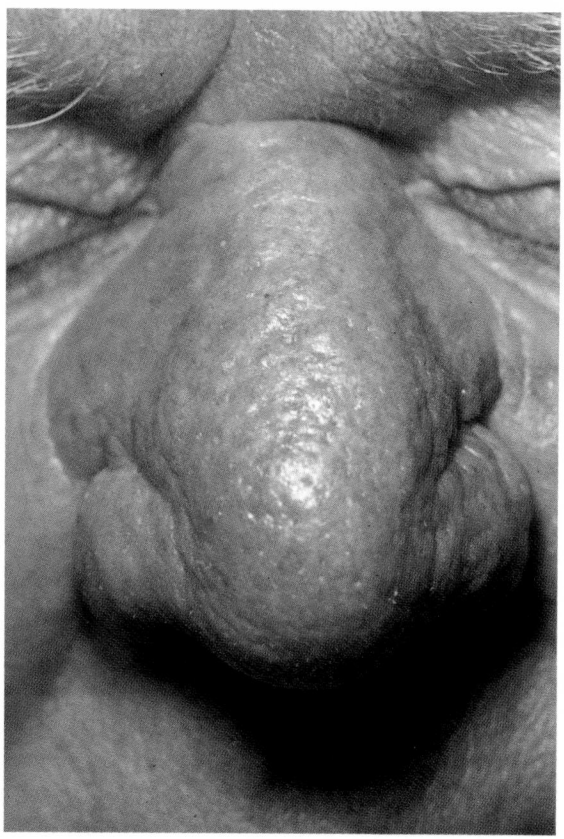

59 Rhinophyma. Increase in soft tissue, sebaceous gland hypertrophy and secondary acne may result from increased vascularity in the centre of face.

60 Sebaceous cysts. Giant sebaceous cysts on the scalp of an elderly man. Most of these are retention cysts caused by plugging of the orifice with sebaceous material. Suppuration is a frequent complication.

60

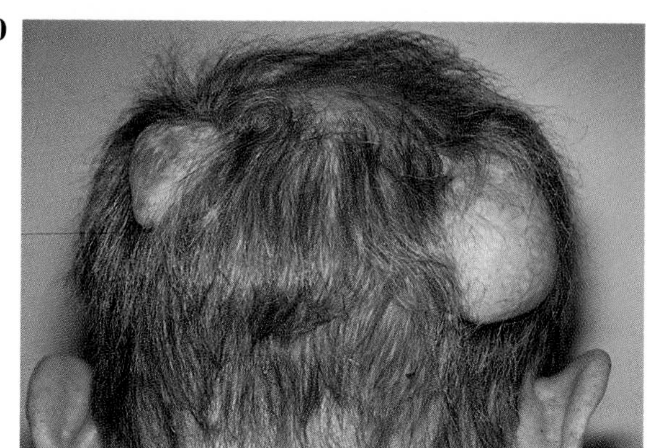

61 Arcus senilis (Gerontoxon). A common finding in the elderly but of no pathological significance. It is formed by lipids being deposited at the periphery of the cornea. This condition is also found in familial hypercholesterolaemias.

62 Cataract. A mature, senile cataract contributing to the patient's disability and lack of independence.

61

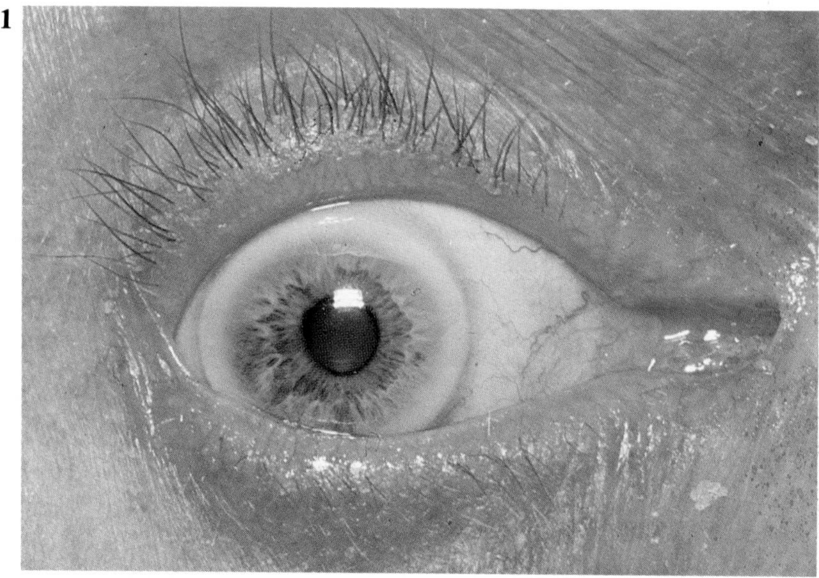

2

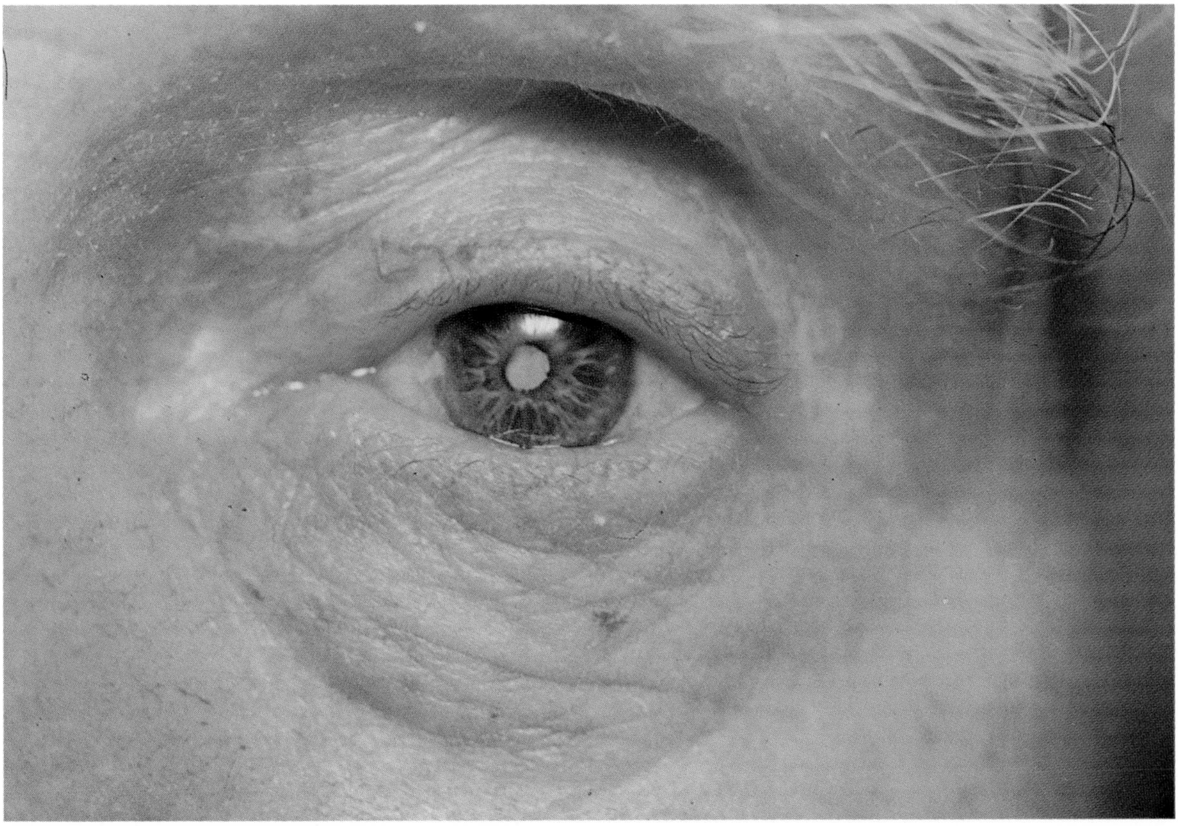

3

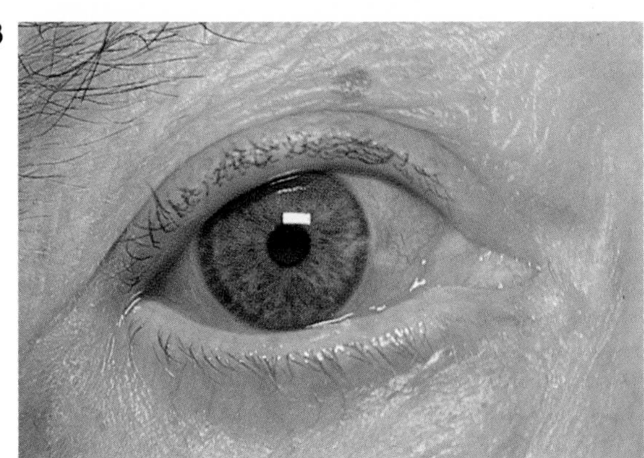

4

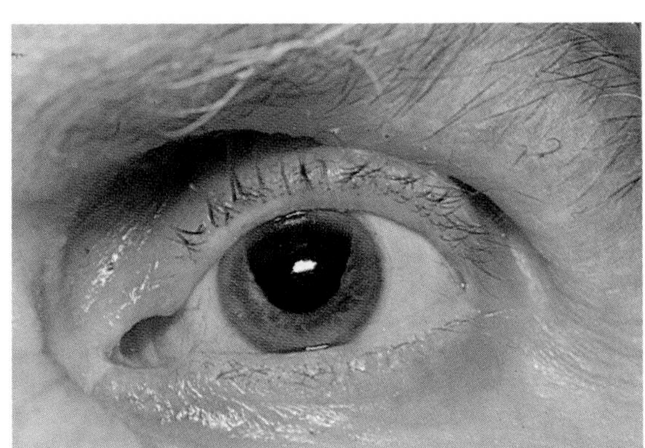

63 Conjunctivitis. A common eye complaint in the elderly, especially residents of long-stay wards. It is usually a keratoconjunctivitis and the aetiologic agent in most cases is an adenovirus.

64 Iridectomy. Irregular pupil after an iridectomy for cataract. This irregularity must be differentiated from other causes of pupillary abnormalities.

Some important causes of visual impairment in older patients

Cataracts
Glaucoma
Senile macular degeneration
Out-dated spectacles
Temporal arteritis
Cerebrovascular accident
Retinal vein thrombosis
Retinal artery thrombosis
Retinal detachment
Old keratitis or uveitis
Papilloedema
Intracranial tumours
Paget's disease
Optic nerve atrophy

65

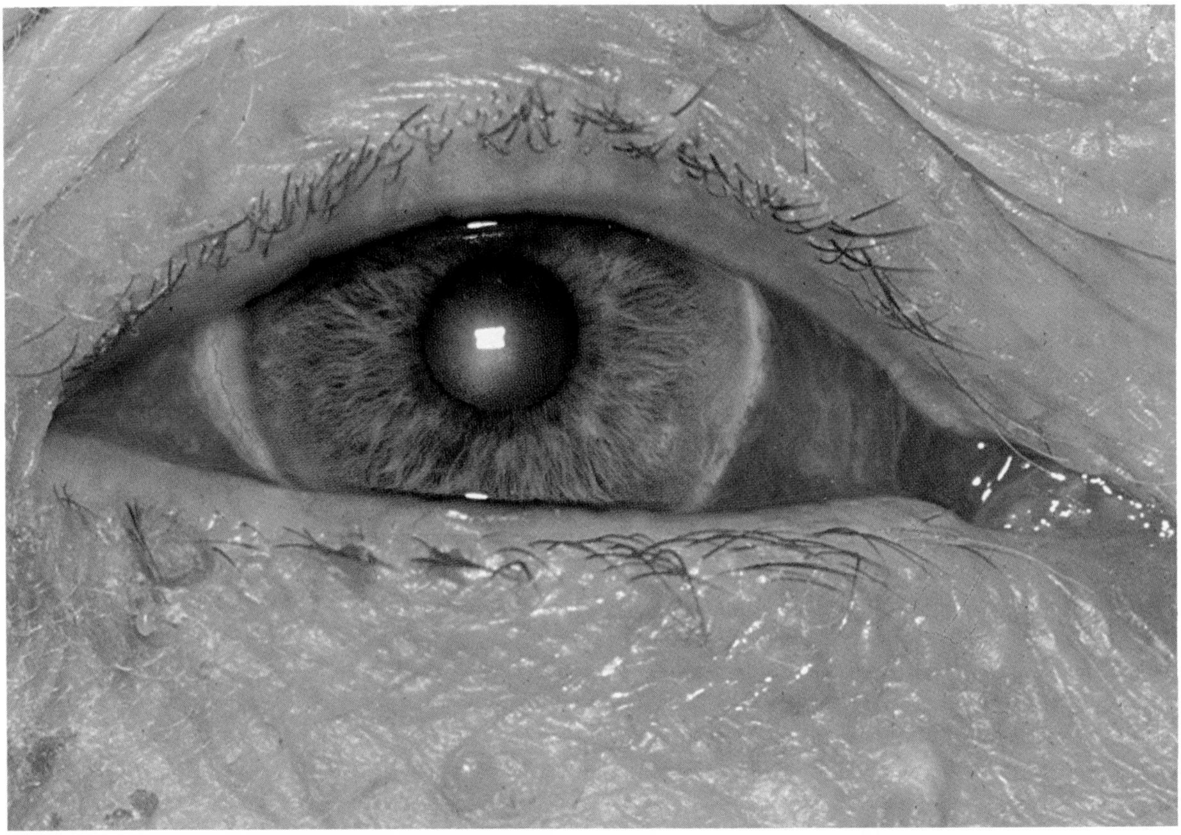

66a

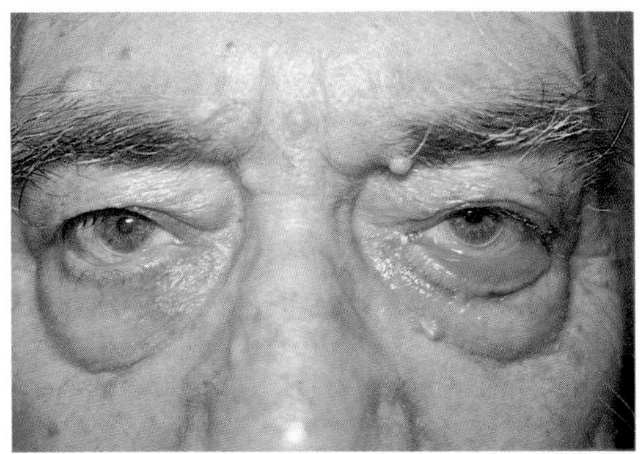

65 Subconjunctival haemorrhage. Alarming in appearance but harmless and self-resolving. In this case it was induced by straining at stools.

66a Ectropion. Chronic ectropion of left lower eyelid resulting in epiphora.

66b Ectropion. Laxity of eyelids is an important mechanism in ectropion of lower eyelid. Wedge resection of lower eyelid with application of skin graft is the method of treatment. This patient also had chronic conjunctivitis.

66b

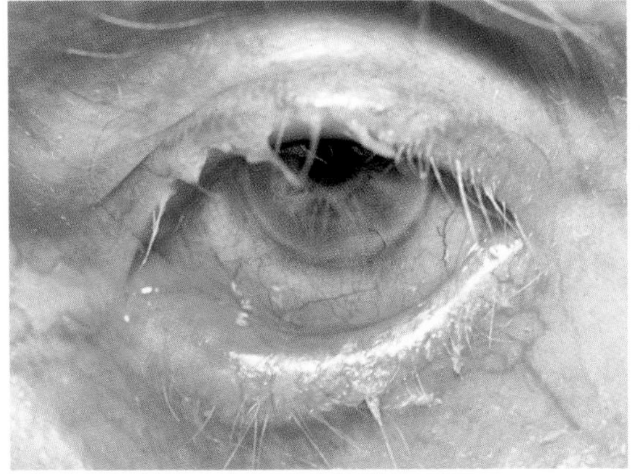

Painful red eye

Stye
Foreign body
Conjunctivitis
Corneal ulcer (e.g. herpetic)
Keratitis
Acute glaucoma
Uveitis

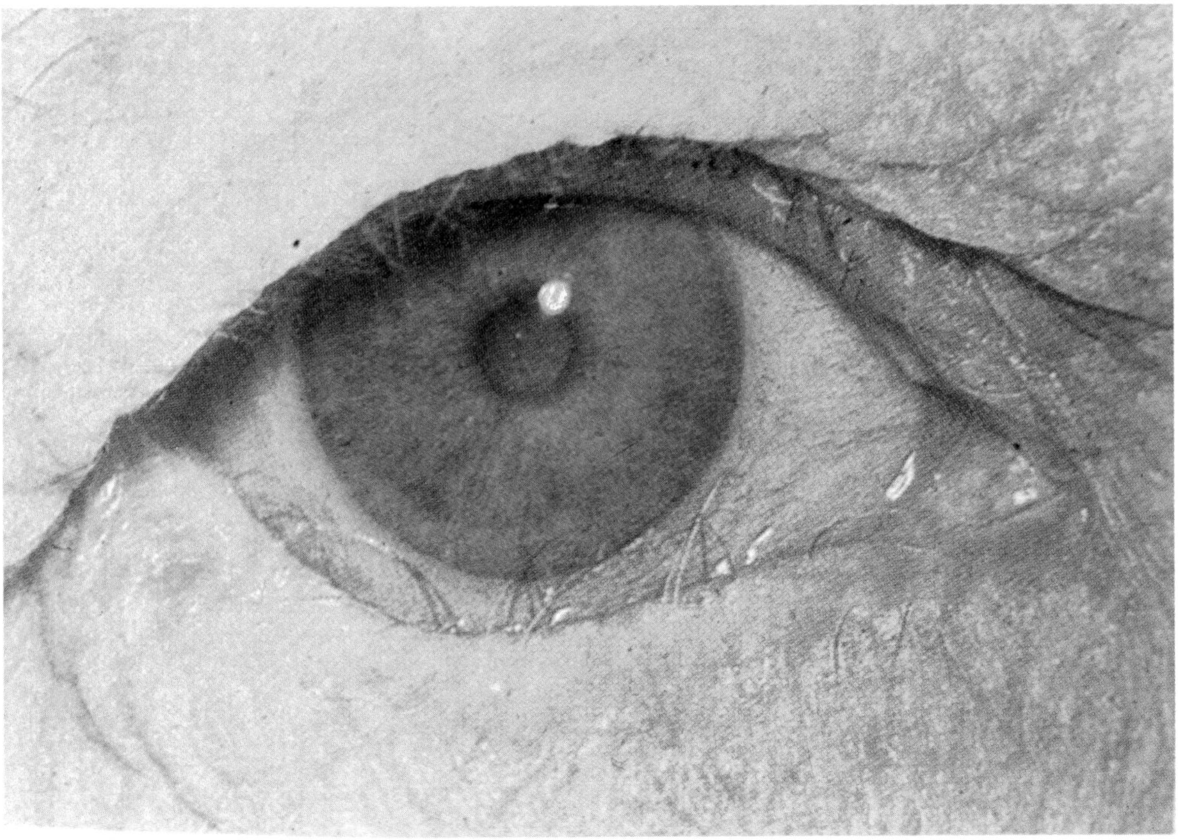

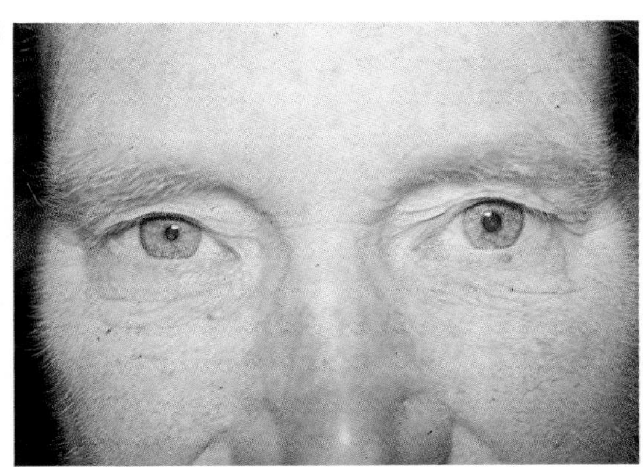

67 Senile entropion. The margin of the lower eyelid has rolled backwards and the eyelashes are brushing against the conjunctiva and cornea.

68 Unequal pupils. The right pupil is dilated in a patient with intracerebral haemorrhage. This pupillary dilatation is less than what one might expect in a younger person.

Pupillary abnormalities occur in:

Lesions of sympathetic fibres
Midbrain lesions
Pontine haemorrhage
Tabes dorsalis
Multiple sclerosis
Diabetes mellitus
Holmes-Adie's pupil
Drugs e.g. atropine, morphine
Local eye disorders

69

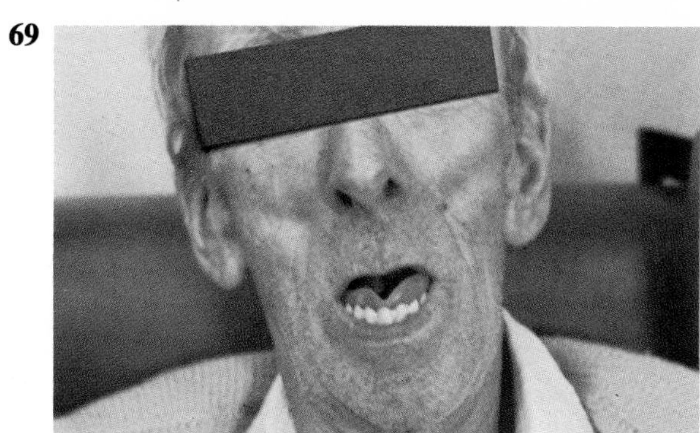

70

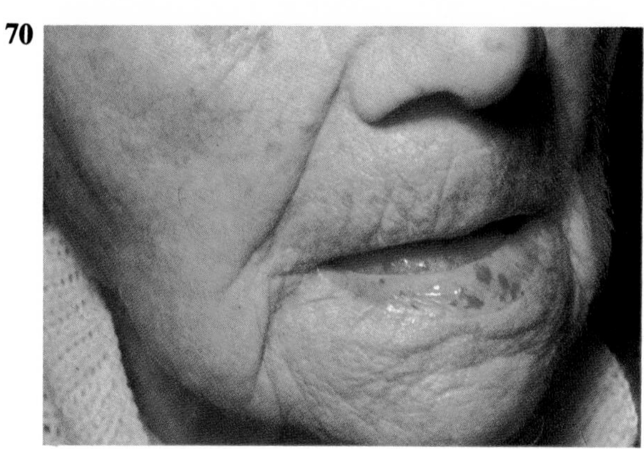

71

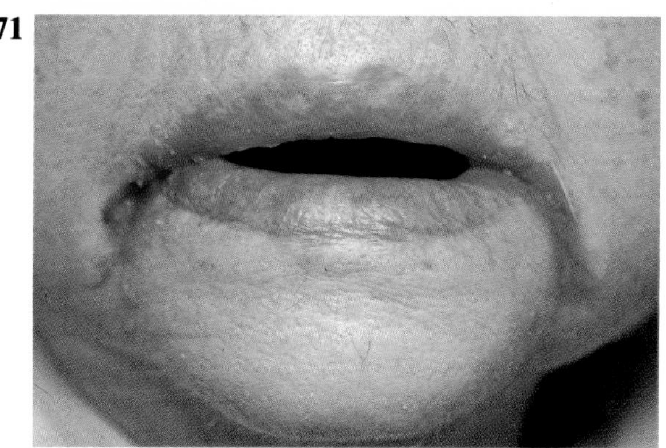

72

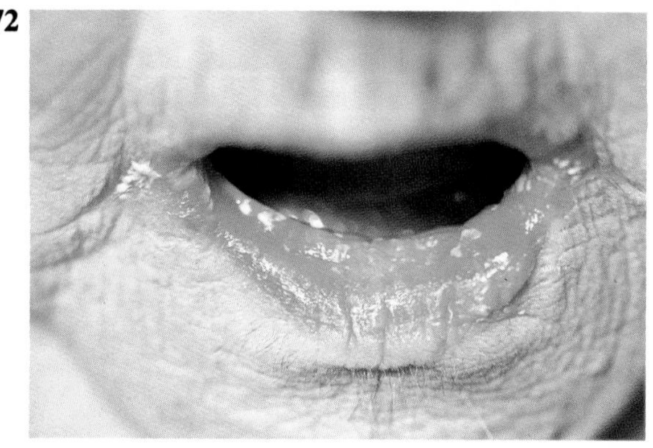

73

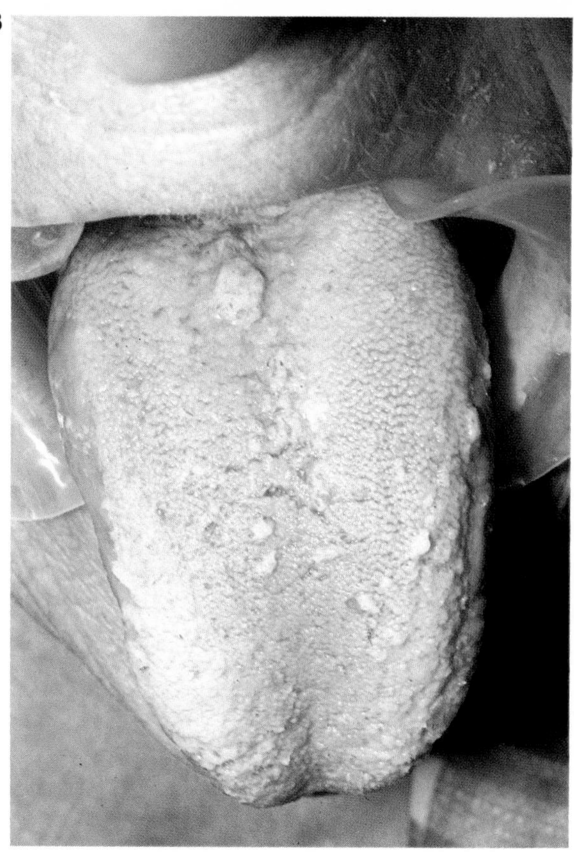

69 Ill-fitting dentures. Caused by shrinkage of gums and jaw with advancing age. May also occur after a stroke with facial paralysis. Ill-fitting dentures can lead to poor nutrition in the elderly. One-third to two-thirds of patients complain of looseness or soreness.

70 Telangiectasia. A case of hereditary haemorrhagic telangiectasia in an elderly man. The telangiectasia are visible in the mucous membrane of lips and increase in number as age advances. Epistaxis is a common complaint.

71 Angular stomatitis. This elderly patient, a spinster, was undernourished and had multivitamin deficiency.

72 Angular stomatitis. Note the associated cheilosis. The patient had iron-deficiency anaemia.

73 Dry-coated tongue. This patient was dehydrated, with high blood urea and low urinary output. Dry tongue may also occur in mouth breathers and is a nonspecific finding.

74

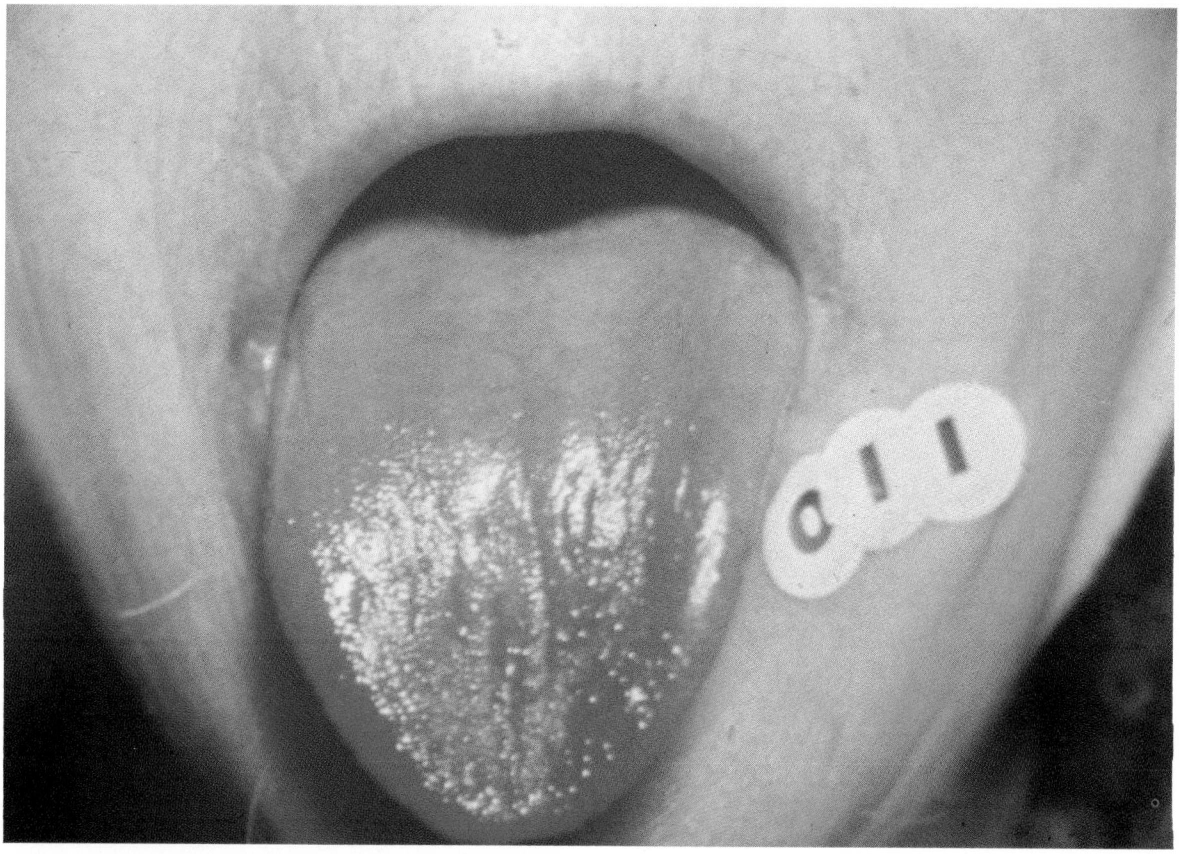

75

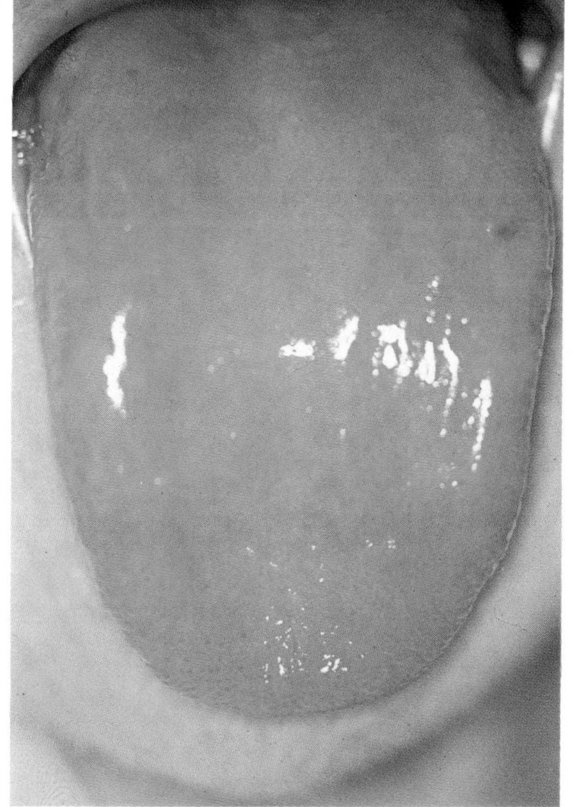

74 Glossitis. Sore, inflamed tongue in a case of Vitamin-B_{12} deficiency anaemia.

75 Smooth, glazed tongue. Atropic glossitis in an elderly lady with chronic iron-deficiency anaemia.

Causes of stomatitis (oral ulceration)

Aphthous ulcers
Debility
Smoking
Alcoholism
Herpes simplex, candidosis
Pyorrhoea and alveolar abcess
Stevens-Johnson syndrome
Neutropenia and leukaemia
Iron deficiency, Vitamin-B complex including Vitamin-B12 and folate deficiency
Pemphigus vulgaris and benign pemphigus of mucous membranes
Lichen planus
Cytotoxic drugs, antibiotics, emepronium bromide, and potassium supplements
Leukoplakia, neoplasm
Ill-fitting dentures

76

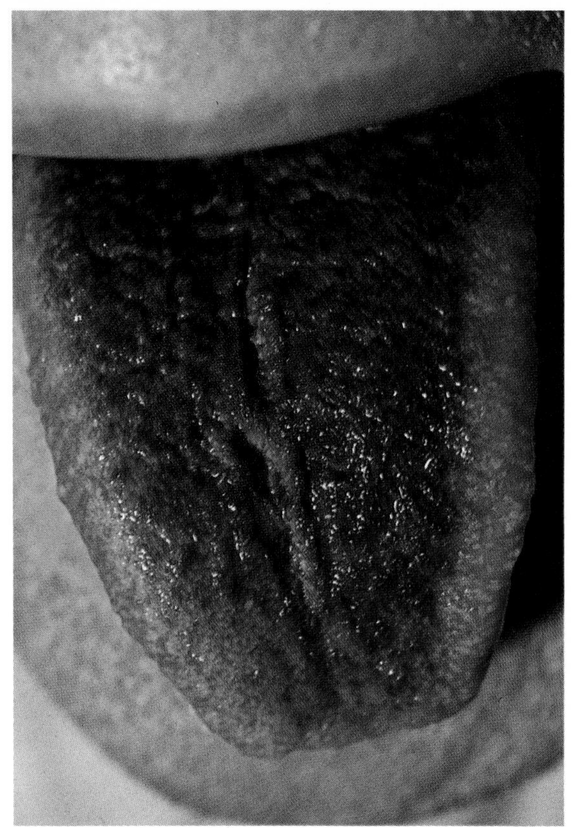

77

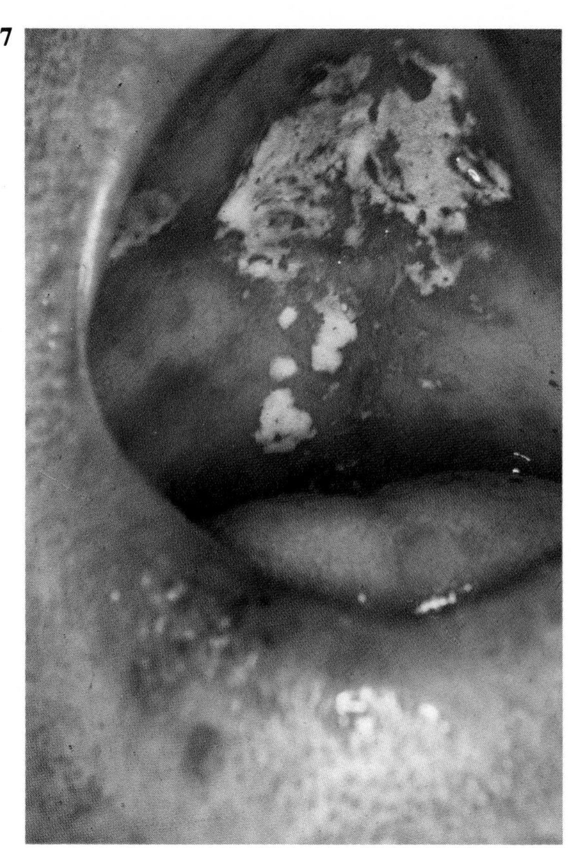

78

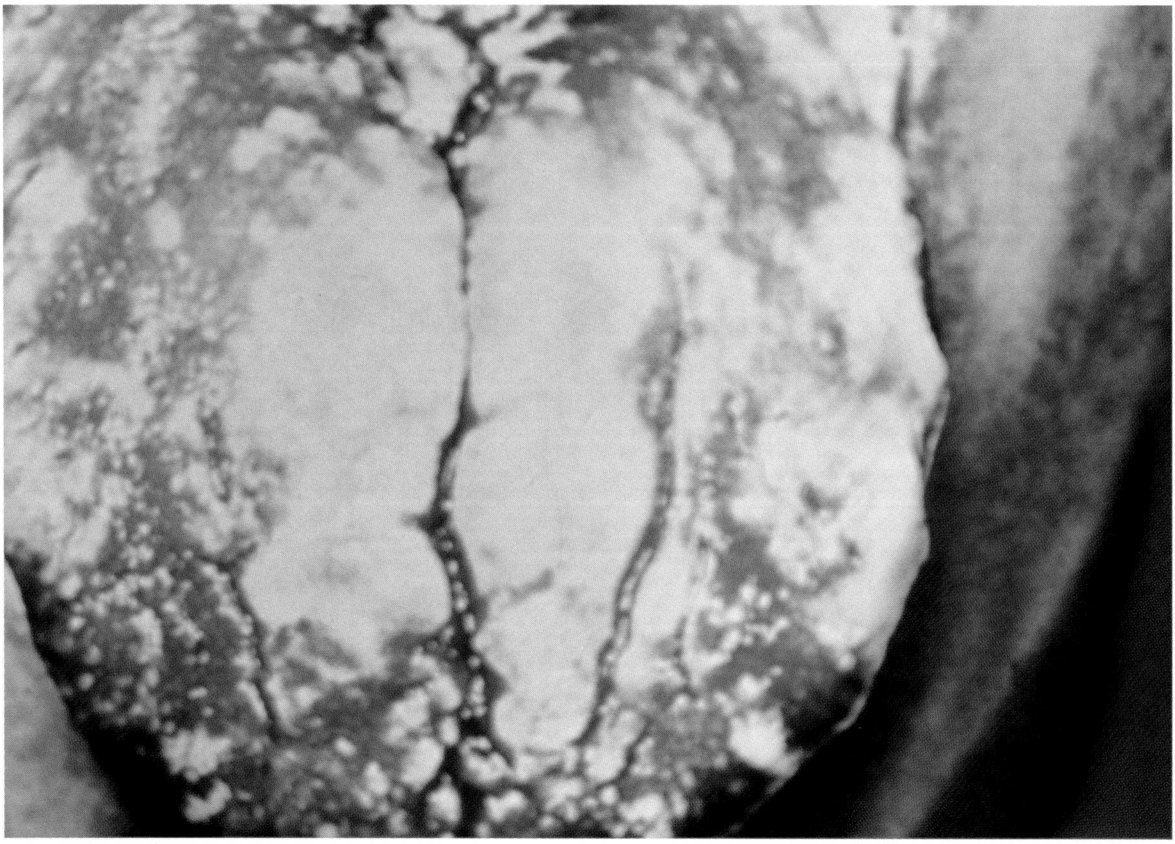

9

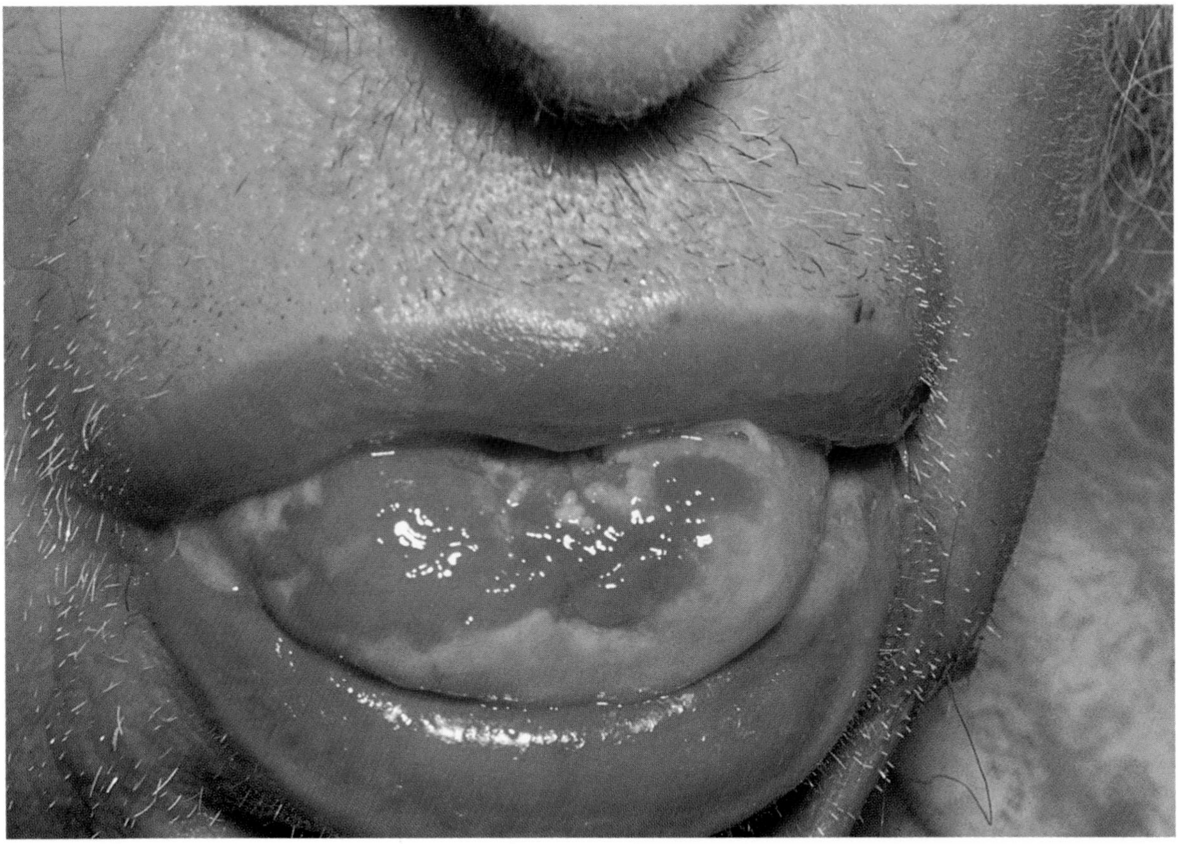

76 Hairy (black) tongue. Elongation of filiform papillae of the medial dorsal surface area caused by failure of keratin layer of the papillae to desquamate normally; brownish, black colouration may be caused by tobacco staining, food, or chromogenic organisms.

77 Leukaemia. Thrush and petechiae in the oral cavity in a case of leukaemia.

78 Candidiasis (thrush). Involving the oral cavity and mainly the tongue, in this case. The adherent and painful white patches are typical of the condition.

79 Drug-induced stomatitis. This ulcer on the tongue was induced by emepronium bromide, after the patient had kept the tablet in her mouth for too long.

80 Carcinoma of the tongue. A small, painless ulcer on the tongue which failed to heal within a few weeks. Squamous-cell carcinoma is the most common malignant oral tumour; half of these involve the tongue.

81 Sublingual varicosities. A common finding in the elderly but of no particular significance.

80

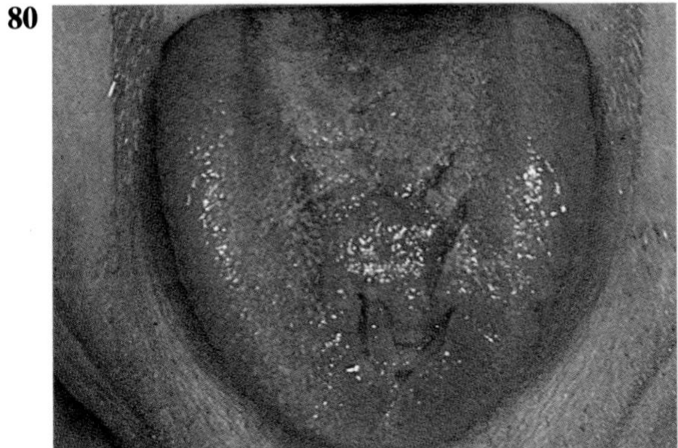

81

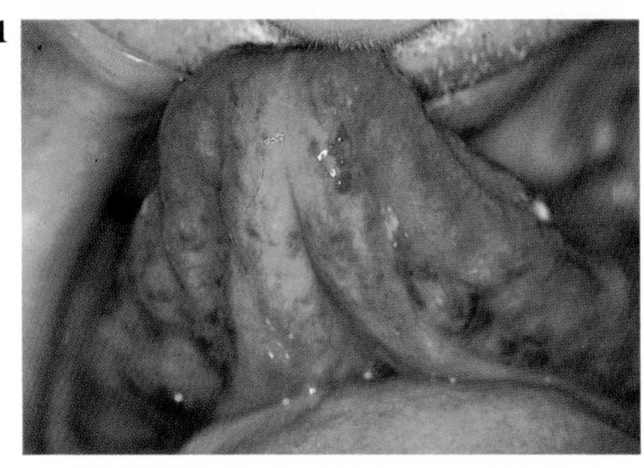

82
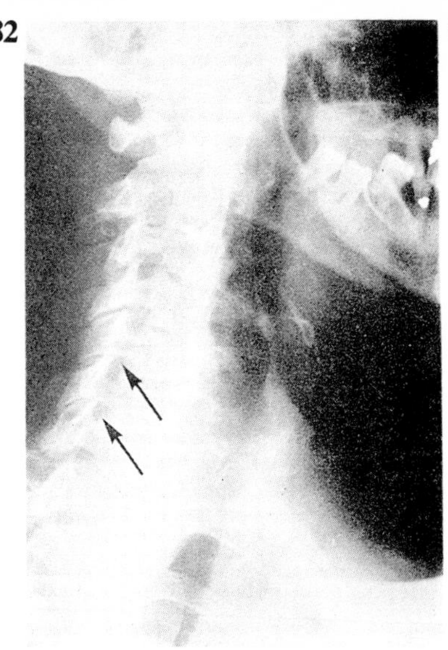
83
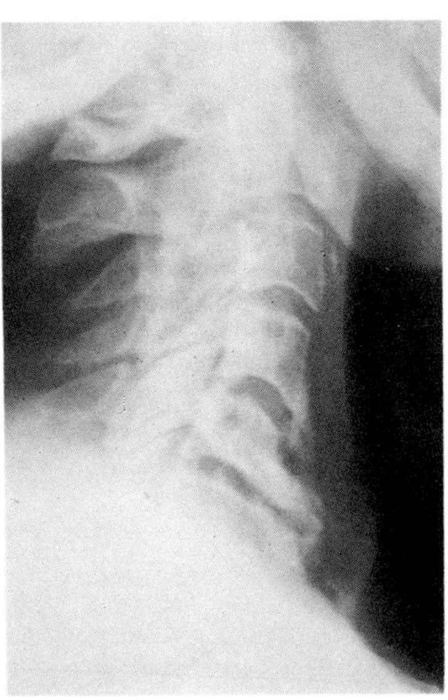
84
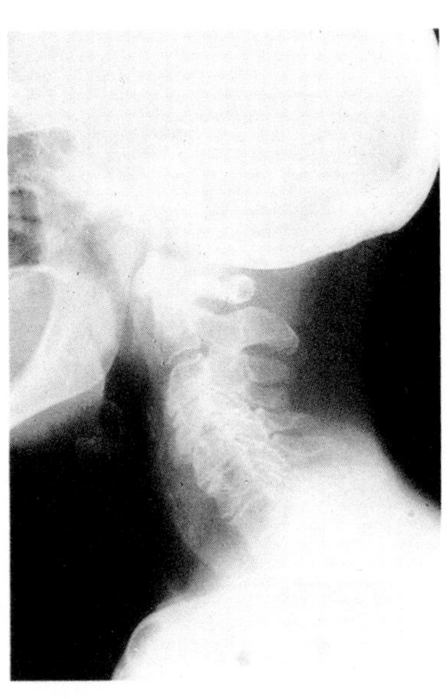

82 Cervical spondylosis. Degenerative changes are present with particular narrowing of the disc faces between C6/7. There is associated osteophyte formation with encroachment on the intervertebral foramina.

83 Cervical spondylosis. There are advanced degenerative changes affecting most joints. The normal curvature is lost and the patient may present with neckache, paraesthesia in upper limbs, dizziness, and drop-attacks.

84 Cervical spondylosis. Note that the atlas has shifted forward on the axis (2nd cervical vertebra). This is an emergency. Urgent orthopaedic attention is required because there is danger of the patient developing quadriplegia.

Cervical spondylosis

Radiological changes of cervical spine degenerative disease are almost universal after 70 years of age. The relation between symptoms and xray changes is very poor.

There is an association between cervical spondylosis and postural imbalance caused by disturbance of cervical articular mechanoreceptor function.

Cervical spondylosis frequently coexists with vertebrobasilar insufficiency.

Clinical features

Brachial radiculitis – pain and paraesthaesia
Headache, giddiness and faints
Drop attacks
Diplopia
Facial sensory disturbances
Dysarthria
Weakness of legs and unsteadiness
Paraplegia or quadriplegia in severe cases

5 Disorders of the brain

Clinical manifestations of cerebrovascular disease

1 Transient cerebral ischaemic attacks (TIAs)
2 Stroke – completed or in evolution
3 Multi-infarct dementia
4 Pseudobulbar palsy
5 Epilepsy

Transient cerebral ischaemic attacks (TIAs)

Disorder of cerebral function caused by vascular causes in which full recovery occurs within 24 hours. If neurological disability lasts for more than 24 hours, then it is classified as completed stroke. TIAs are important to recognise because they presage a full-blown CVA. Many of the conditions contributing to development of TIAs can be treated.

Aetiology

Main pathological abnormality is atheroma and hypertension. Precipitating factors:
Microemboli from platelet aggregates on an atheromatous ulcer.
Hypotension – myocardial infarction, heart failure, dysrhythmia, postural hypotension, 'steal' syndrome.
Miscellaneous – anaemia, polycythaemia, giant-cell arteritis, cervical spondylosis, drugs, for example, sedatives.

Clinical features of carotid TIAs

Hemiparesis, paraesthesiae, hemianopia, blindness (amaurosis fugax), dysphasia, dysphagia, confusion, carotid artery bruit.

Clinical features of Vertebrobasilar TIAs

Vertigo, nystagmus, drop-attacks, diplopia, dysarthria, dysphagia, amnesia, weakness.

Completed stroke

In completed stroke the neurological damage reaches its peak in 6 to 24 hours and results in prolonged disability.

Aetiology

Major cause is cerebral infarction due to a combination of thrombosis and inadequate perfusion of brain tissue. Hypertension and other factors that contribute to the development of atheroma are aetiologically important, in both TIAs and strokes. Cerebral damage may also result from embolus from heart or great vessels, cerebral haemorrhage and subarachnoid haemorrhage.

Clinical features

Symptoms and signs depend on extent and site of brain damage. The carotid territory is most often involved.

The onset is usually sudden or rapid:
Impairment of consciousness
Hemiparesis with extensor plantar reflex
Ipsilateral sensory loss
Hemianopia
Cortical sensory loss when there is damage to parietal lobe
Disturbance of attention
Loss of recognition of body image

In left-sided lesions – dyslexia, agraphia, acalculia.
Lesions involving thalamus may produce persistent pain, hypersensitivity and involuntary movements.
Lesions involving dominant hemisphere may produce loss of postural control and gait disorders.
Ischaemia in vertebrobasilar territory may produce a tendency to lean and fall backwards.

Complications of a CVA

Intellectual failure
Urinary incontinence
Spasticity and contractures
Pressure sores
Epilepsy
Depression
Frozen shoulder
Hypothermia
Bronchopneumonia

Diffuse cerebrovascular disease

It is the second most important cause of dementia in old age – the first being Alzheimer's disease. The underlying pathology consists of multiple small lacunar infarcts.

Clinical features

Stepwise course of both physical and mental deterioration, usually associated with acute recurrent cerebrovascular episodes. Dementia develops slowly with unpleasant changes in personal habits and behaviour. Patient becomes agitated, restless, cantankerous and paranoid. General picture resembles parkinsonism. There is increased rigidity especially of legs, resulting in shuffling gait and recurrent falls. Eventually the patient becomes completely immobile and bedfast.

Pseudobulbar palsy

Occurs during the course of diffuse cerebrovascular disease. The clinical picture is the result of bilateral upper motor neurone lesions:

Nasal dysarthria, increased jaw jerk, no wasting of tongue, gross emotional lability, dysphagia, and eventually aspiration pneumonia.

Brain failure

Classification and aetiology

1 *Acute*
Toxic confusional states
Infections, myocardial infarction
Heart failure, drugs, alcohol
Sudden environmental change
Faecal impaction, etc.

2 *Chronic Dementias*
Senile dementia – Alzheimer's disease
Multi-infarct dementia
Huntington's chorea
Dementia with parkinsonism
Jakob-Creutzfeldt disease
Pick's disease
Kuru
Multiple sclerosis

3 *Organic Brain Disease*
Myxoedema, Vitamin-B_{12} and folate deficiencies, drugs like barbiturates, head injury, tumours, alcoholism, neurosyphilis, chronic renal failure, normal pressure hydrocephalus, non-metastatic complication of carcinomas, pellagra, hypercalcaemia, prolonged hypoglycaemia

Dementia

Diffuse impairment of the intellect and personality, of insidious onset and usually progressive.

Non-medical causes of dementia and confusion in old age

Eccentricity
Exaggeration of symptoms by patient, relatives or staff
Social and cultural barriers
Pseudodementia or depression
Diogenes syndrome

Clinical features of senile dementia
(chronic brain failure)

Almost normal behaviour in early stages
Forgetfulness, nocturnal restlessness
Habits deteriorate, difficulty in handling memory
Patient faulted on current events and time
Confusional episodes, disorientation
Deterioration of personal care
Incorrect responses
Antisocial behaviour
Complete incapacity to look after self

Incidence

Over 65 years – 10% affected
5% severe
Over 75 years – 13% affected
Over 80 years – 22% affected

Epilepsy

Epilepsy appearing for first time in old age is likely to be caused by cerebrovascular disease. Sometimes an epileptic attack may herald a stroke.

The following diseases may present in older people with symptoms and signs similar to a stroke.

1 Intracranial tumour – primary or secondary
2 Subdural haematoma
3 Cerebral abscess
4 Post-traumatic encephalopathy
5 Meningitis and meningoencephalitis
6 Epilepsy (Todd's paralysis)
7 Meningovascular syphilis
8 Giant-cell arteritis

Intracranial tumours

Types

Meningioma – most common in elderly
Gliomas
Metastasis
Acoustic neuroma
Pituitary tumours

Clinical features

General symptoms:
Headache, confusion, behaviour disorders, epilepsy, dementia.

Localising features:
Hemiparesis, hemianopsia, diplopia, cranial nerve palsies.

False localising signs:
Secondary to raised intracranial pressure, 6th nerve palsy, cerebellar ataxia.

Parkinsonism

Parkinsonian syndrome consists of different pathological conditions with marked clinical similarities. It is a common disease of the central nervous system starting during the sixth or seventh decades.

The basic defect consists of dopamine deficiency in the pigmented nuclei of the brain stem.

Aetiology

Idiopathic
Post encephalitic
Head injury
Cerebral tumours with midbrain compression
Manganese poisoning
Carbon monoxide poisoning
Drugs – phenothiazines, butyrophenones, reserpine, methyldopa

Clinical features

Pill-rolling tremor – not common in older patients.
Tremor of tongue, lips, lower jaw and head.
Hypokinesia – this is the most important cause of disability.
Immobile face, infrequent blinking, impaired chest expansion, difficulty in protruding tongue, loss of synergic movements, loss of balance, positive glabellar tap.
Muscular rigidity – appears early in neck, cogwheel or lead pipe rigidity, characteristic posture with adducted flexed limbs.
Festinant gait, micrographia, turning in bed becomes difficult, stooping posture, impairment of postural control and righting reflexes, falls, complete immobility.
GIT symptoms – dysphagia, excessive salivation, constipation, hiatus hernia, weightloss.
Mental disturbances – depression and irritability, dementia in advanced cases.
Other features – feeble and monotonous speech with loss of phonation, contractures, increased flushing, and sweating.

Prognosis

Idiopathic parkinsonism in the elderly is a chronic progressive incurable disease. About 60 per cent of patients are dead within 10 years of first being diagnosed. The causes of death are bronchopneumonia, pressure sores, urinary tract infections, fractured femur, and other complications of postural instability, wasting and falls.

85 and 86 Atheroma. Aortic arch with great vessels of the neck and Circle of Willis showing common sites of arteriosclerosis.

85

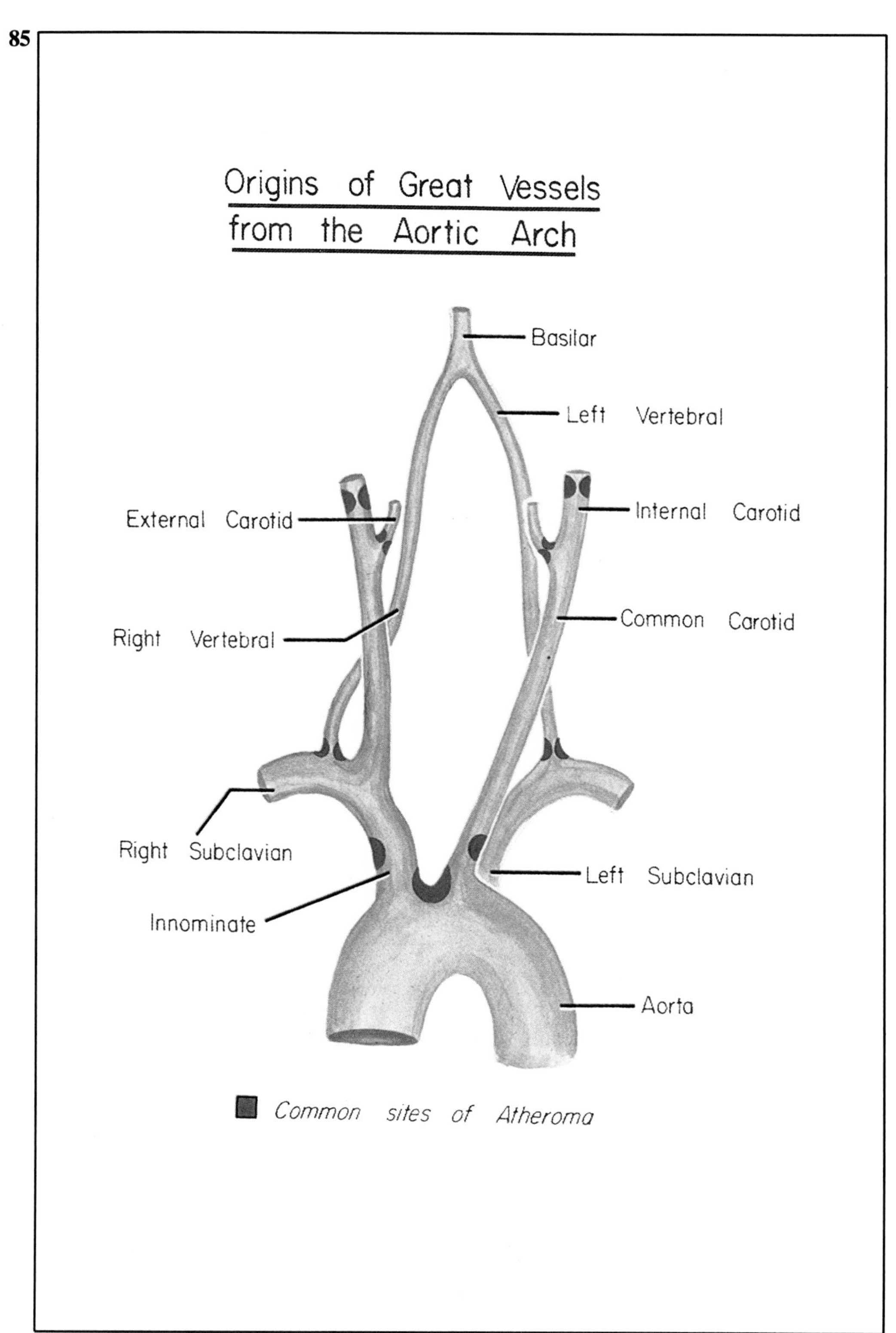

6

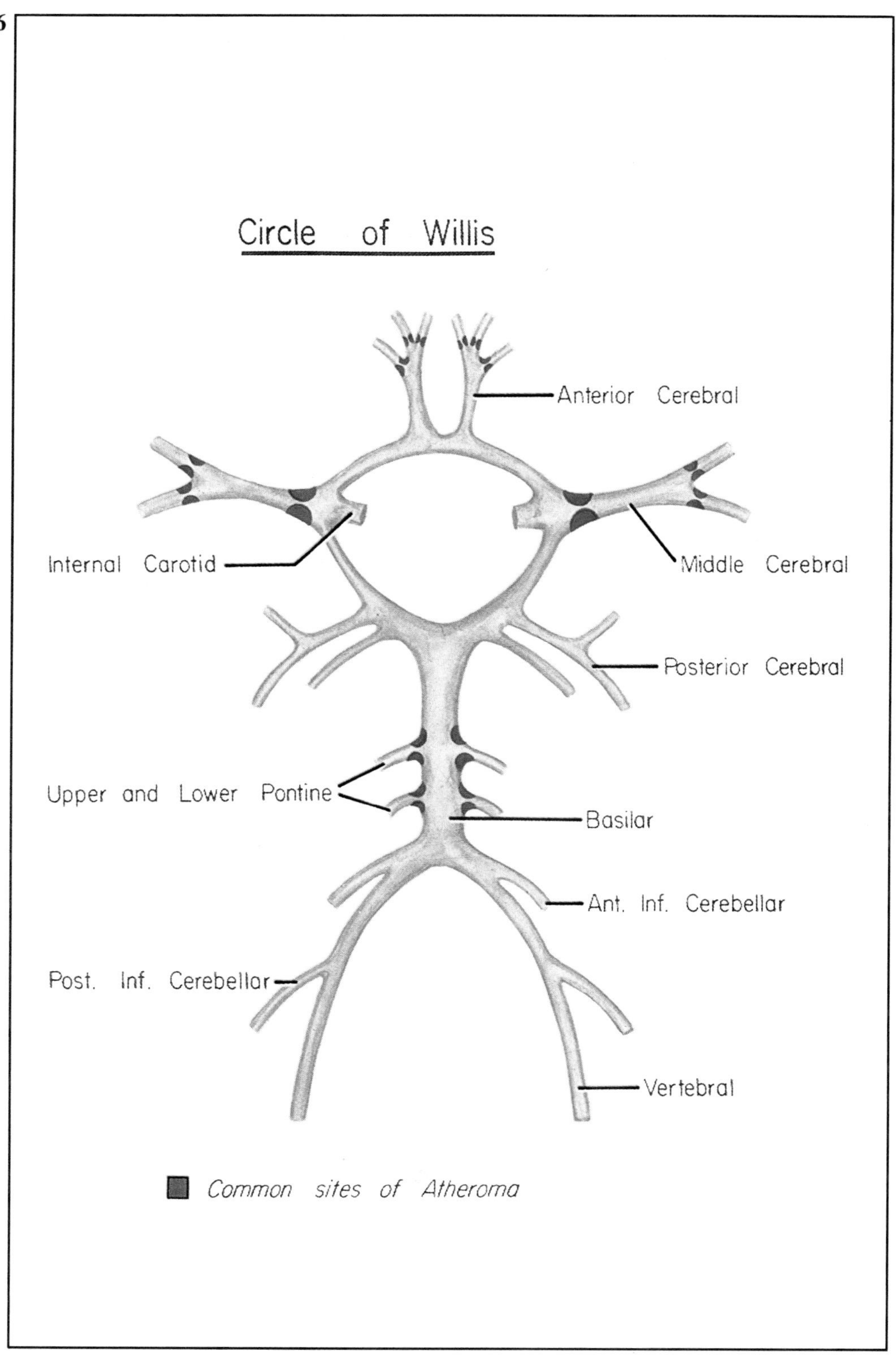
Circle of Willis
Anterior Cerebral
Internal Carotid
Middle Cerebral
Posterior Cerebral
Upper and Lower Pontine
Basilar
Ant. Inf. Cerebellar
Post. Inf. Cerebellar
Vertebral
Common sites of Atheroma

87

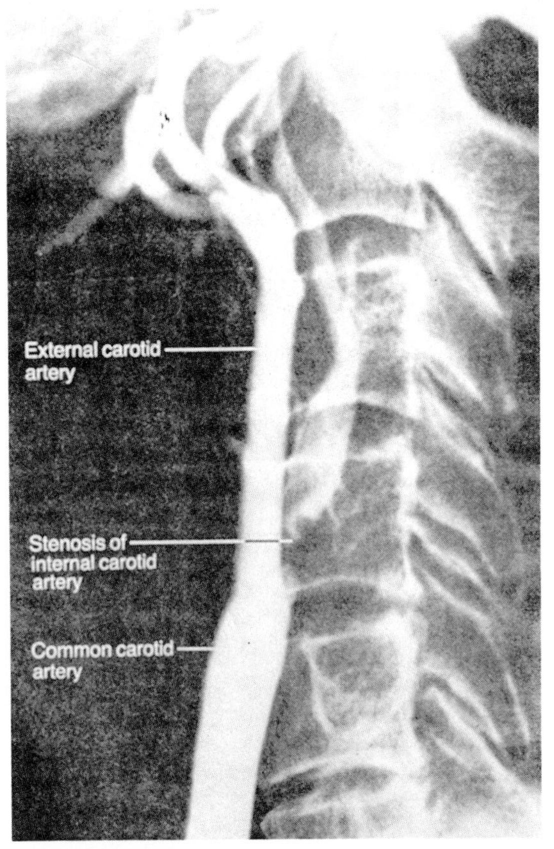

87 Stenosis of internal carotid artery. Revealed by arteriography. A bruit in the neck may be audible and there is risk of a cerebrovascular accident.

88 Stenosis of internal carotid artery. A more severe case shown by arteriography.

88

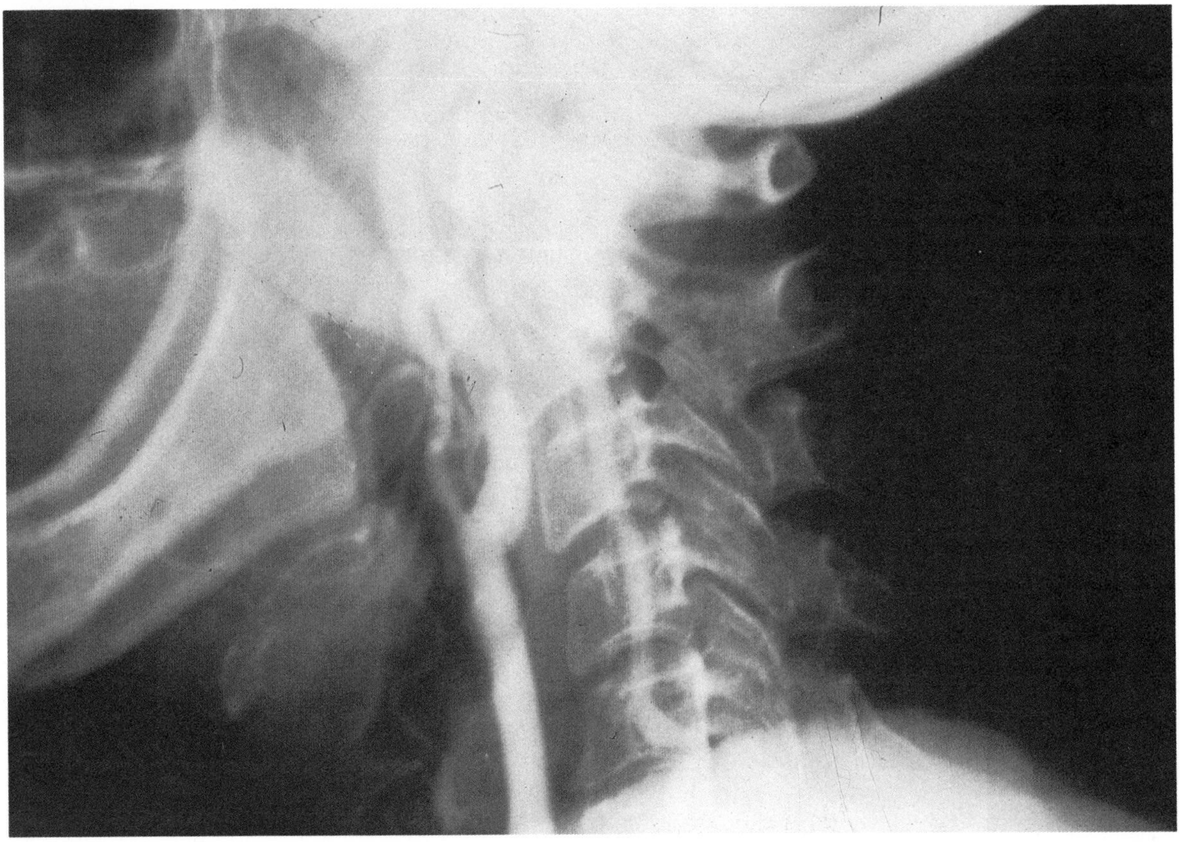

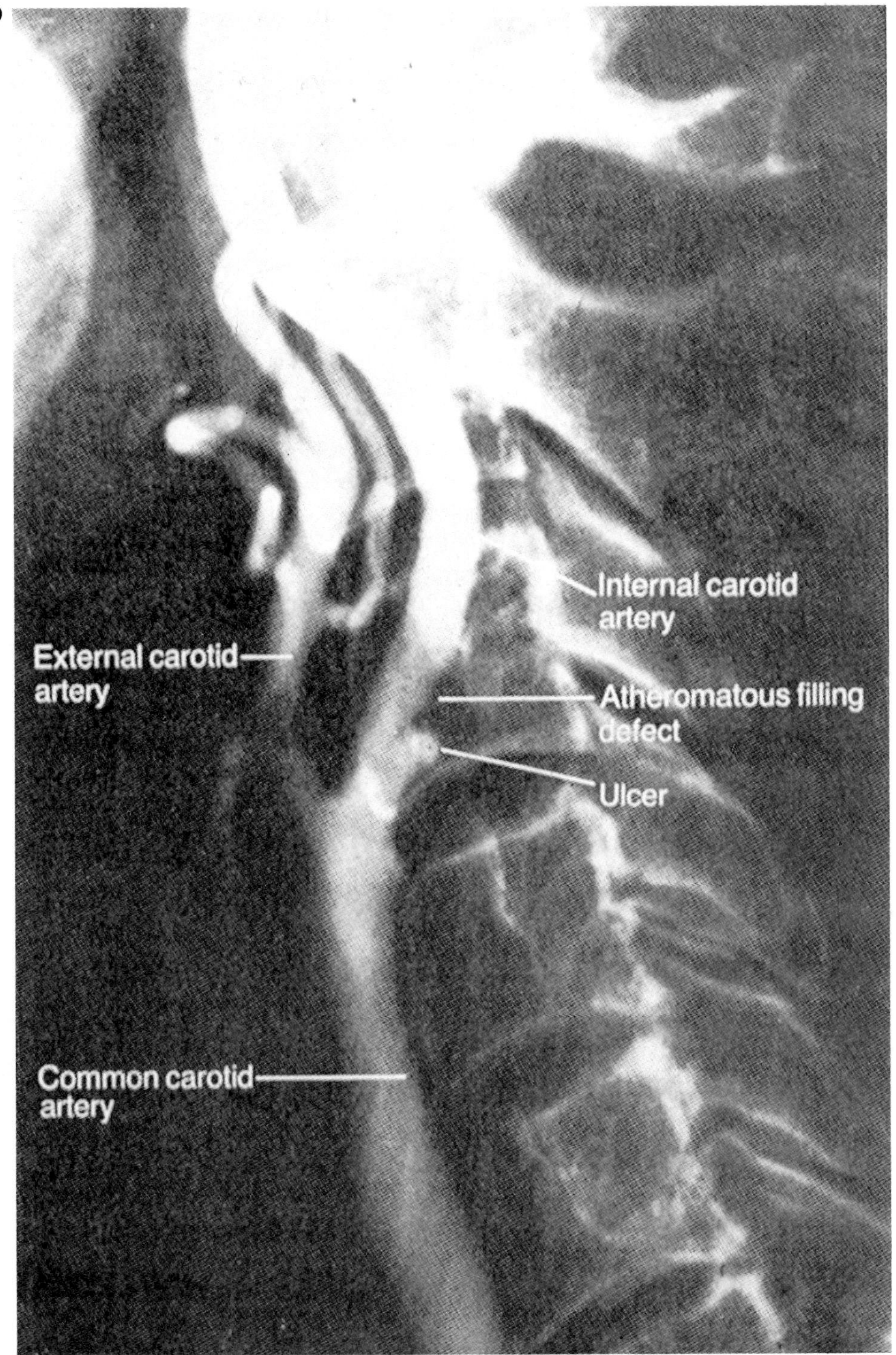

89 Atherosclerosis. Carotid angiogram showing an atheromatous filling defect in the internal carotid artery. Such lesions may cause transient cerebral ischaemic attacks.

90

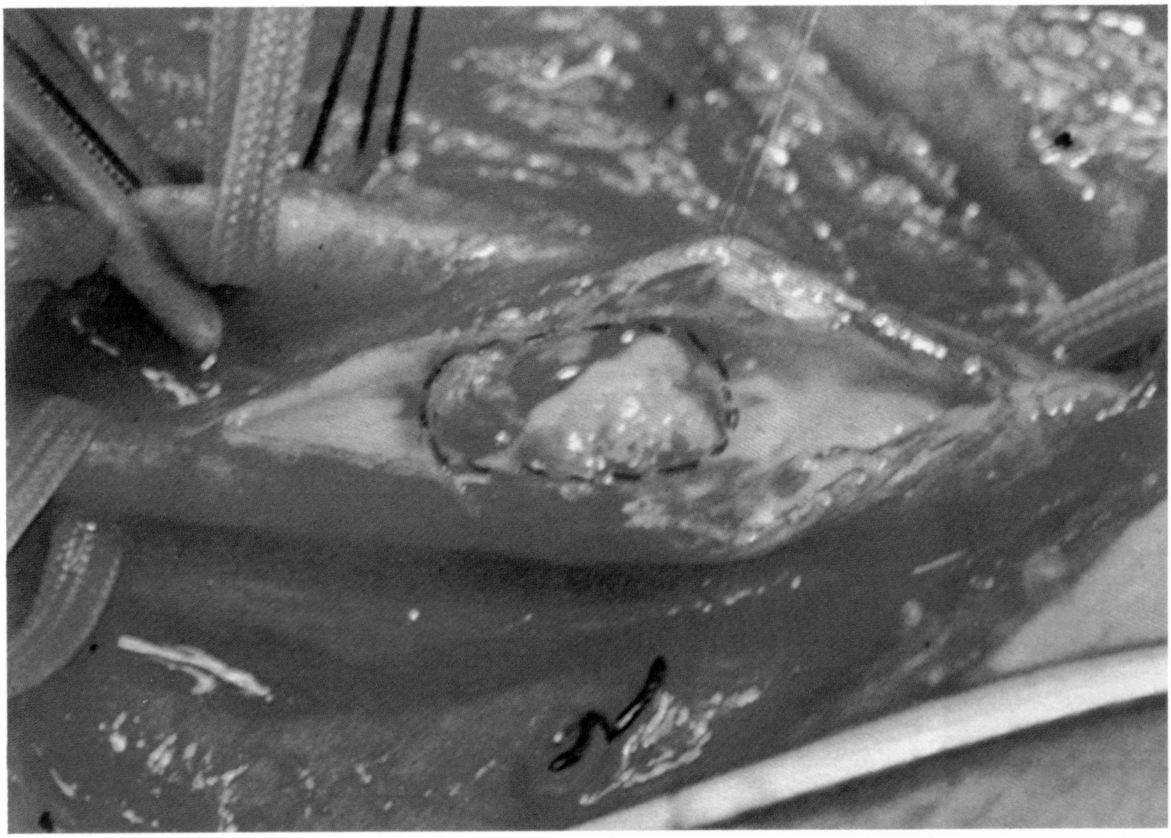

90 Carotid thrombosis. Thrombus in the internal carotid artery revealed at surgery.

91 Cerebral infarction. Isotope scan showing a middle cerebral artery infarct. The classical picture consists of contralateral hemiplegia, hemianaesthesia, and homonyous hemianopia. Aphasia is present when the dominant hemisphere is involved. There may be past history of hypertension and transient cerebral ischaemic attacks.

91

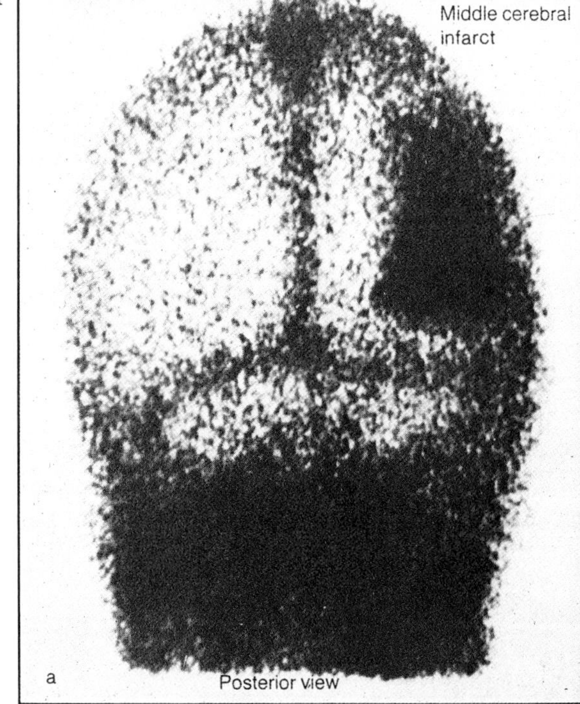

92

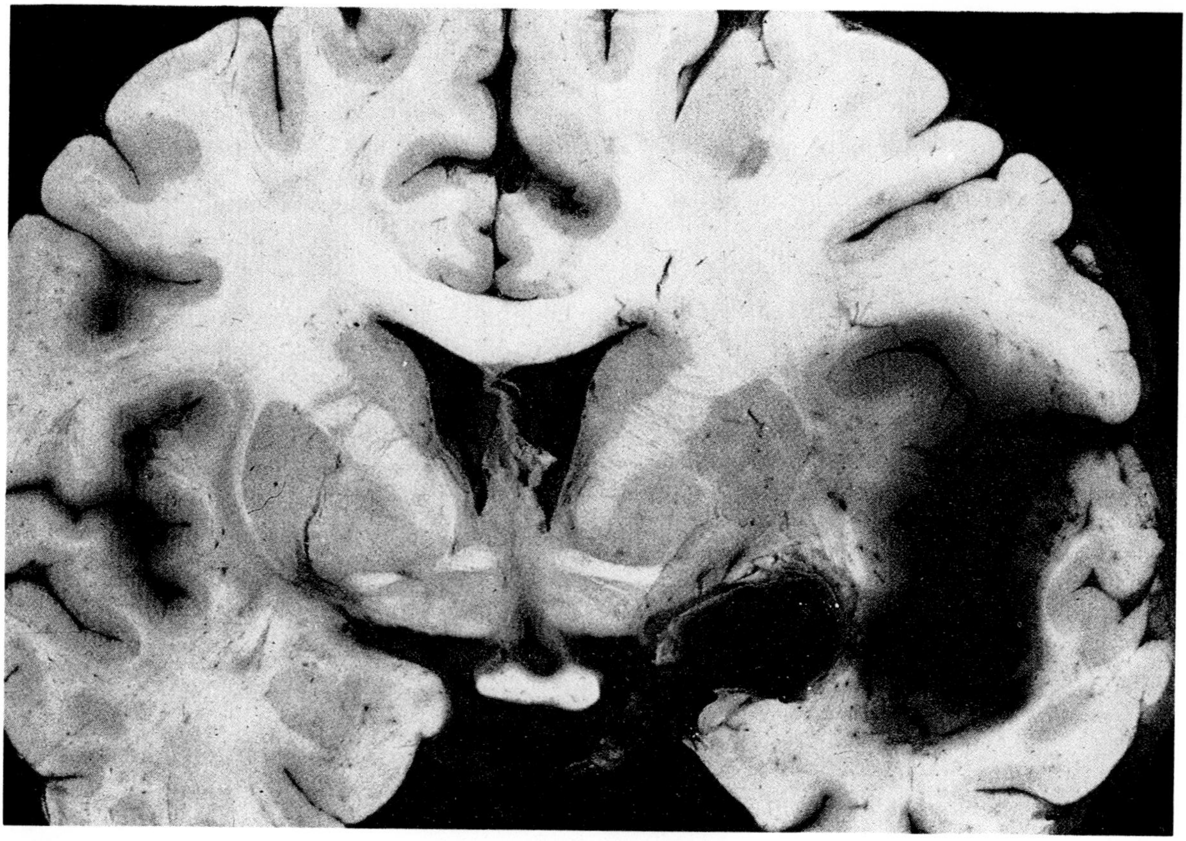

93

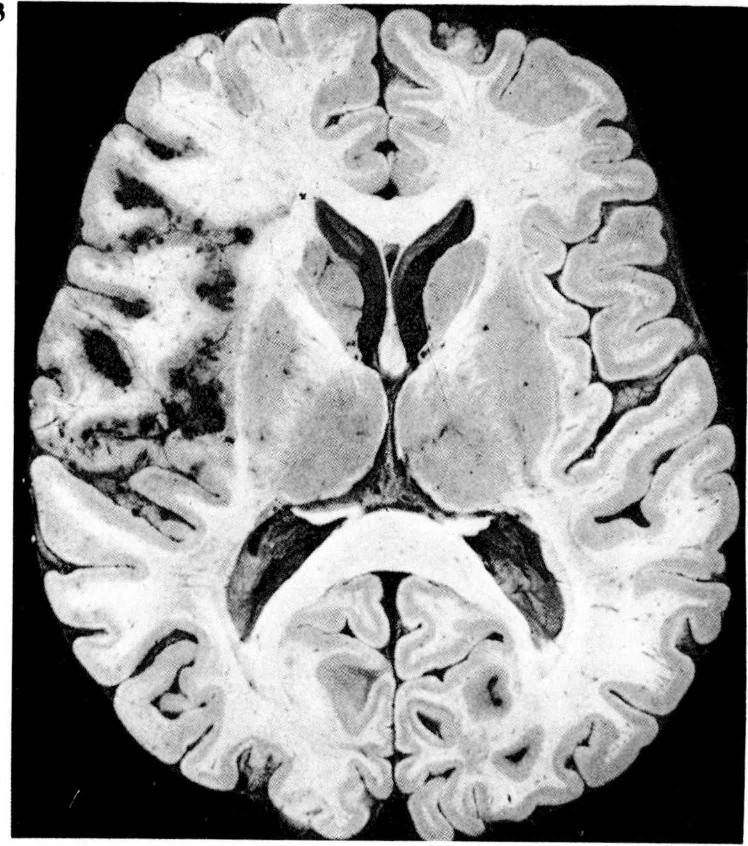

92 Meningocerebral haemorrhage. Subsequent to rupture of a middle cerebral artery aneurysm.

93 Haemorrhagic infarct. An infarct in the territory of the supply of the middle cerebral artery. Usually presents with a sudden hemiplegia.

94

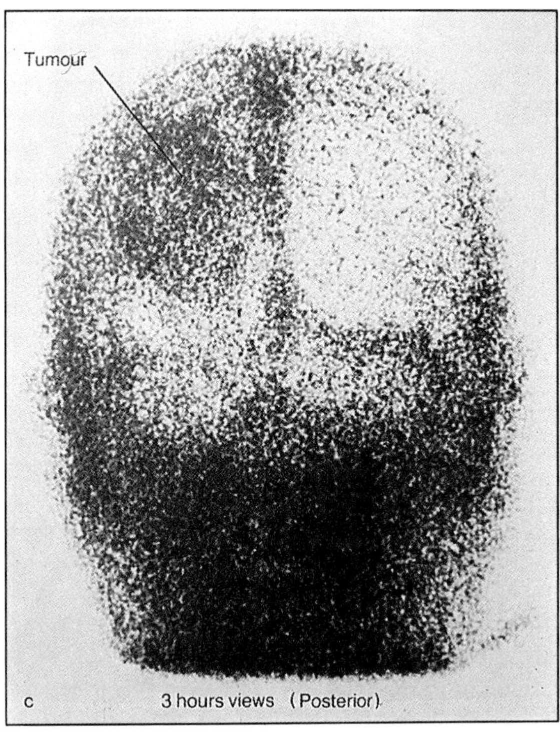

94 Brain tumour. An isotope scan showing space-occupying lesion in the left cerebral hemisphere. Sudden haemorrhage into such a tumour may present as a cerebrovascular accident.

95 and 96 Meningioma. Isotope scans showing anterior and right lateral views of a dense round lesion, which is very suggestive of a meningioma. The patient presented with confusion, falls, incontinence, dysphasia, and ataxia.

97 Parasagittal meningioma. Slow-growing tumour presenting with neurological signs in the trunk and lower limbs.

98 Astrocytoma Grade IV. Highly malignant brain tumour. Occasionally seen in the elderly and may present with stroke-like illness or dementia.

95

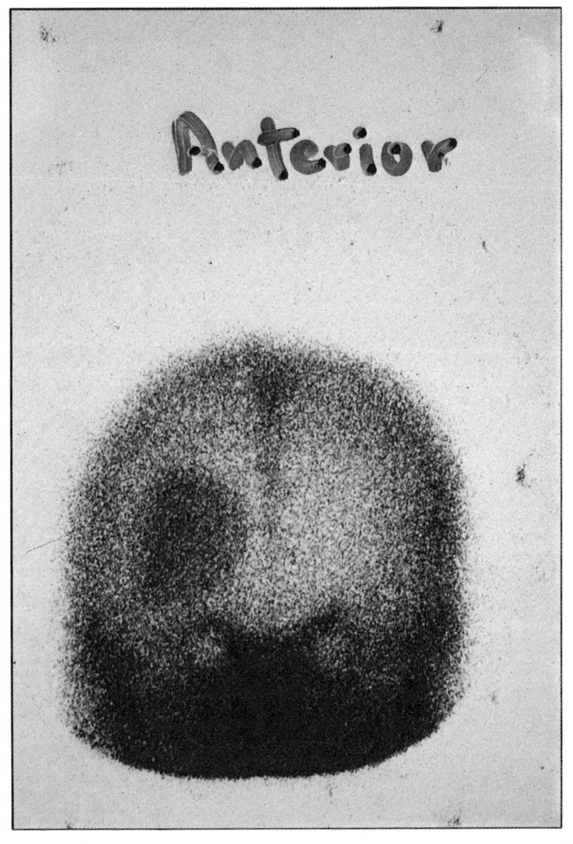

96

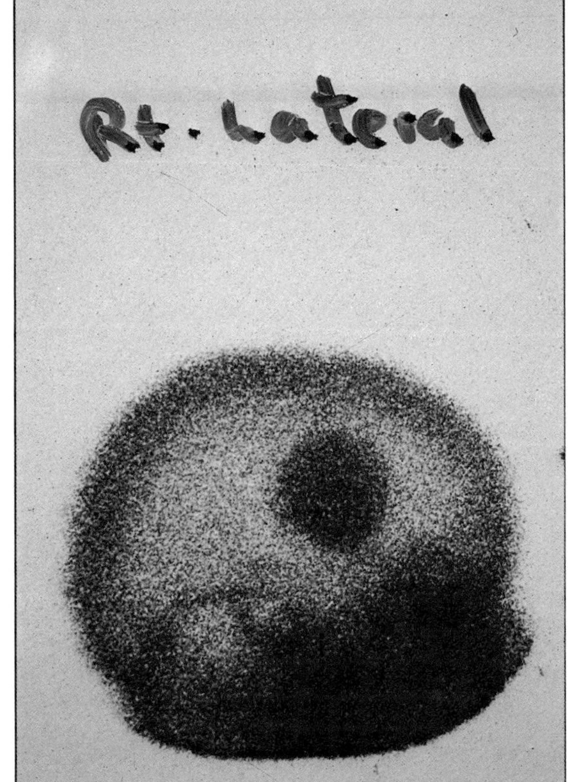

7

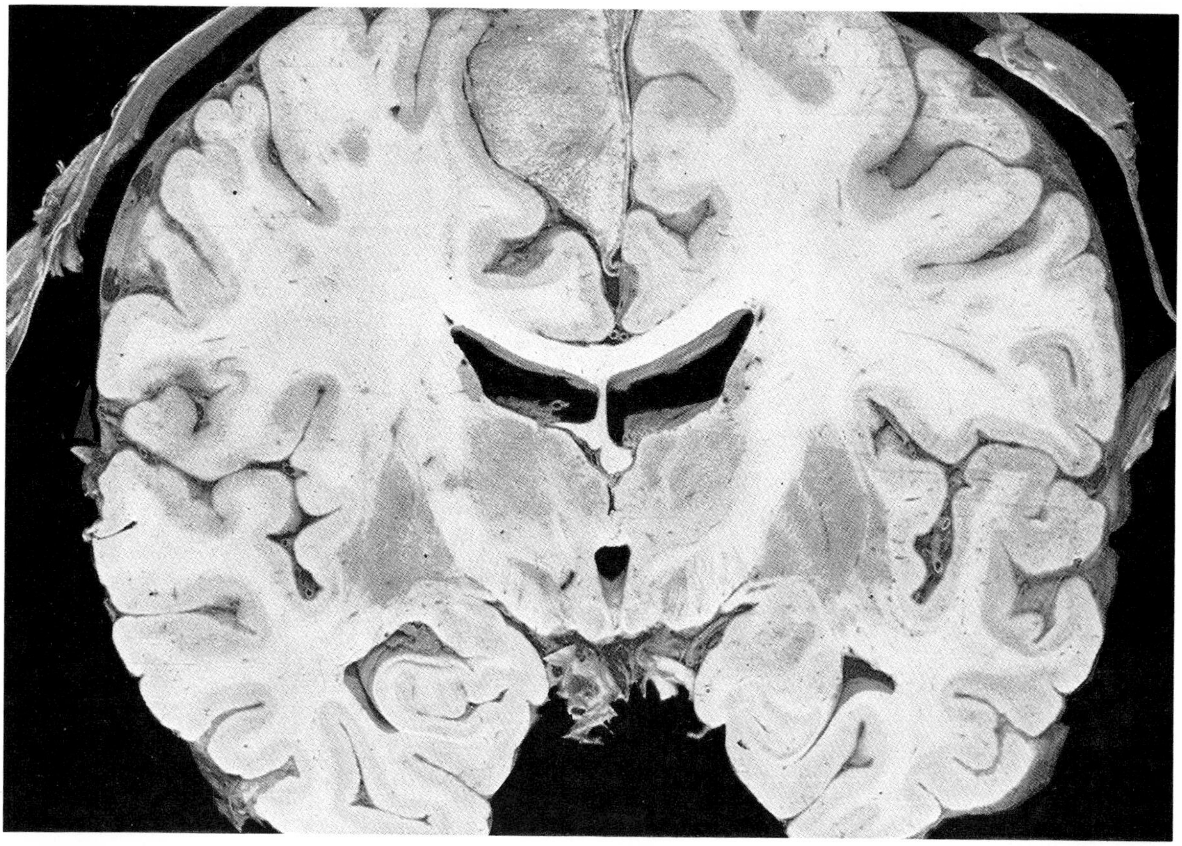

8

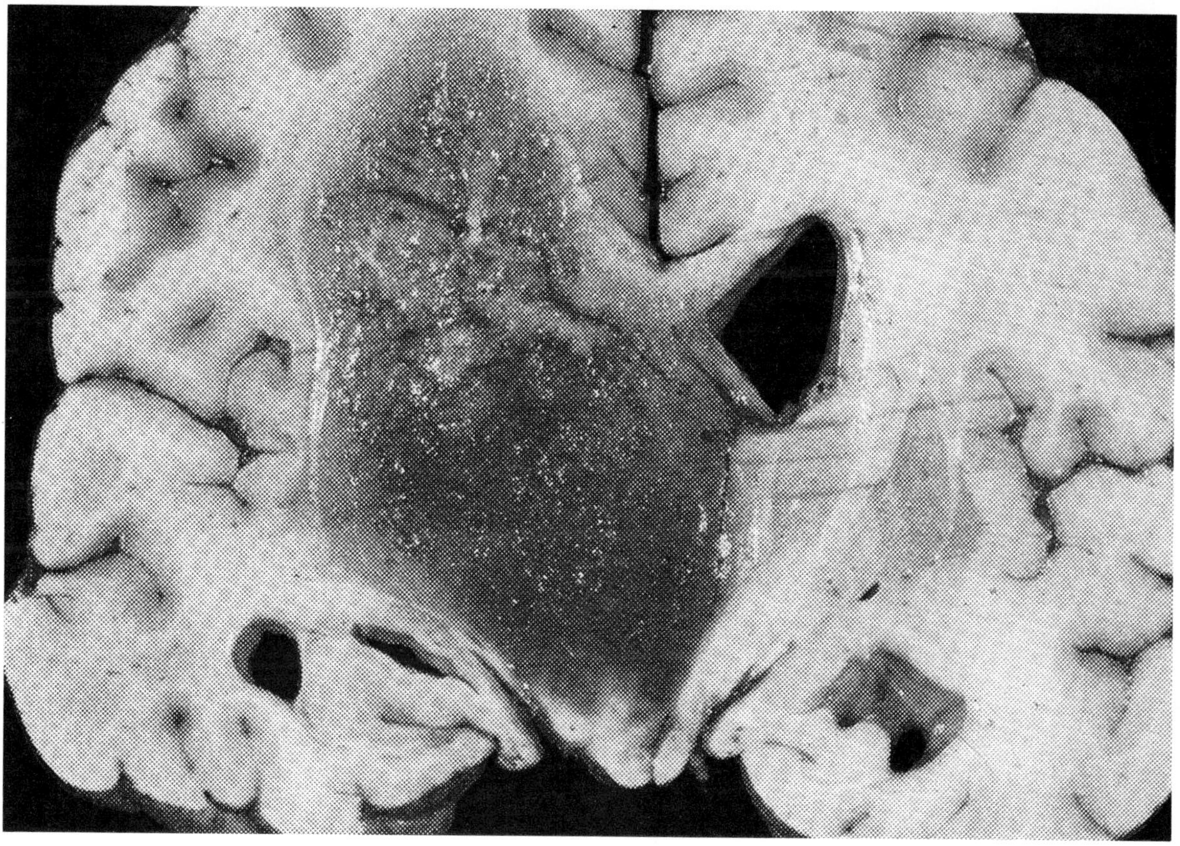

99

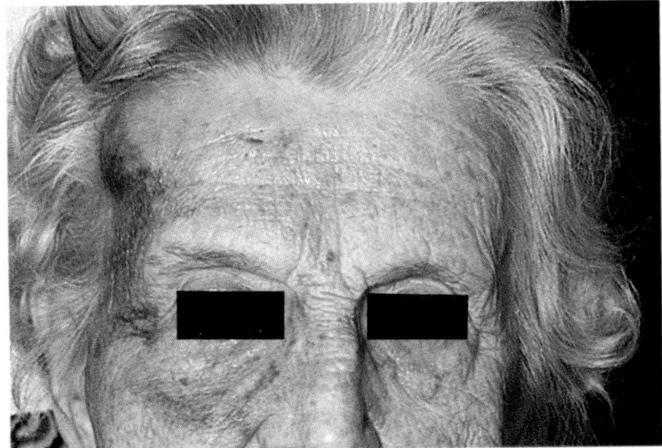

100

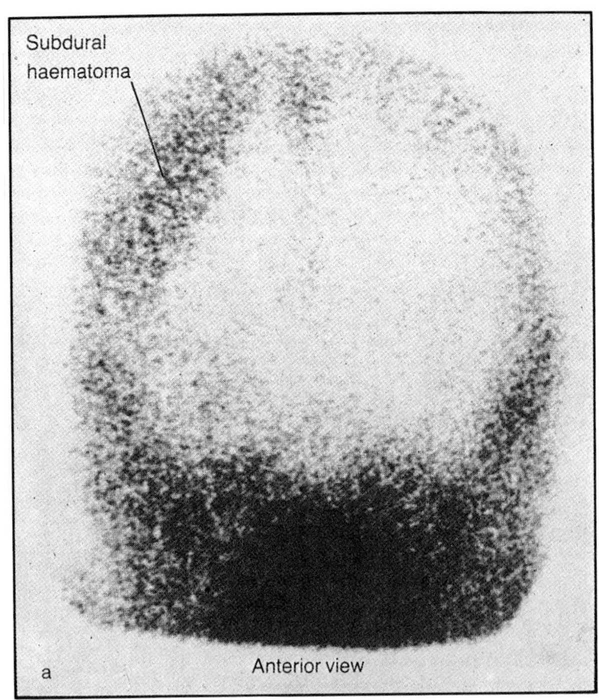

99 Head injury. An area of bruising on the right temporal region. The patient felt well and xrays revealed an intact skull. After a few days the patient developed symptoms suggestive of subdural haematoma.

100 Subdural haematoma. An isotope scan showing area of subdural haematoma.

101 Subdural haematoma. The dura and clot have been removed from the specimen and the compression of brain by a subdural haematoma is apparent.

101

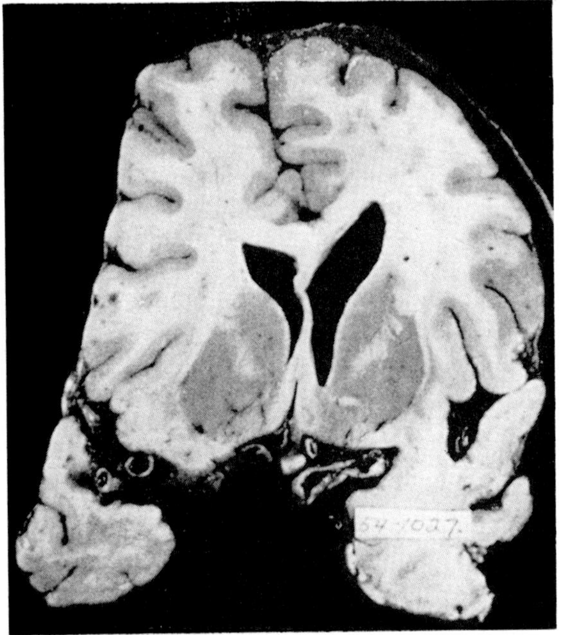

Subdural haematoma

Collection of blood between dura and arachnoid space caused by trauma or spontaneously.

The head injury, in the elderly may be trivial.

Clinical features

Fluctuating level of consciousness
Confusion
Headaches
Hemiparesis
Ptosis and dilated pupil on affected side
Lateralising signs
Dementia-like picture
Skull xrays may show a fracture displaced pineal, or displaced choroid plexus
Computer assisted tomography will localise the haematoma
CSF may be clear or xanthochromic

2

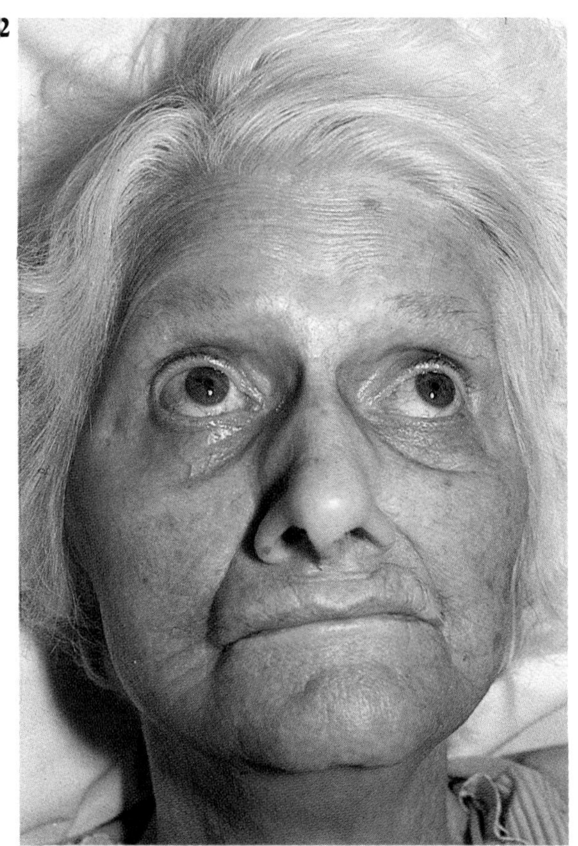

102 Fixed gaze. The eyes are fixed in an upward direction and there is paralysis of gaze. This is thought to be caused by brain-stem compression and can occur with intracerebral haemorrhage.

103 Babinski's reflex. Upgoing plantar reflex, a typical sign of a recent upper-motor neurone lesion. May sometimes be absent in elderly hemiplegics.

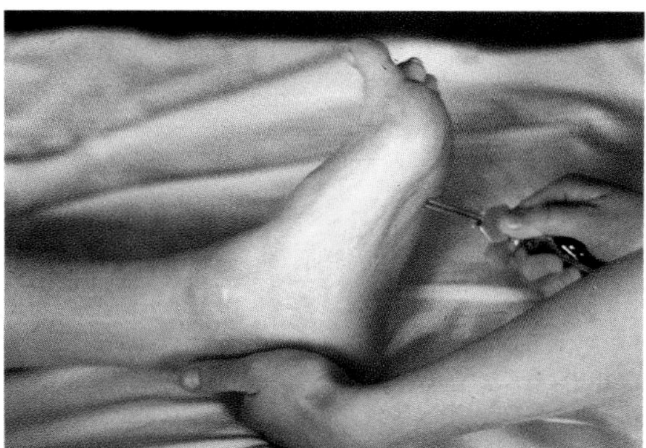

4

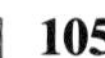

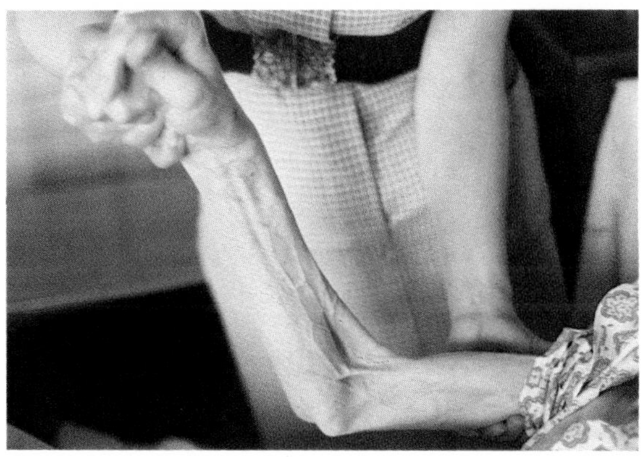

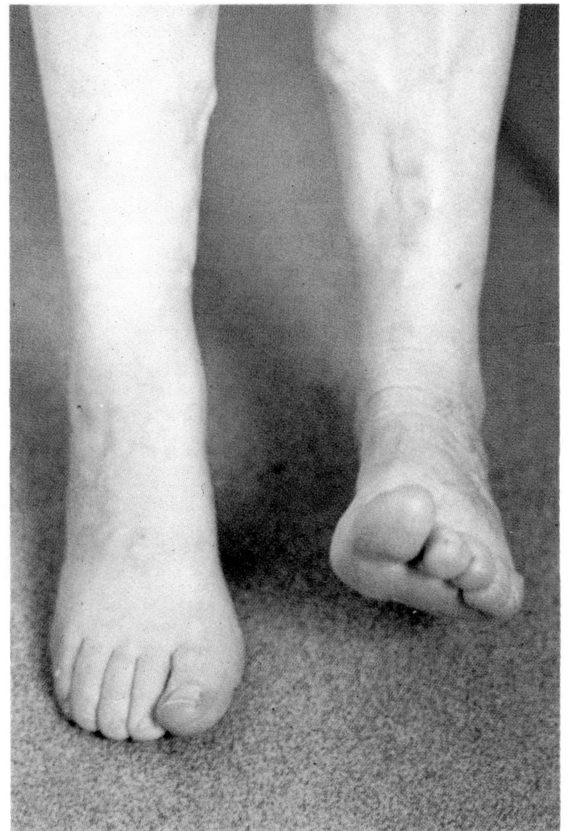

104 Foot drop. In a case of right hemiplegia. The patient is unable to dorsiflex the right foot and will require a footboard or other support to prevent permanent disability.

105 Increased spasticity. Spasticity of the arm after recent hemiplegia. Early physiotherapy is required to prevent contractures and further disability.

106

106 Loss of postural stability. In cerebrovascular accidents involving the sub-dominant hemisphere, walking apraxia and loss of postural control is usually apparent. The patient is unable to sit upright and tends to fall sideways. Patients should not be left in that position.

Expert geriatric nursing care and active physiotherapy is essential in such cases. Special chairs and other aids may be required in improving the balance and posture. This patient is in danger of developing contractures, but with good geriatric care this risk can be minimised.

107

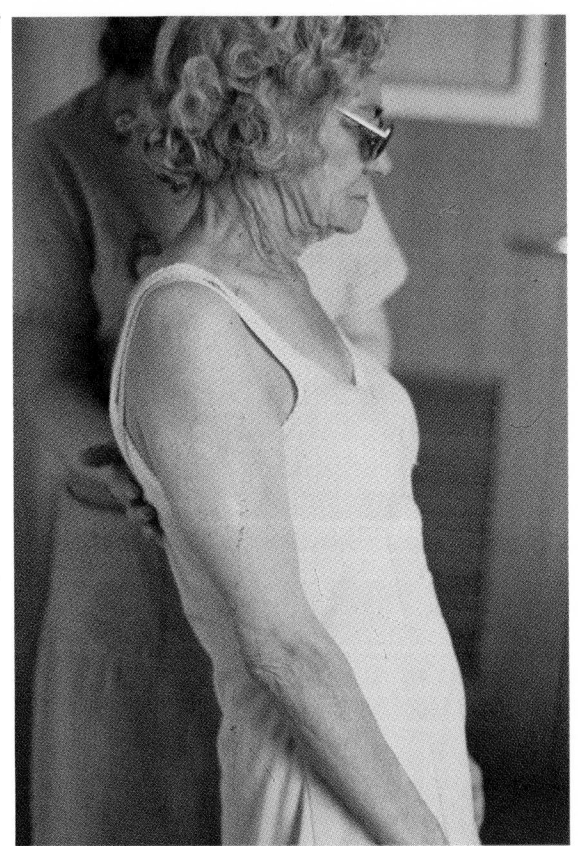

107 Backward falling. A tendency to lean and fall backwards is a frequent problem in vertebrobasilar ischaemia and global cerebral syndromes.

This patient should improve with regular physiotherapy and walking exercises. A special weighted walking frame may reduce the tendency to lean backwards.

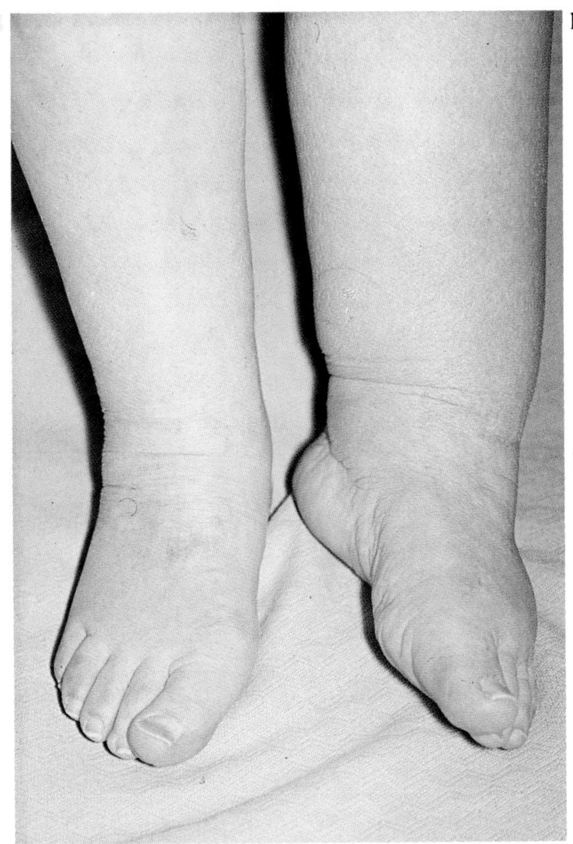

109a

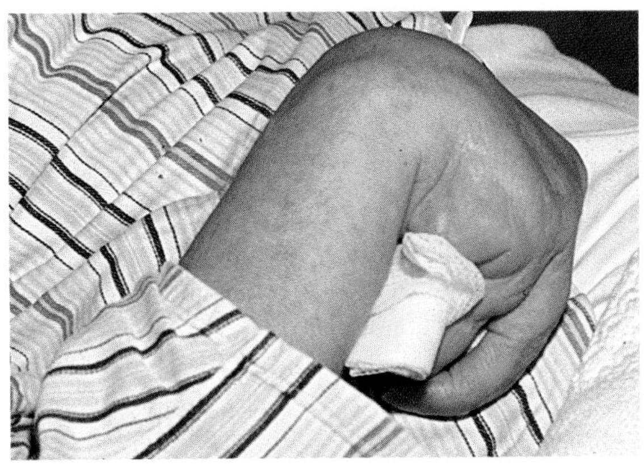

109b

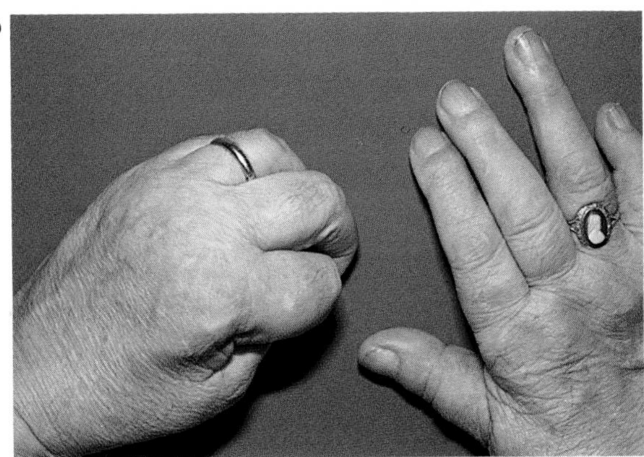

110

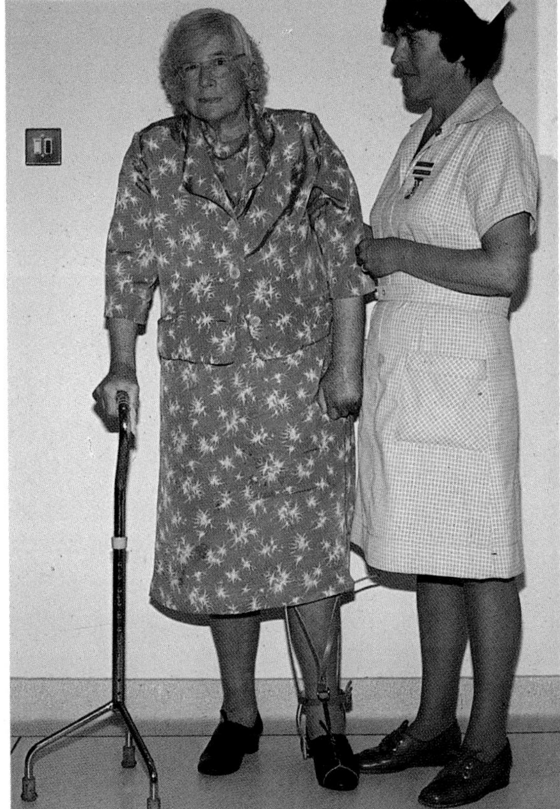

108 Hemiplegic oedema. Oedema of the left foot. Prescribing diuretics is of little benefit but physiotherapy, mobilisation and limb elevation should improve the condition.

109a Hemiplegic hand. Severe contracture of the right hand several months after a dense hemiplegia.

109b Hemiplegic hand. Another case of hemiplegic contracture of the left hand. Such disability can be prevented with early physiotherapy.

110 Left hemiplegia. Showing good recovery with prolonged physiotherapy and rehabilitation.

The patient is now able to walk with the help of a tripod and a calliper. She has also become independent in self-care and activities of daily living.

111 and 112 Perceptual disturbances – spatial neglect. Assessment of spatial neglect in patients with non-dominant hemisphere stroke is most satisfactorily done by getting the patient to draw and the neglect of the left side will be apparent from the drawing. This syndrome is usually accompanied by hemianaesthesia, hemianopia, inappropriate emotions, loss of righting reflex, and apathy.

111

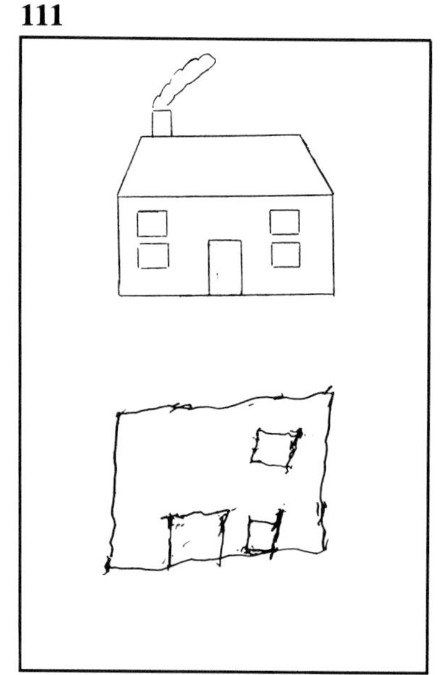

112

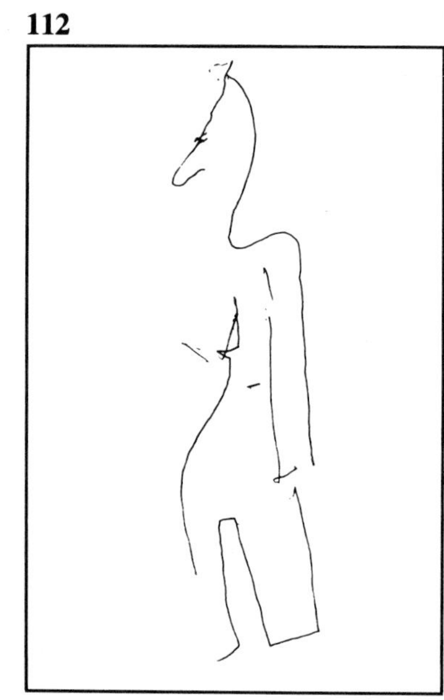

113

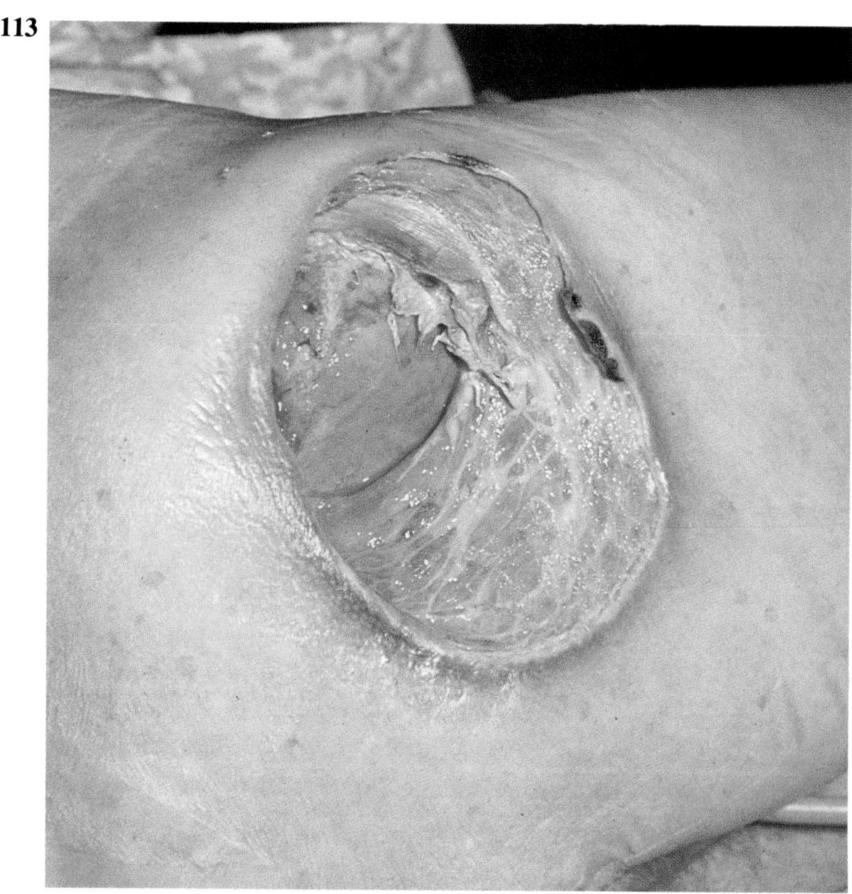

113 Ischial pressure sore. One of the serious but preventable complications of immobility in an elderly patient caused by cerebrovascular accident.

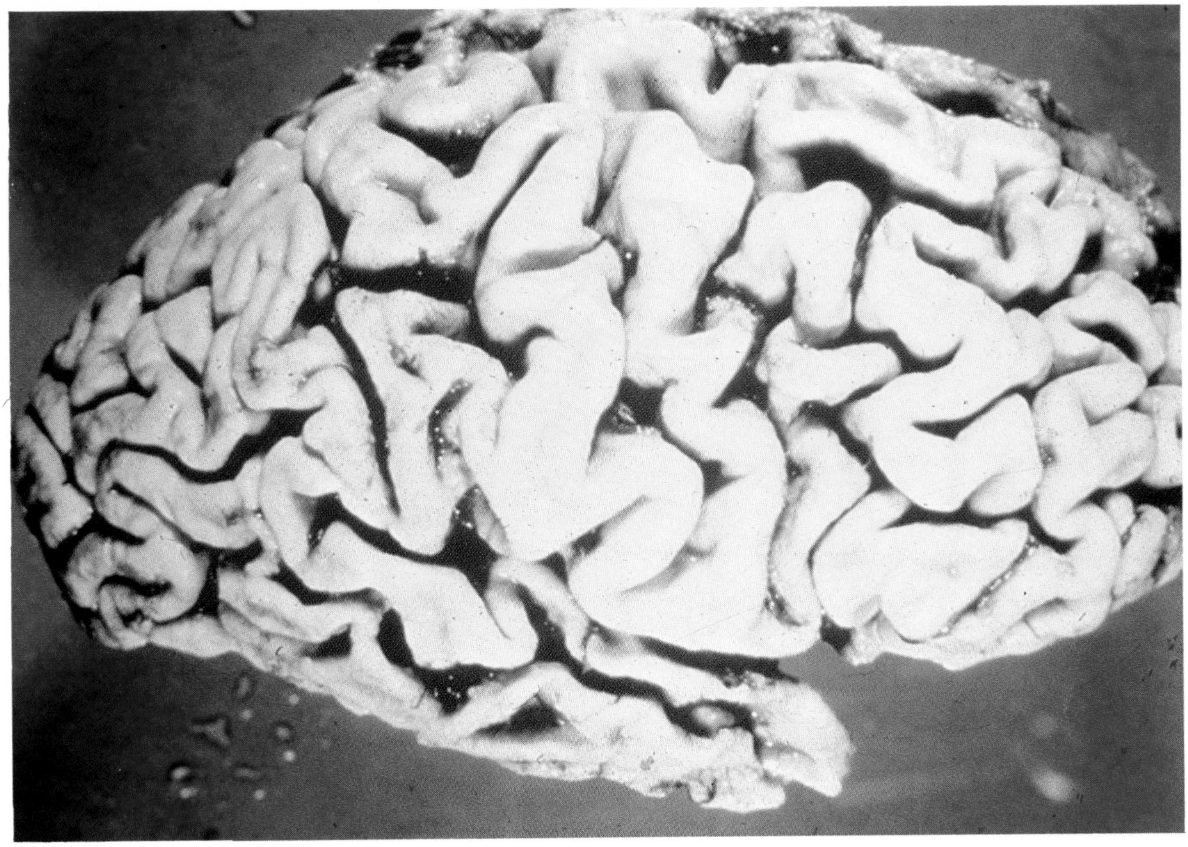

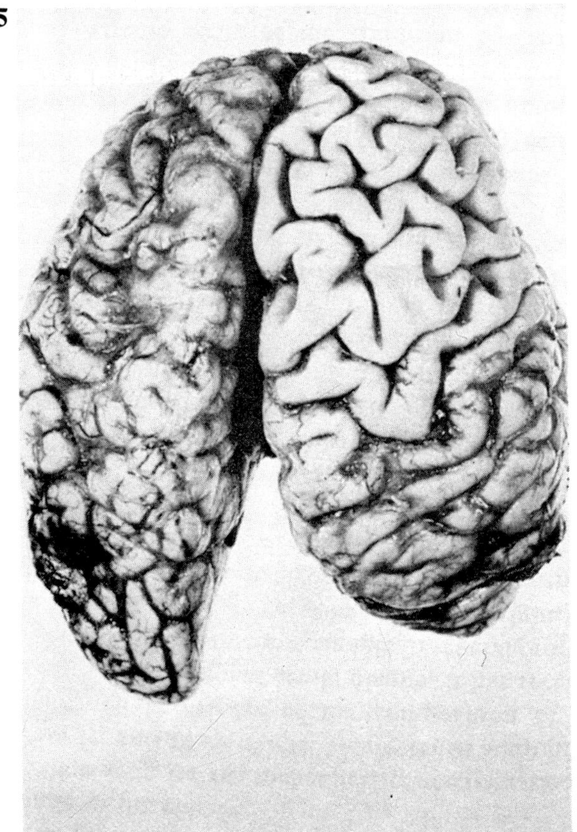

114 Cerebral atrophy. Side view of a fixed brain showing extreme shrinkage of temporal lobe as well as generalised cerebral atrophy more marked anteriorly.

115 Cerebral atrophy (senile dementia). View from above of an atrophic cerebral hemisphere on the right and control from subject of same age on the left. Note the shrunken gyri and gaping sulci in the affected brain, and opalescence of the leptomeninges in the control. Such atrophy occurs over a period of years, but the clinical picture may show only minimal brain failure. An acute physical illness may trigger the onset of dementia.

116

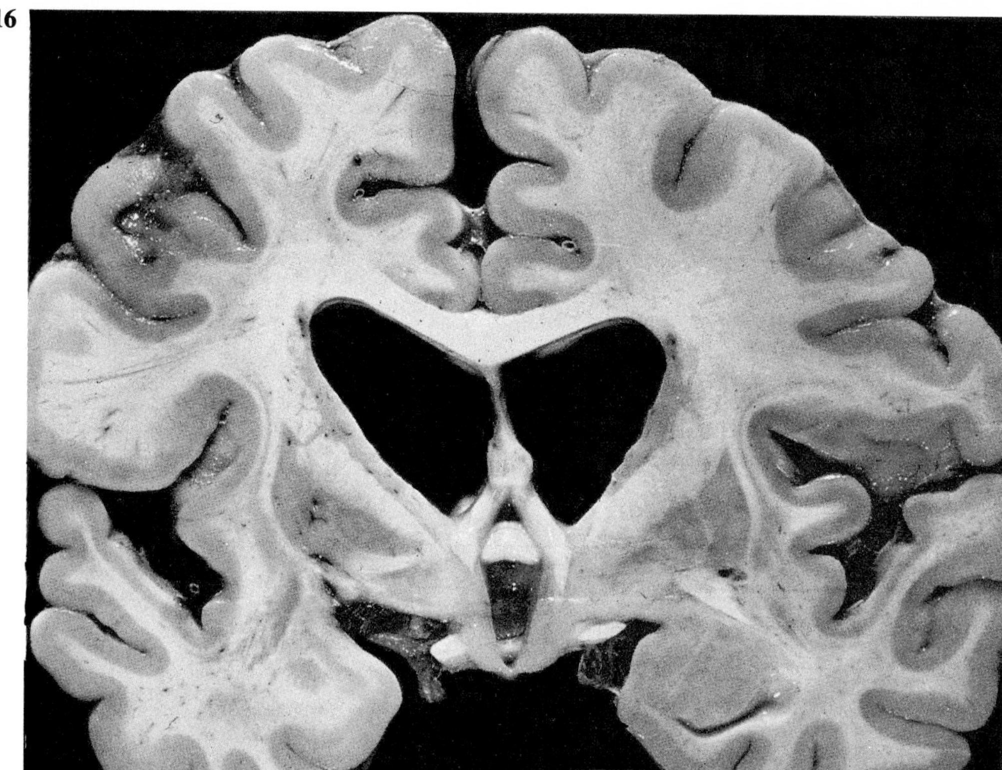

117

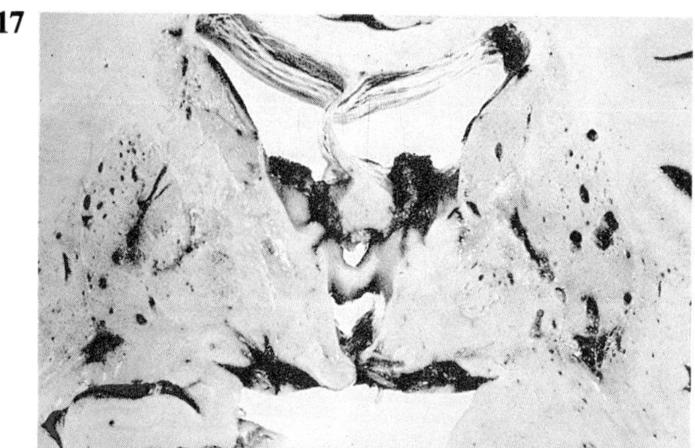

118

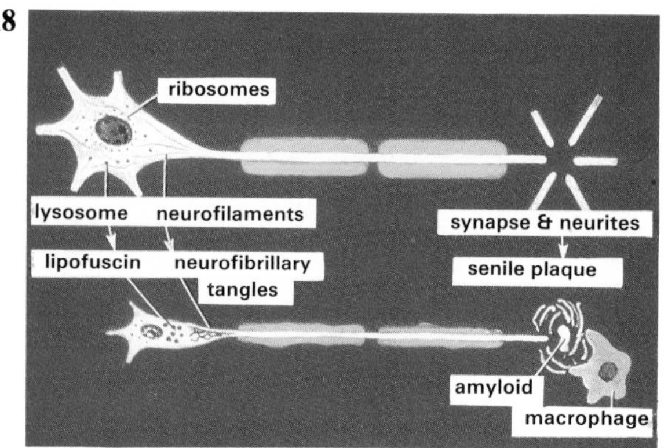

116 Huntington's chorea. There is diffuse cerebral atrophy but the caudate nuclei are most affected.

117 Multi-infarct dementia. Dilated perivascular spaces (etats lacunaires) and scars of small old infarcts in basal ganglia.

118 Senile dementia. Evolution of senile plaques and neurofibrillary tangles. Senile plaques may be found in very small numbers in very old, non-demented patients.

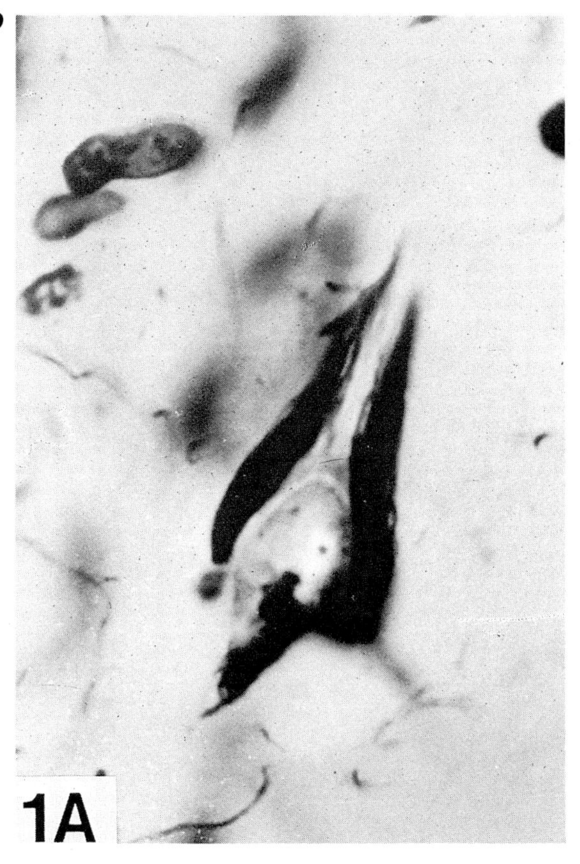

119 Neurofibrillary tangle. Composed of thick strands of argentophilic material largely filling the neuronal cytoplasm and extending into apical dendrite. (*Bodian stain ×560*)

120 Neurofibrillary tangles. Composite picture of neurofibrillary tangles; the almost triangular dense intraneuronal structures. Argyrophilic plaques are also present as larger and more fragmented areas of staining.

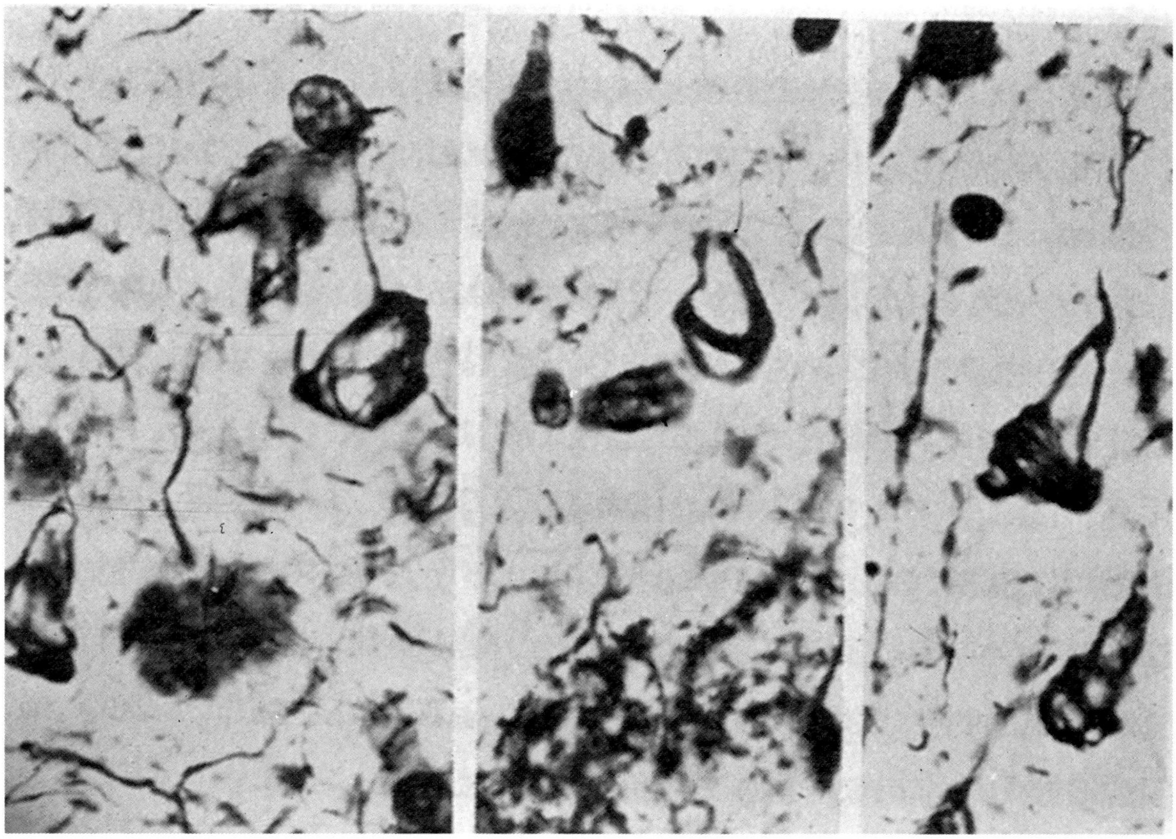

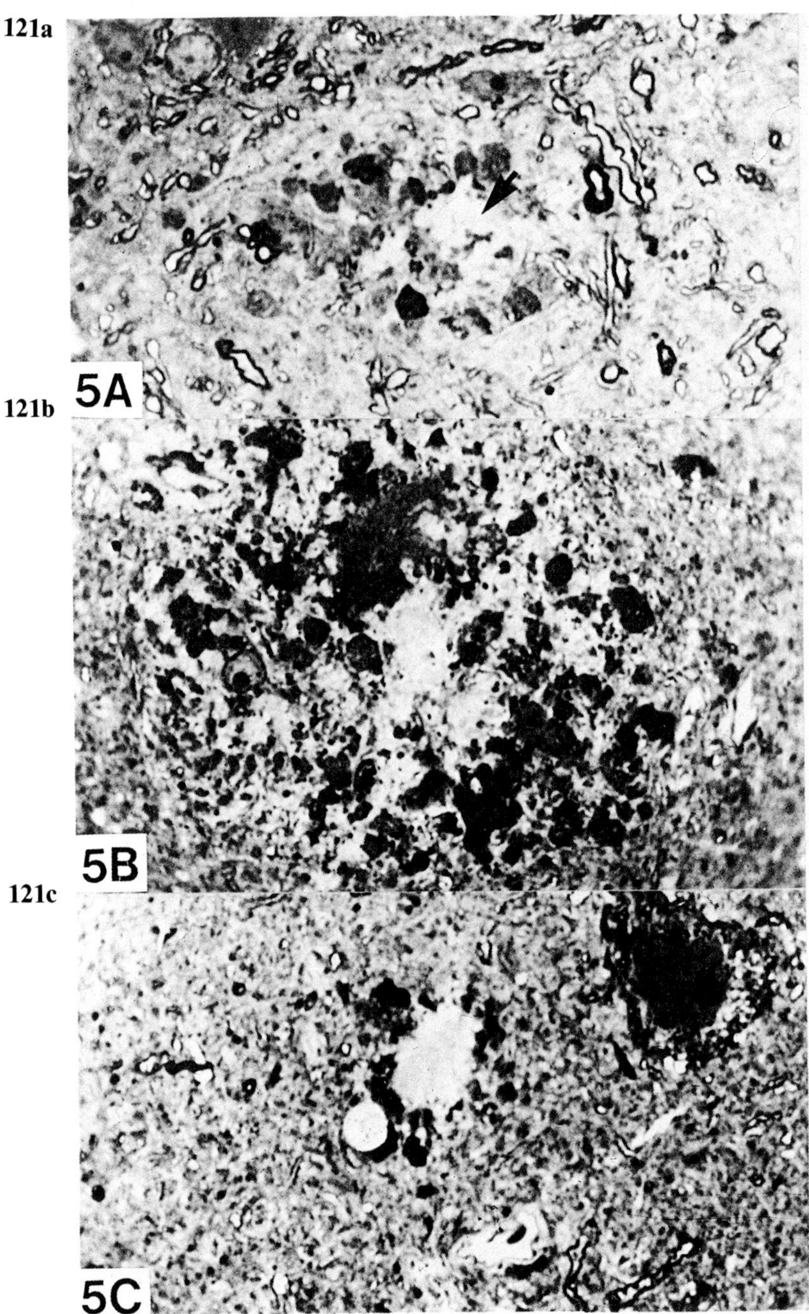

121a Plaque. A typical plaque in thick section reveals its central amyloid core (arrow) surrounded by degenerating neurites.

121b Plaque. Another typical plaque reveals much dense material derived from degenerating mitochrondria and lysosomes in neuritis. The lighter components around the central core were processes with fibrillar material and wisps of amyloid.

121c Plaque. A compact or burned out plaque consists almost entirely of amyloid. (*Toludine blue ×560*)

122 and 123 Primitive reflexes. Disease of the frontal lobes – particularly senile and multi-infarct dementia allow the emergence of primitive reflexes among which the most easily tested are the grasp reflex and forced groping. In forced groping the patients hand follows a moving stimulus inside the palm. In the grasp reflex a pressure applied by the examiner's fingertips moving towards the patient's fingertips on the flexor tendons causes a grasp which will not be released even if the patient is pulled clear of the bed. Other primitive reflexes seen in dementia are sucking reflex, snout reflex, palmomental reflex, and glabellar tap.

122

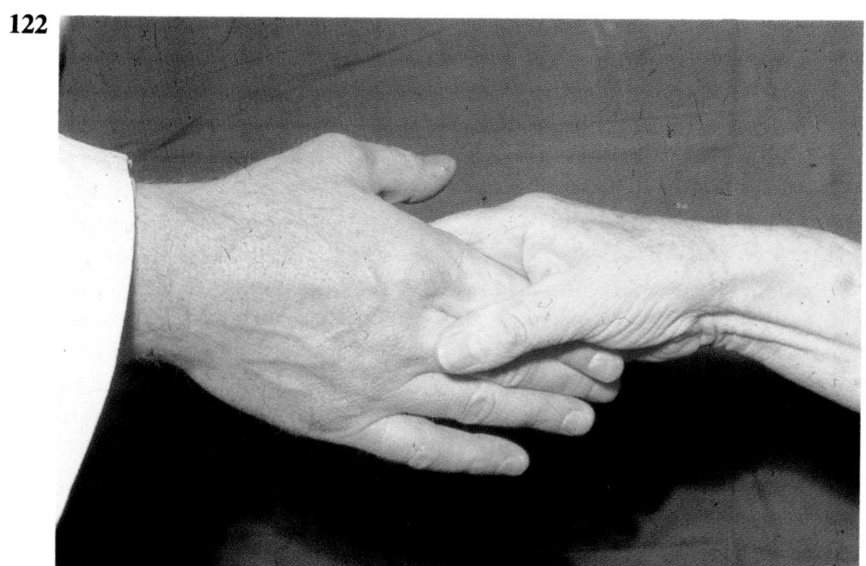

123

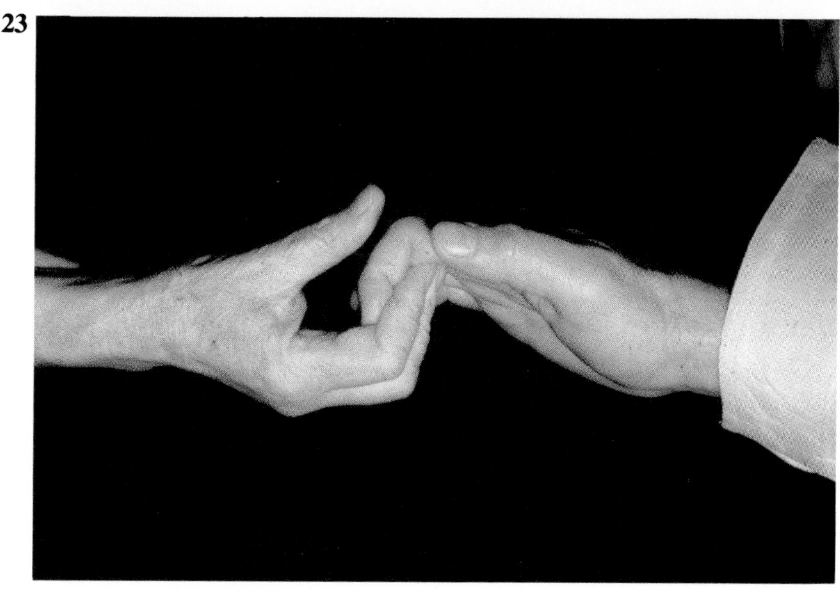

124

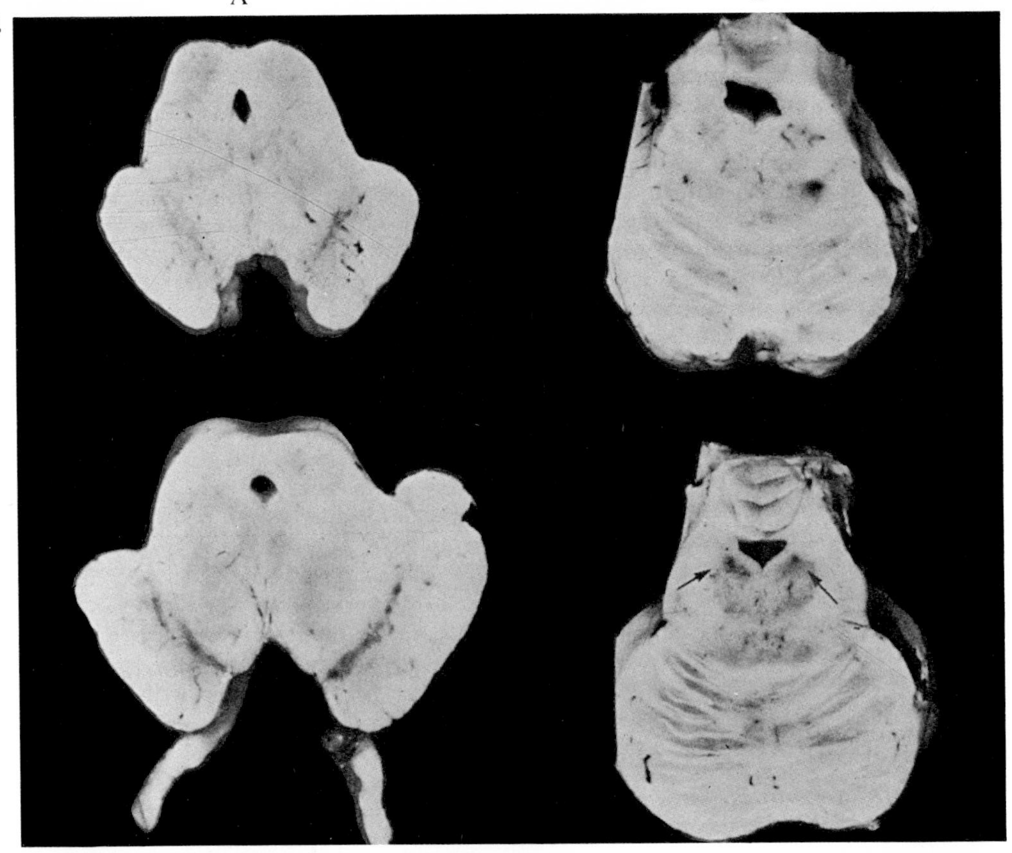

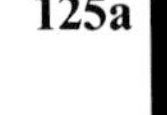

125a

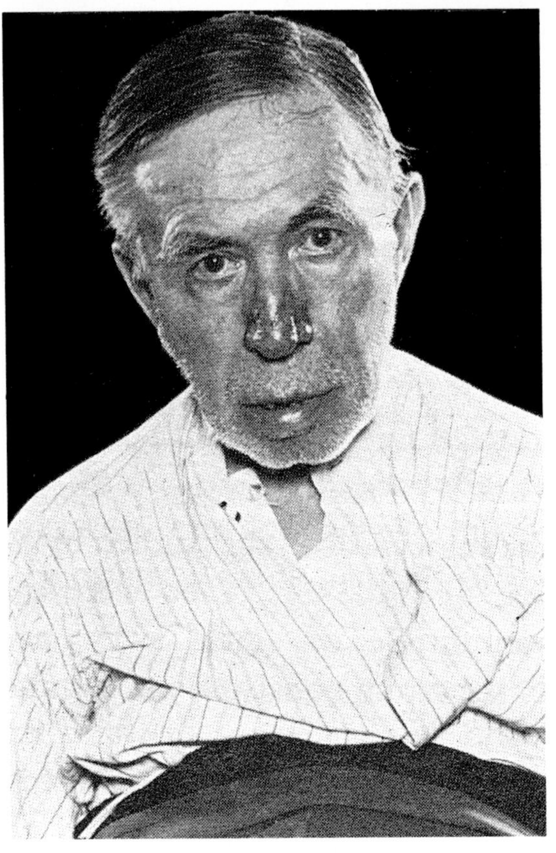

125b

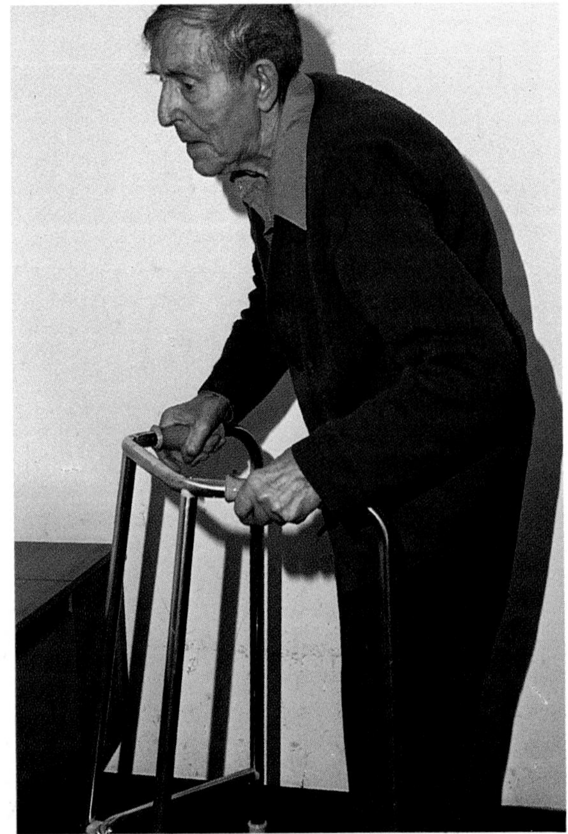

124 Parkinsonism. Patient's brain above, normal control below.
(A) Severe pallor of substantia nigra.
(B) Disappearance of pigmented neurones of locus caeruleus.

125a Parkinsonism. Showing the classic expressionless face and unblinking stare.

125b Parkinsonism. Typical stooped posture with considerable akinesia and shuffling gate.

126 Advanced Parkinsonism. With increased muscle tone, dementia and permanent flexion of upper and lower limbs.

127 Advanced Parkinsonism. The arms are flexed with increased rigidity and there is complete akinesia. Such patients are in danger of suffering from pressure sores, faecal impaction, urinary incontinence, dehydration, and broncho-pneumonia.

126

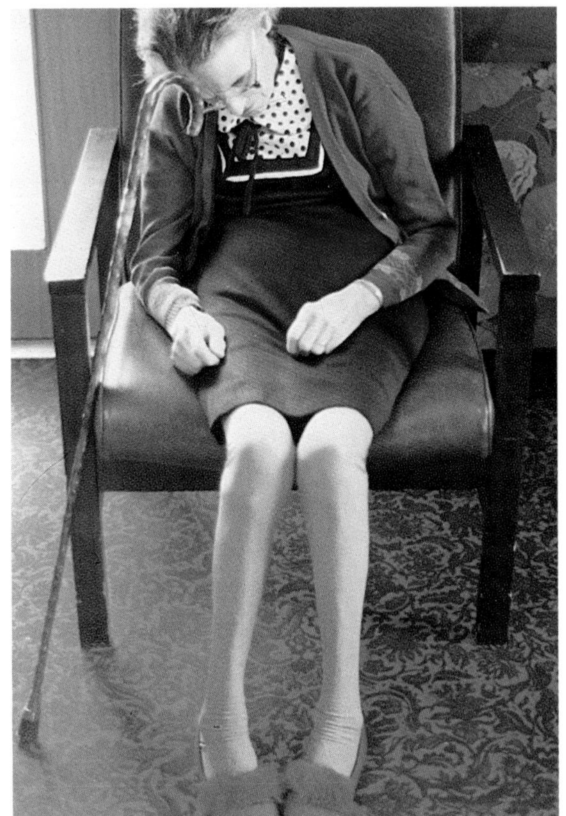

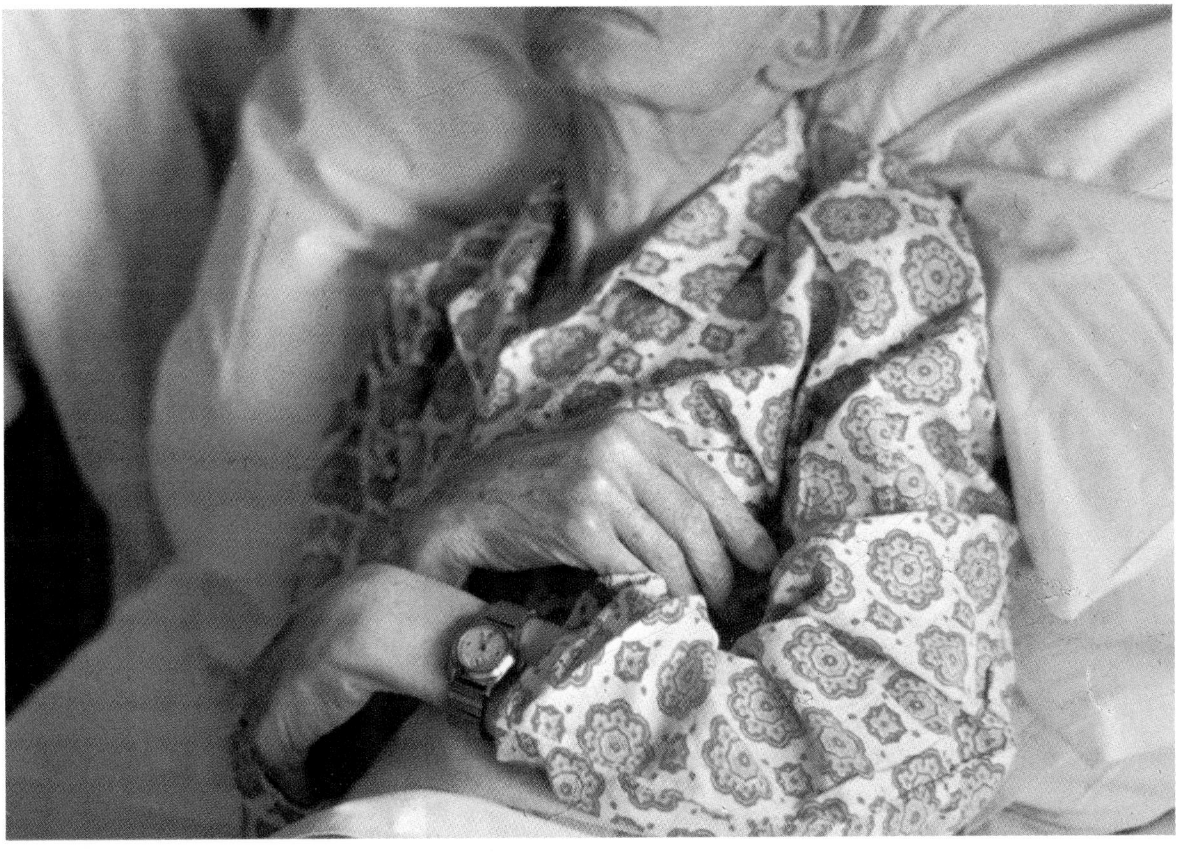

128 Oculogyric crisis. The eyes are deviated and fixed upwards and the patient has pronounced generalised rigidity.

129 Progressive supranuclear palsy. The patient has dementia, upper motor neurone signs, and an inability to look upwards.

128

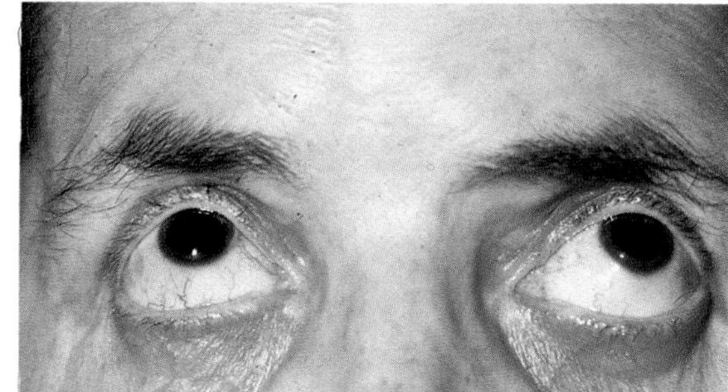

129

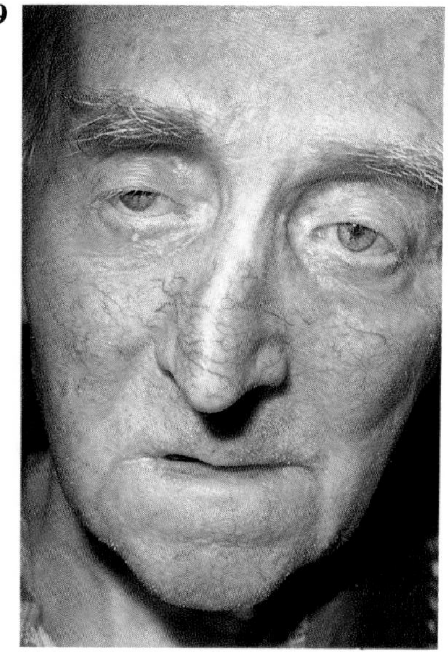

Progressive supranuclear palsy
(Steel-Richardson-Olszewski syndrome)

Clinical Features:

Mild dementia
Parkinsonism-like picture
Difficulty in walking and frequent falls
Dystonic rigidity of face, neck and trunk
Supranuclear ophthalmoplegia affecting vertical gaze
Pseudobulbar palsy

129a

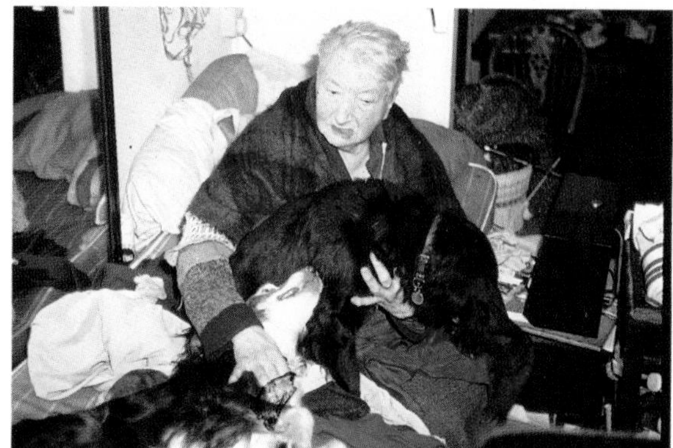

129b

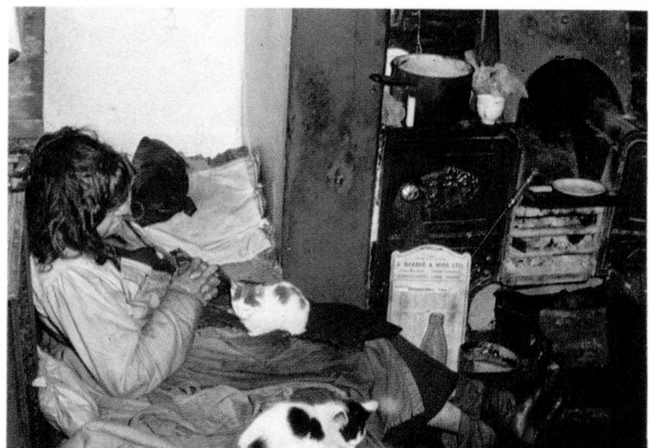

129a and b Diogenes syndrome. A form of severe self-neglect occasionally seen in the elderly. The patients are usually single and spend their money on pets or buying food and other household items which they never use. They may have an odd personality but there are no signs of dementia. Prolonged self-neglect eventually leads to physical illness and hospitalization.

6 Disorders of the chest

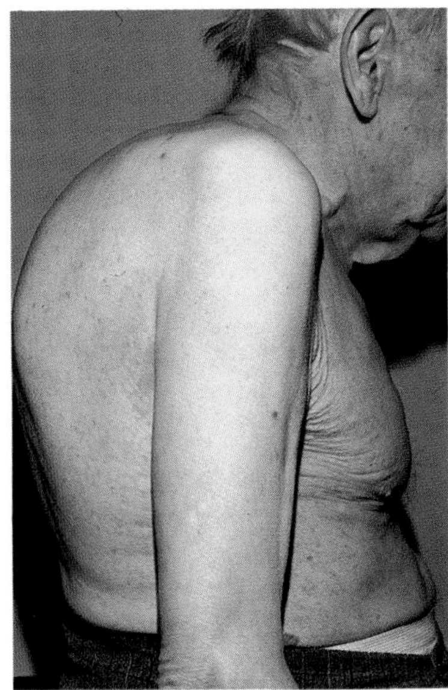

131

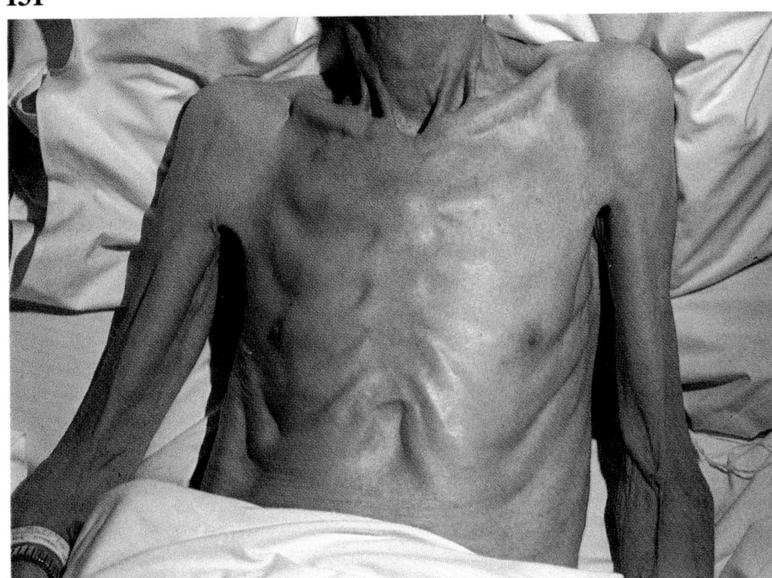

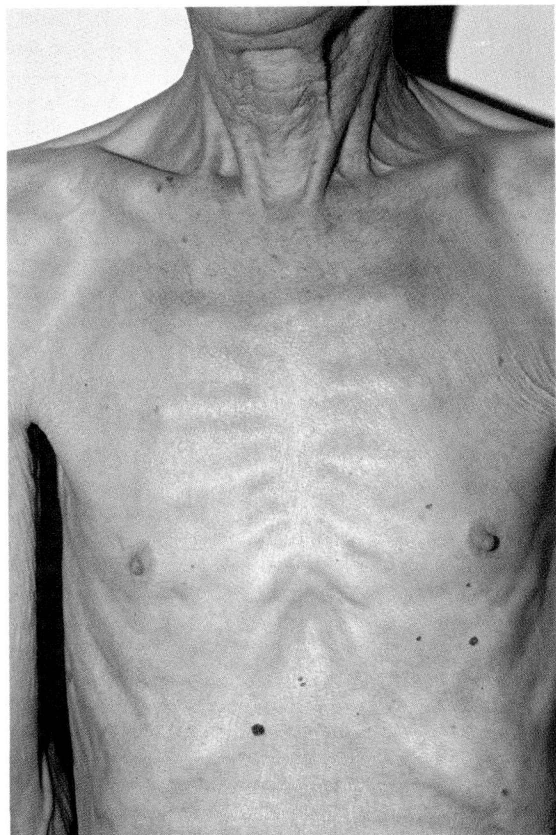

130 Barrel-shaped chest. This elderly man had chronic obstructive airways disease and suffered with persistent dyspnoea. Note the dorsal kyphosis.

131 Cachexia. Wasted chest with weightloss caused by carcinoma of stomach.

Common causes of wasting in elderly
(weakness and general ill health)

Malignant disease
Depression and bereavement
Tuberculosis
Bacterial endocarditis
Anaemias
Chronic renal failure
Osteomalacia
Hypothyroidism
Severe social deprivation

132 Dyspnoea. Chest of a patient with chronic asthma. Breathing required considerable effort and the accessory muscles of respiration are being fully used.

133
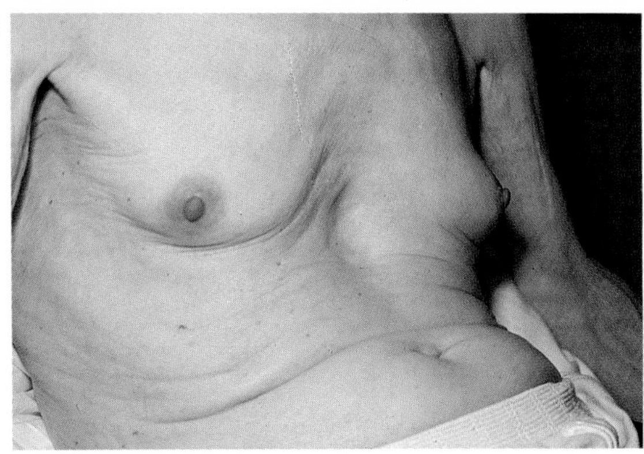

134
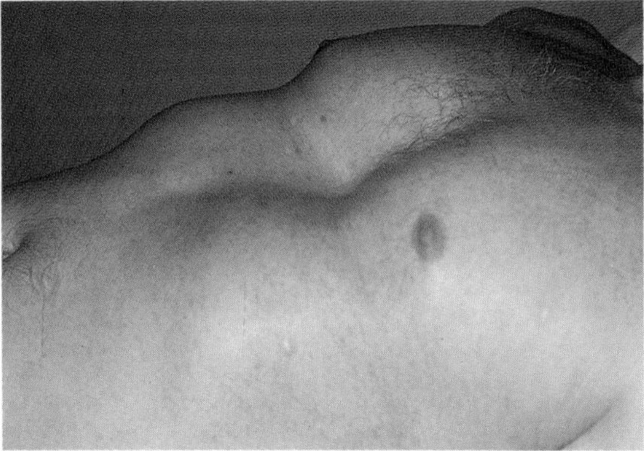

135
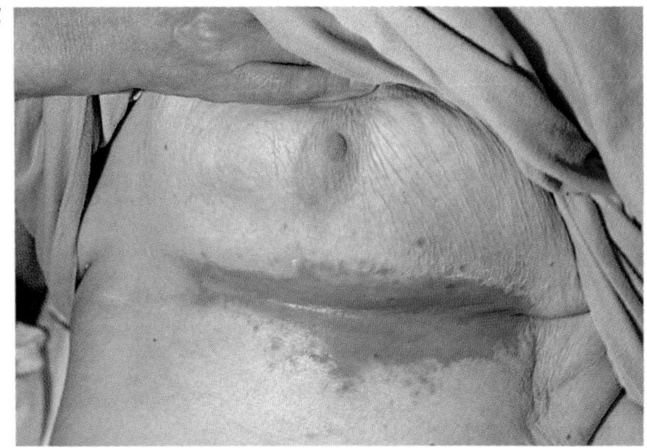

136
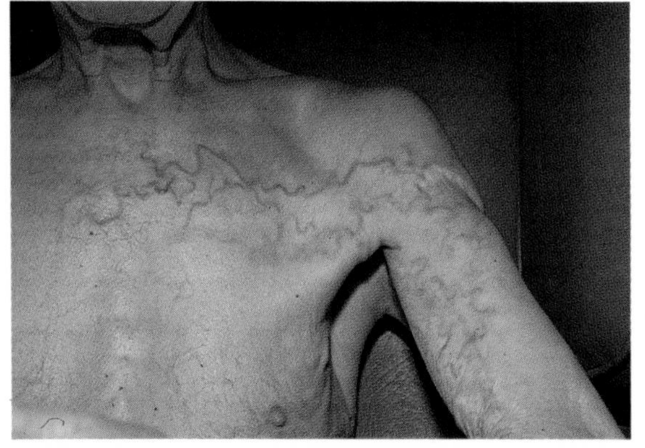

133 Gynaecomastia. Enlargement of breasts in an elderly male who was found to have bronchogenic carcinoma.

134 Pectus excavatum. Depressed sternum, caused by an association of rickets and whooping cough in childhood. The patient had no respiratory problems.

Causes of gynaecomastia

1 Endocrine
   Hypothyroidism and thyrotoxicosis
   Acromegaly
   Hypothalamic lesions
   Testicular and adrenal tumours
2 Drugs
   Oestrogens
   Spironolactone
   Reserpine
   Methyldopa
3 Cirrhosis of the liver
4 Carcinoma of the bronchus and lymphoma
5 Chronic renal failure treated with dialysis
6 Longstanding paraplegia

135 Submammary intertrigo. Sore area under the breast of an obese elderly lady. Poor personal hygiene is an important contributory factor.

136 Superior vena cava obstruction. Obstruction caused by malignant enlargement of lymph nodes in the superior mediastinum causing dilatation of the superficial veins in the upper chest wall and arm. The patient was found to have carcinoma of the lung.

137

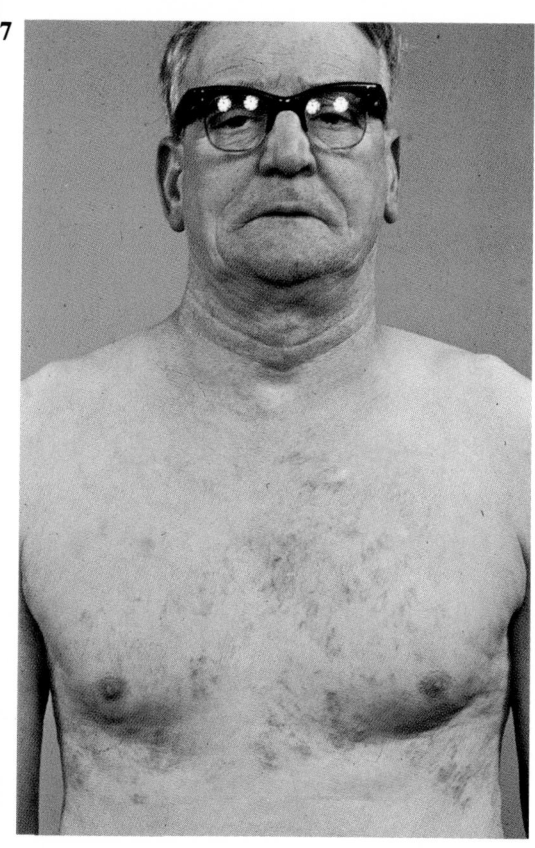

137 Superior vena cava obstruction. Note the prominence of veins on the chest, and facial congestion.

138

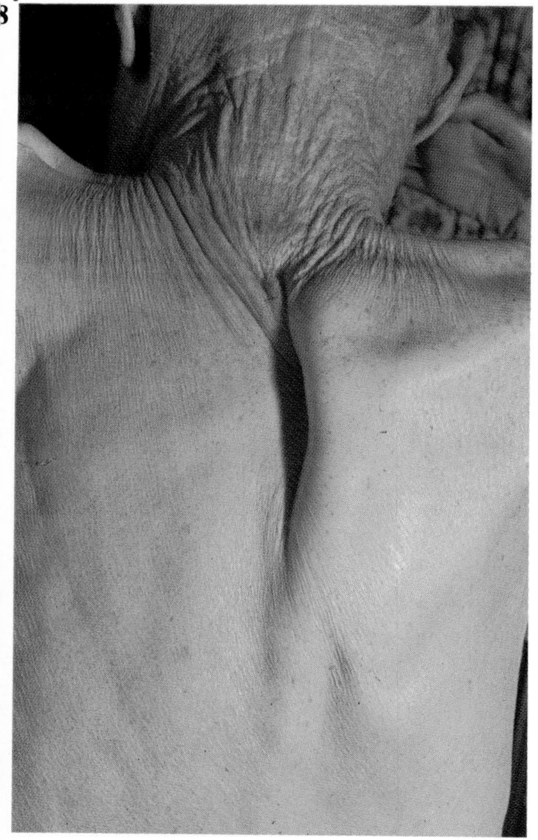

138 Winging of scapula. Result of paralysis of serratus magnus muscle caused by a lesion involving the long thoracic nerve. There is inability to raise the arm over the head from a forward position, with winging of medial border of scapula on pushing forward against resistance. The patient had diabetes mellitus.

Causes of mononeuritis multiplex:

Diabetes mellitus
Carcinoma
Rheumatoid arthritis
Polyarteritis nodosa
Sarcoidosis

139a

139b

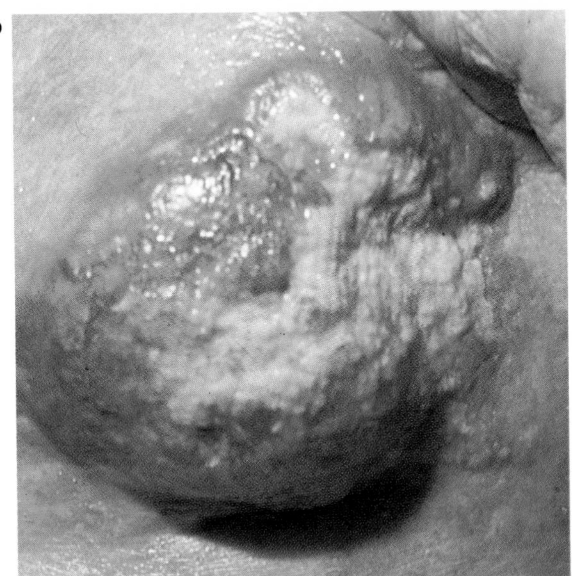

140a

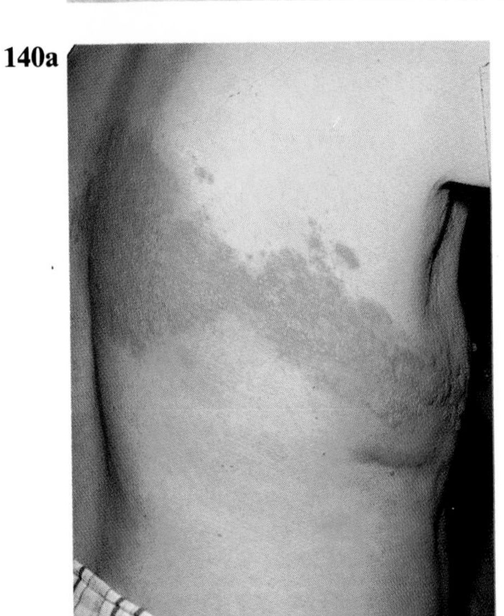

141

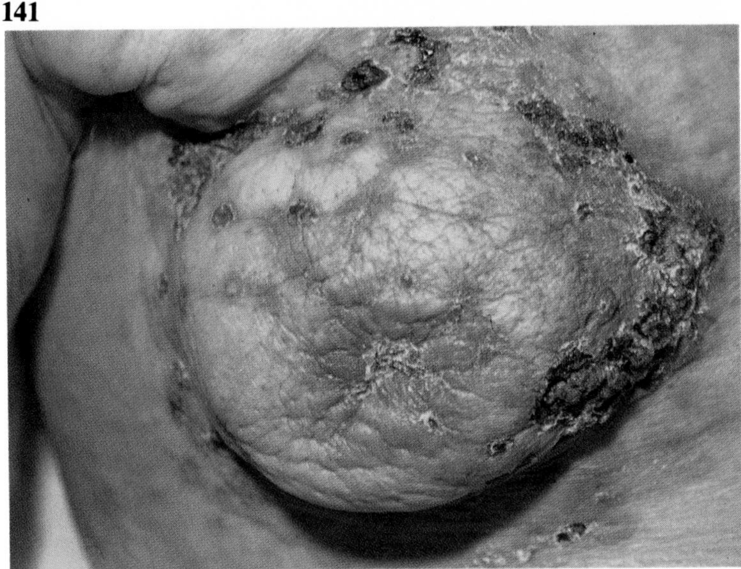

140b

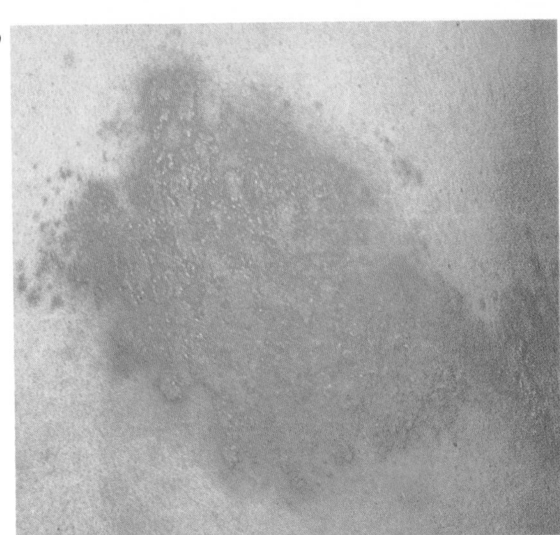

139a Herpes zoster. An early case of Herpes zoster showing painful bullons eruption on the chest wall. Local application of idoxuridine and oral treatment with steriods may modify the course of illness.

139b Carcinoma of the breast. Painless fungating carcinoma in an 85-year-old woman. The condition had been present for several months, but the patient simply ignored it. Carcinoma of the breast tends to run a chronic course in the very elderly. The approximate incidence is 190 per 100,000 per year in females.

140a and b Herpes zoster. Herpes on the lateral chest wall involving the mid-thoracic dermatomes. The patient had chronic lymphatic leukaemia and subsequently developed post-herpetic neuralgia.

142

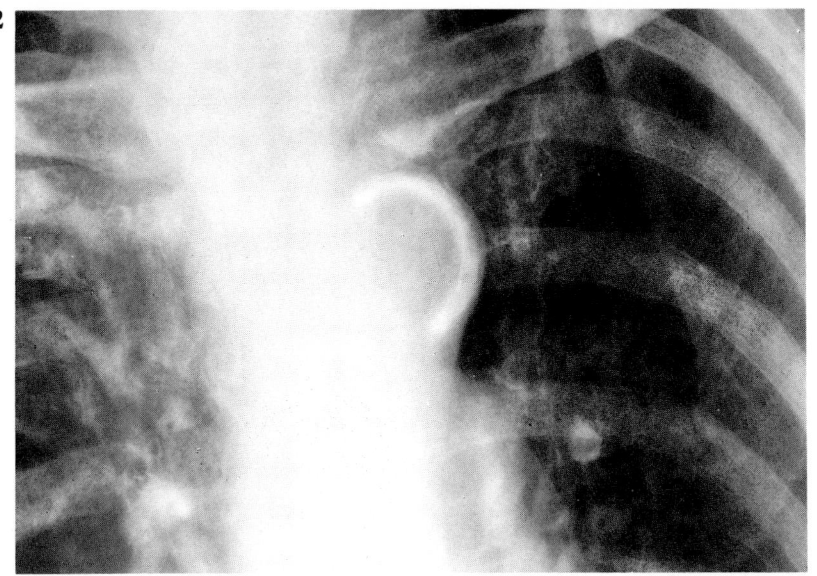

142 Calcified aortic knuckle. A common, benign appearance associated with advancing age and aortic valve sclerosis. Should be distinguished from calcification of ascending aorta.

143a

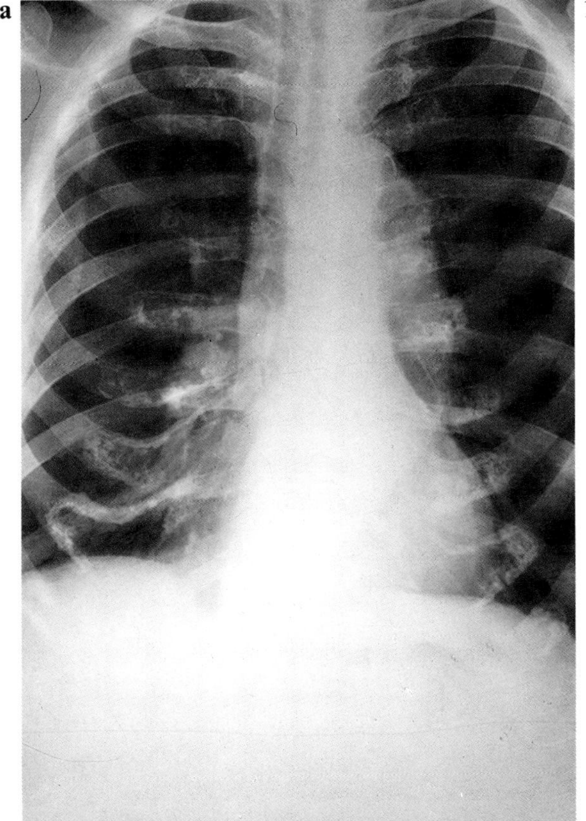

143b

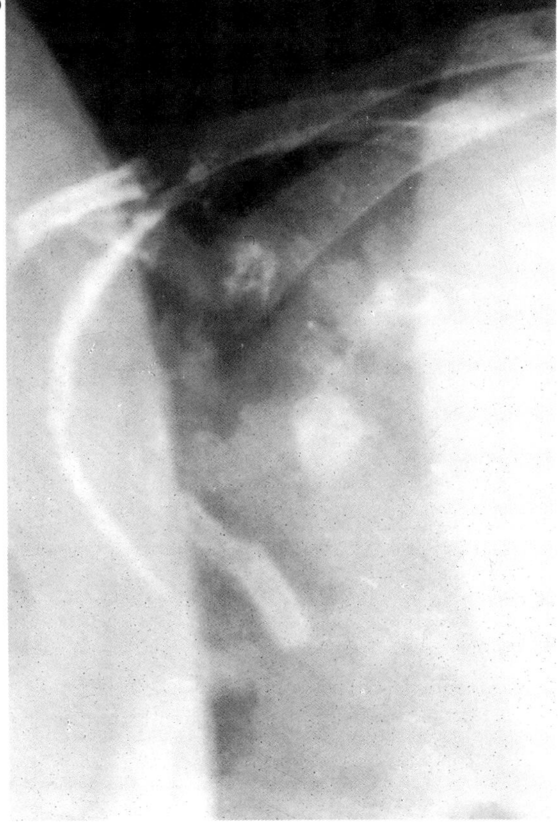

141 Carcinoma of the breast. In this case there is more widespread infiltration by the malignant tissue. The lesion was again painless and there was no evidence of metastases.

143a Calcified costochondral cartilages. A common, radiological finding in the elderly. May be confused with intrapulmonary or pleural calcification.

143b Calcified costochondral cartilages. A close up view.

144 Unfolded aorta. A common radiological finding in the elderly, caused by a combination of arteriosclerosis and hypertension. The condition is symptomless but may be confused with aortic aneurysm.

145 Aortic aneurysm. An aneurysm involving the aortic arch. The patient had previously contracted syphilis and had symptoms of mediastinal obstruction.

146 Aortic aneurysm. An aneurysm involving the descending aorta and caused by arteriosclerotic changes in the vessel wall. Note streaks of calcification in the aortic wall.

Aneurysms of the aorta

Aetiology

Aneurysms of the abdominal aorta

Atherosclerosis plus hypertension

Aneurysms of the ascending aorta

Arteriosclerosis
Cystic medial necrosis
Syphilis

Aneurysms of the descending aorta

Arteriosclerosis
Non-penetrating chest trauma

144

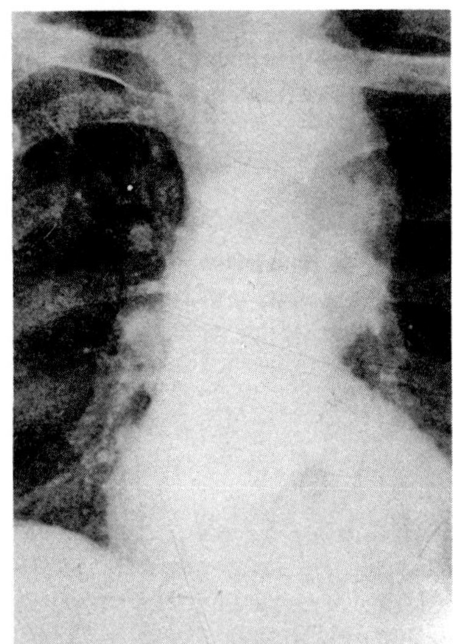

145

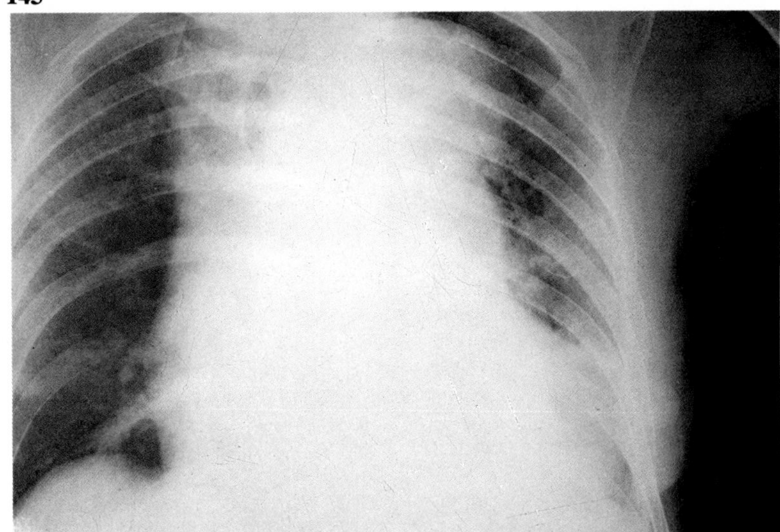

146

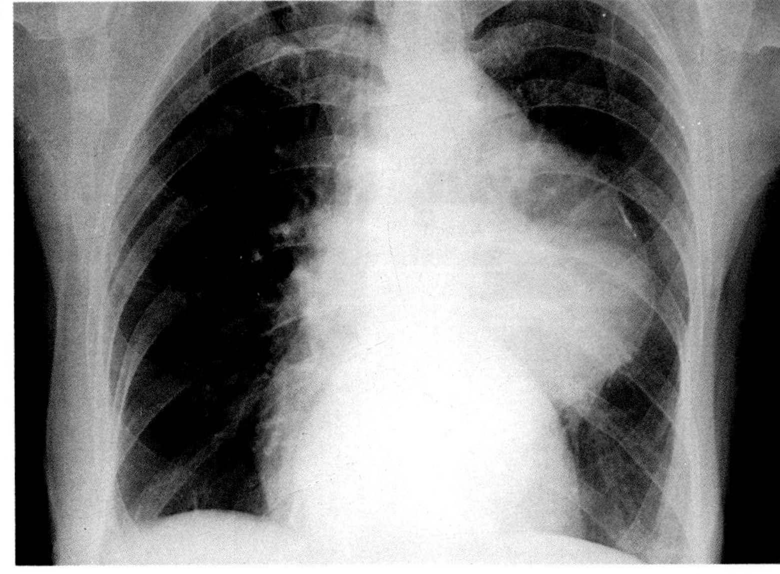

47

48

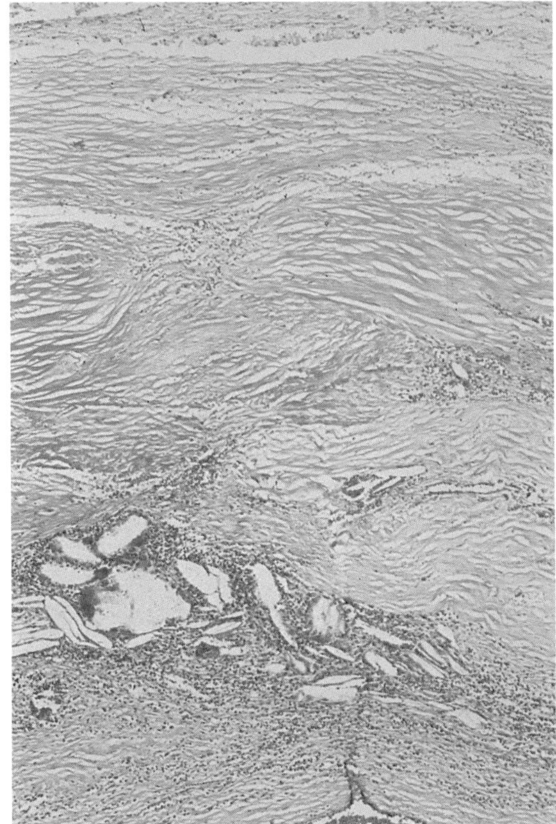

147 and 148 Aortic arteriosclerosis. Early arteriosclerotic changes in the aortic wall. This may eventually lead to the development of an aneurysm. The first picture shows a fatty streak in the aortic wall; the second picture shows a fibrofatty plaque in the aorta.

Arteriosclerosis in the elderly may present as cerebrovascular accident, ischaemic heart disease, ischaemic colitis, peripheral vascular disease, or it may remain completely silent.

149

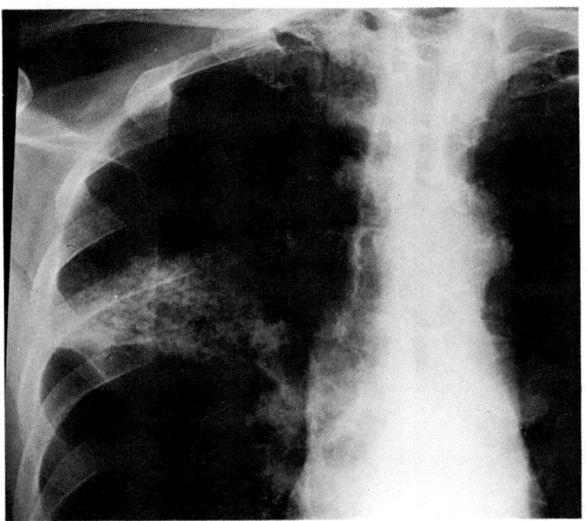

150a

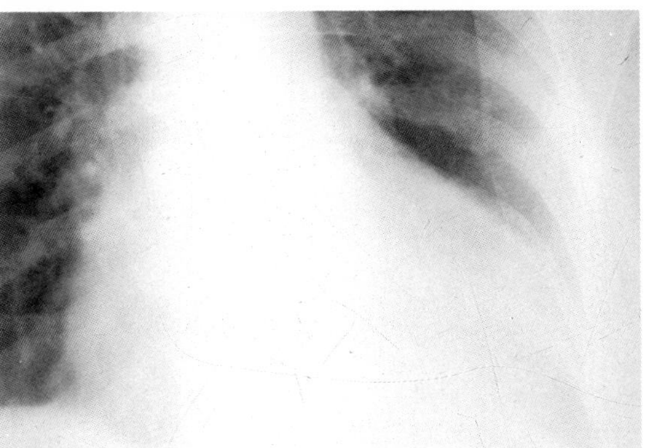

150b

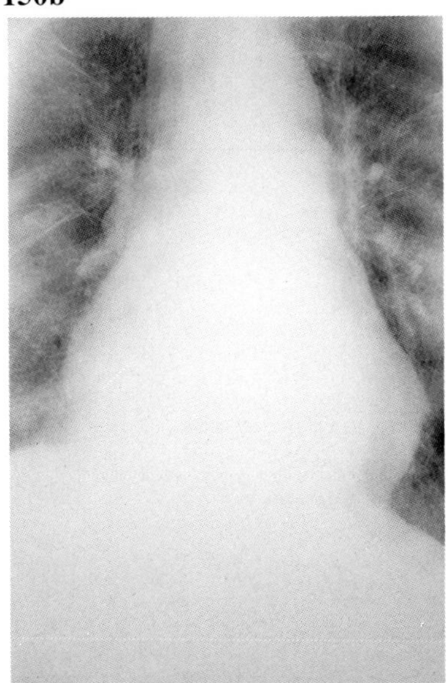

150c

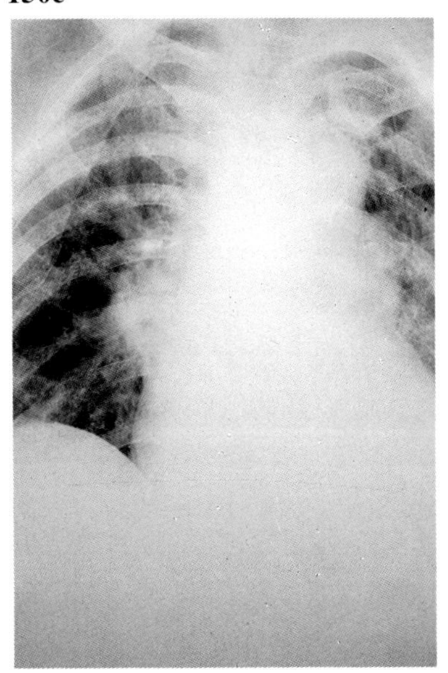

149 Pneumonia. A common disease of old age which carrys a high mortality rate.

150a Cardiomegaly. Routine chest Xray in an elderly patient showing cardiac enlargement with left ventricular prominence. The patient had no symptoms of cardiorespiratory disease.

150b Congestive cardiac failure. A frequent cause of admission to geriatric units. Note the gross cardiomegaly and pulmonary oedema.

150c Congestive çardiac failure. There is pulmonary oedema and the cause is hypertensive heart disease.

Cardiac failure in the elderly

Ischaemic heart disease – 48.5%
Hypertension
Degenerative calcific changes in mitral ring or aortic cusp
Corpulmonale
Senile cardiac amyloidosis
Endocarditis – including non-bacterial thrombotic endocarditis
Calcified aortic stenosis
Rheumatic heart disease
Mucoid degeneration of the mitral valve
Myxoedema
High output failure in chronic anaemia, thyrotoxicosis, Paget's disease, and beri-beri

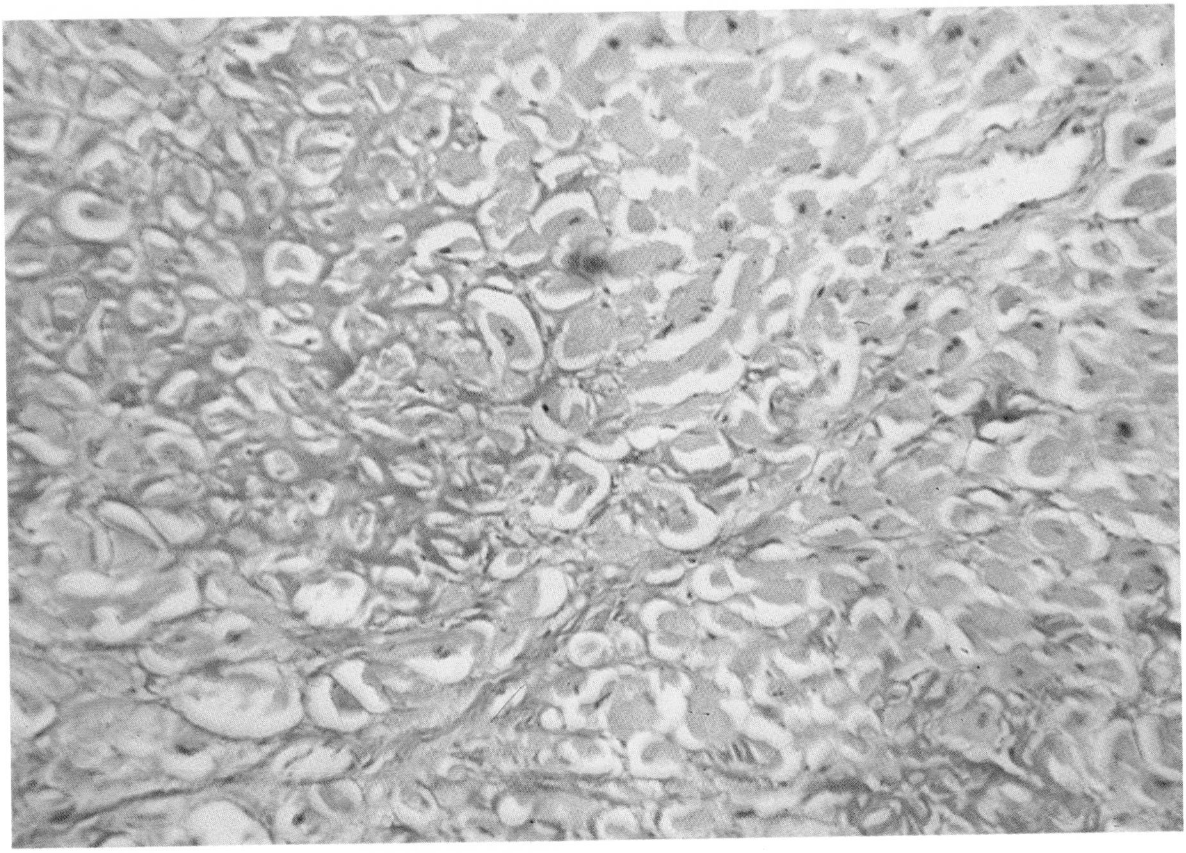

1

52

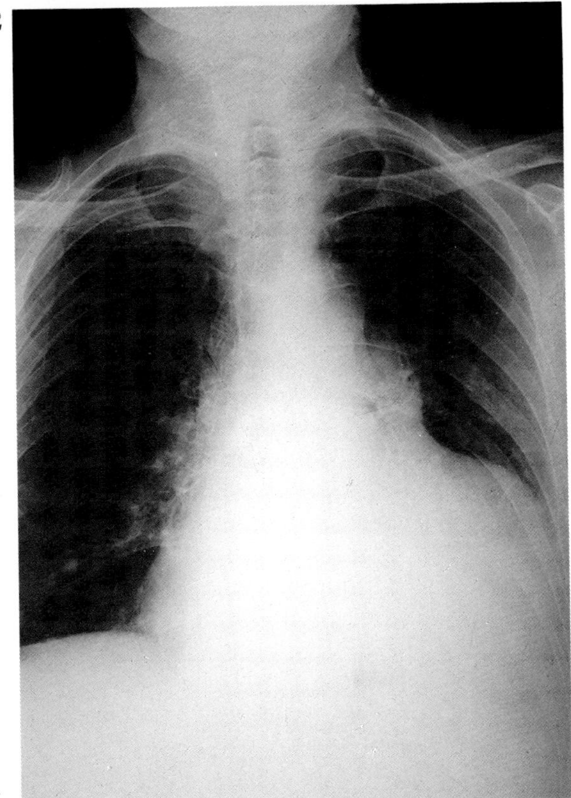

151 Cardiac amyloidosis. Found with increasing frequency in the very old and is said to cause congestive heart failure. In the histology picture the amyloid is stained green, muscle yellow, and fibrous tissue red. (*Sulphonated alcian blue technique*)

152 Left ventricular aneurysm. A complication of previous myocardial infarction, involving the left ventricular wall and producing severe left ventricular failure.

It appears in less than 20 per cent of cases within few months after the infarct and may give rise to systemic embolism.

Complications of carcinoma of the bronchus

1 Local complications:
Brachial obstruction, superior vena cava obstruction, pleural effusion, erosion of large blood vessels, cervical sympathetic, recurrent laryngeal or phrenic nerve involvement
2 Metastasis
Hilar nodes, liver, cerebrum, adrenals, bone
3 Non-metastatic extra-pulmonary effects
Cachexia, anaemia
Clubbing and hypertrophic pulmonary osteoarthropathy
Neuropathy and myopathy
Endocrine syndromes:
Inappropriate ADH production
Ectopic ACTH production
Pigmentation
Inappropriate parathormone production
Carcinoid syndrome
Thyrotoxicosis-like disorder
Gynaecomastia
Hypoglycemia
Red-cell aplasia
Skin changes:
Metastasis, pruritis, various types of skin rashes, dermatomyositis, eczema herpeticum, hyperhidrosis

154

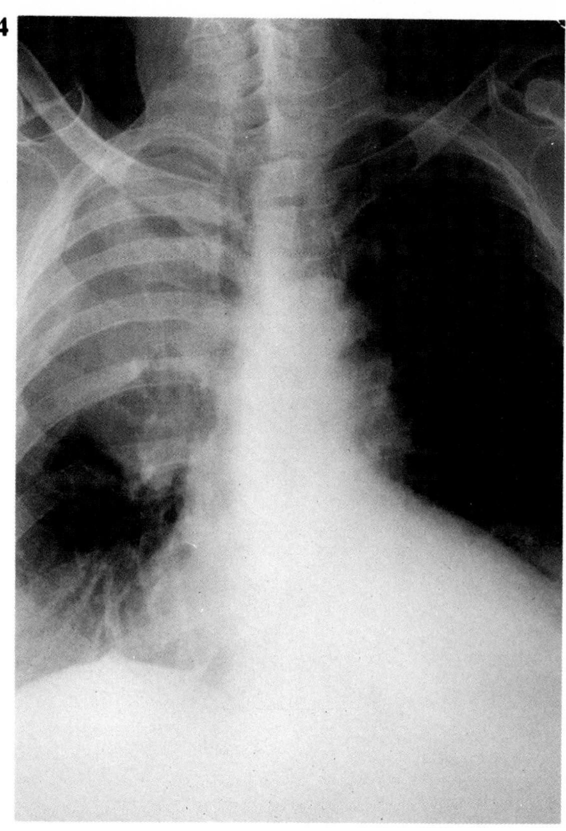

153

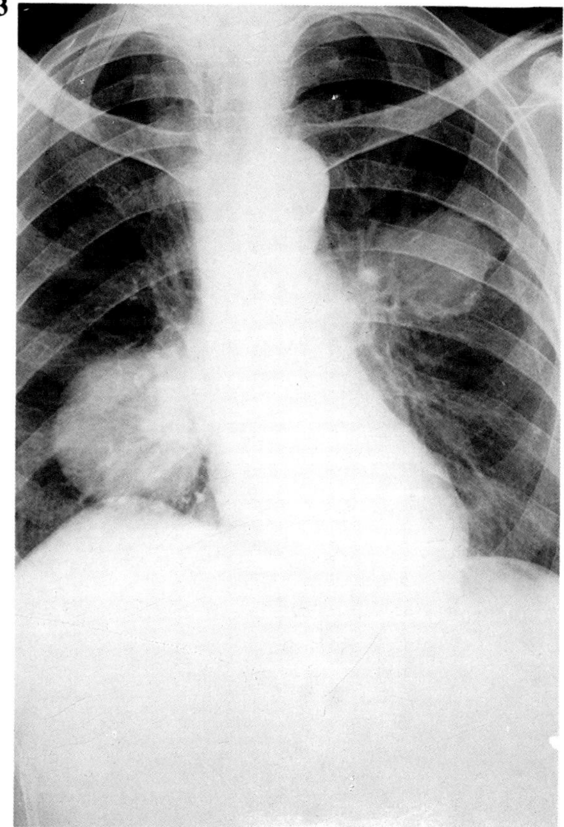

153 Bronchogenic carcinoma. The right upper lung is involved. It is a common malignancy of old age. The incidence is approximately 250 per 100,000 population per year.

154 Pulmonary metastases. Round discrete shadows of secondary deposits from carcinoma of the ovary.

Hypernephromas, melanomas, and tumours of the breast, pancreas, and testicle tend to favour the lungs for the growth of metastases.

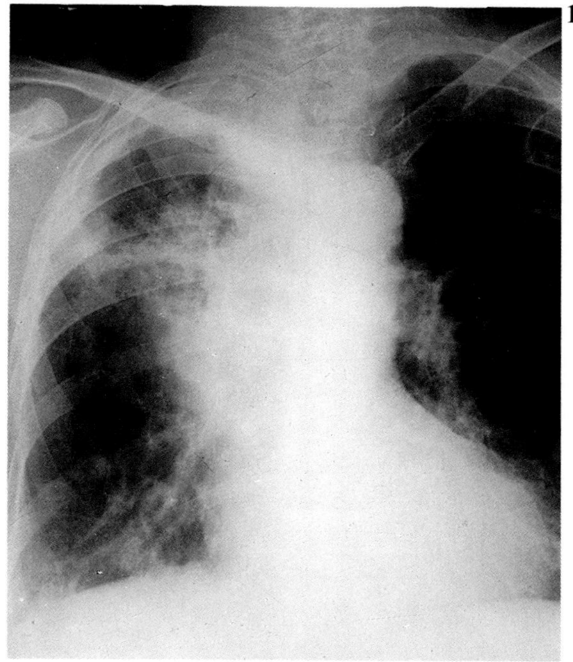

155b

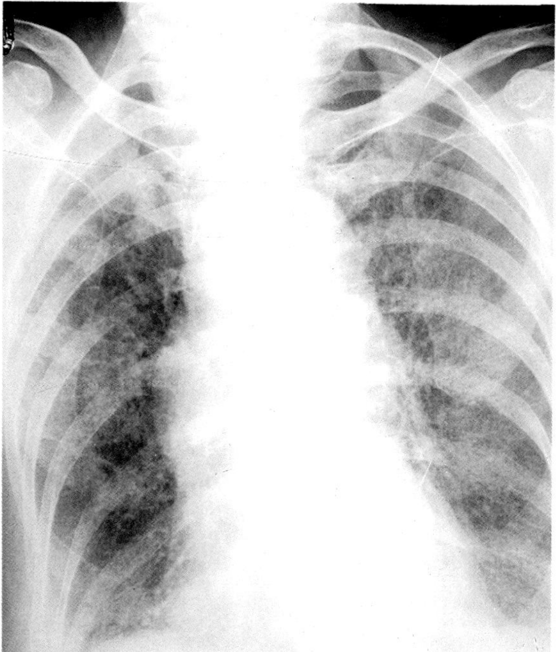

156

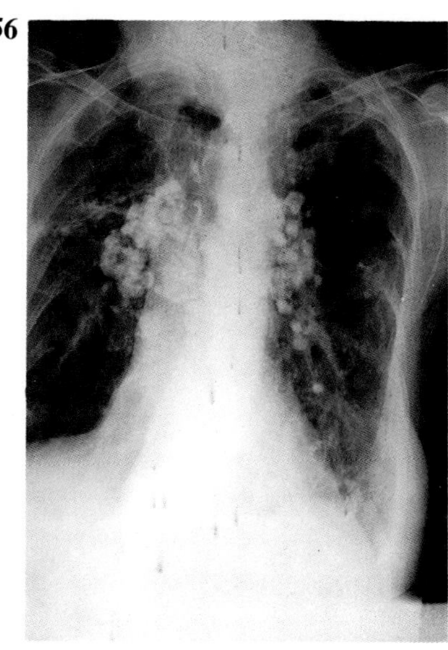

155a Pulmonary tuberculosis. The decline of tuberculosis in the elderly has been much slower than in the younger population. 'Occult tuberculosis' is a frequent finding in geriatric patients. This lady presented with weightloss, weakness, anaemia, and elevated ESR.

155b Pulmonary tuberculosis. Chest xray showing miliary tuberculosis. The elderly patient presented with acute respiratory illness.

156 Sarcoidosis. Chest xray of a 75-year-old patient showing bilateral hilar lymphadenopathy with calcification. The Kviem test was positive for sarcoidosis.

Special features of TB in elderly

There has been a relative increase in the incidence of TB among elderly patients. The reasons are:

1 Failure or delay in making correct diagnosis
2 Reactivation of previously acquired and healed primary TB lesions
3 Poor diet and bad living conditions
4 Other debilitating diseases with increasing age
5 Decline in tuberculin sensitivity with advancing years

Clinical features:

Tend to be modified in the elderly
Non-specific ill health and weightloss
Pyrexia of unknown origin
Xray of the chest may show miliary TB, pleural effusion or may appear normal
Wide variety of blood-cell abnormalities
Tuberculin test may be negative initially and positive later
Confirmation may be obtained by biopsying enlarged glands, scalene nodes, liver or bone marrow
In some cases a therapeutic trial may be necessary

157a

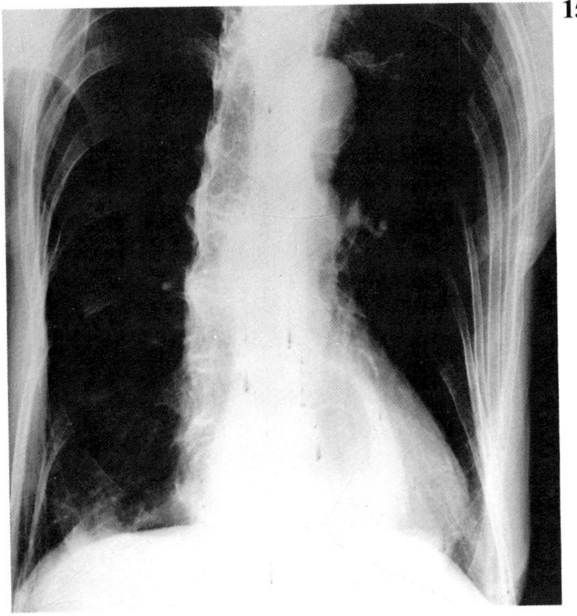

157b

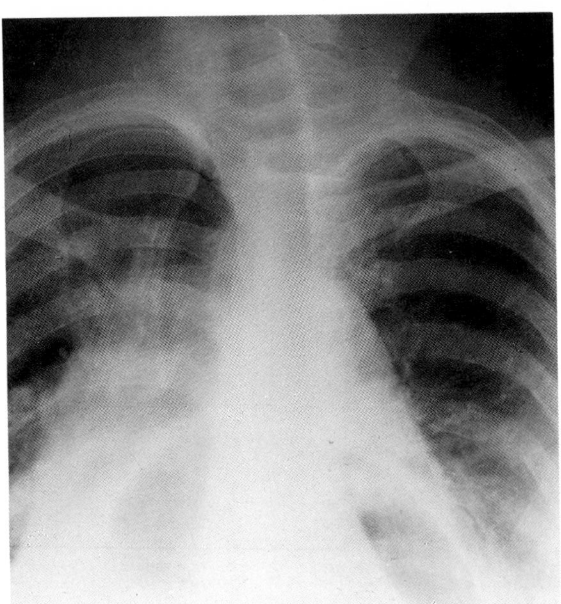

157a and b Hiatus hernia. Incidental finding on routine chest xray. Note the shadow containing an air bubble behind the cardiac silhouette. It is usually silent but can produce symptoms of reflux oesophagitis and iron-deficiency anaemia.

158 Hiatus hernia. Barium meal xray showing a sliding hiatus hernia. This elderly patient had symptoms of reflux oesophagitis.

Hiatus hernia

Types

1 Oesophagastric sliding type
2 Paraoesophageal rolling type
3 Mixed

Clinical features

1 Symptoms caused by oesophagitis
  - Dysphagia
  - Discomfort in chest with bending, stooping or lying down
  - Pain like that of ischaemic heart disease

2 Symptoms caused by hernia
  - Usually asymptomatic
  - Retrosternal discomfort
  - Irritation of diaphragm causing cough and hiccup

3 Symptoms caused by haemorrhage
  - Chronic bloodloss leading to anaemia
  - Rapid bloodloss may result in shock

158

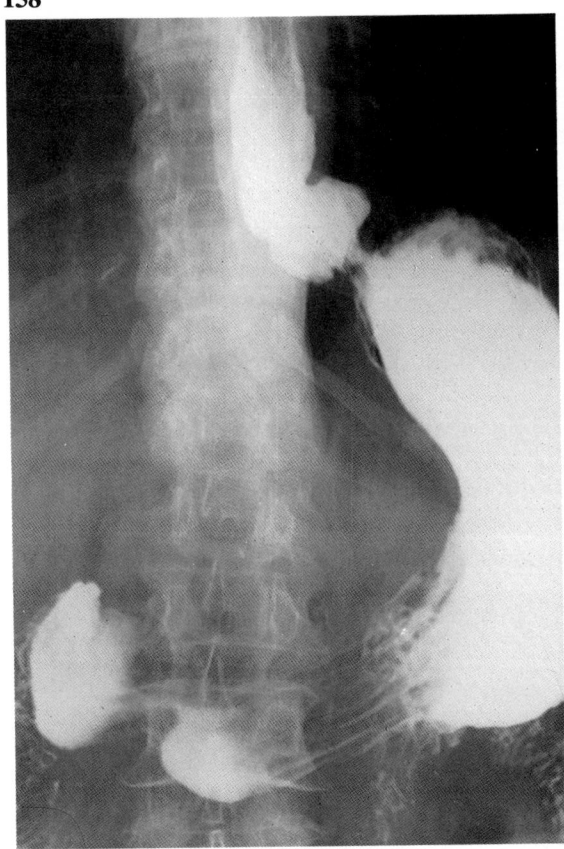

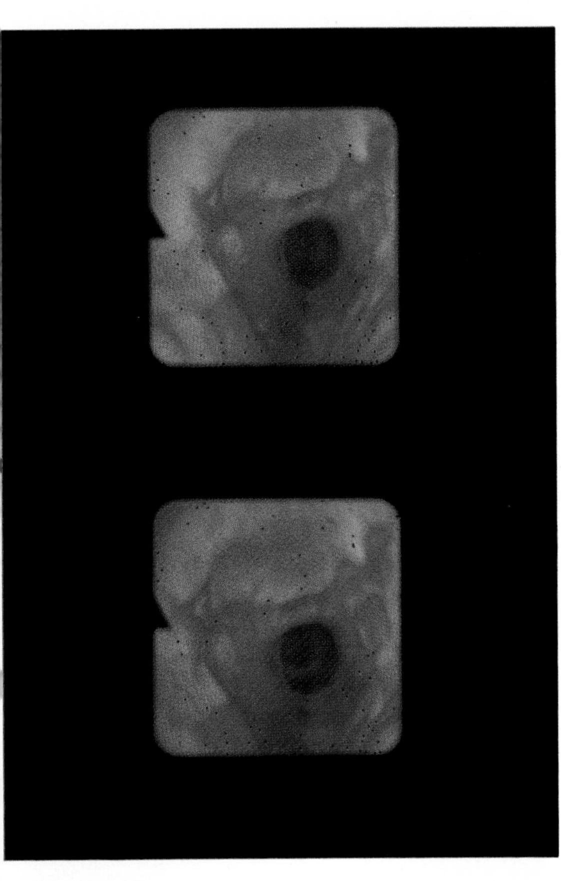

159 Reflux oesophagitis. Endoscopic view of lower oesophagus showing reflux oesophagitis with inflammatory changes in the mucosa. Note open cardia.

160 Oesophageal stricture. Barium swallow xray showing an oesophageal stricture. Endoscopy revealed its malignant nature.

161 Oesophageal candidiasis. Endoscopic view showing typical pale patches of candidiasis. The elderly patient complained of sore throat and dysphagia. Radiologically it may be confused with oesophageal carcinoma.

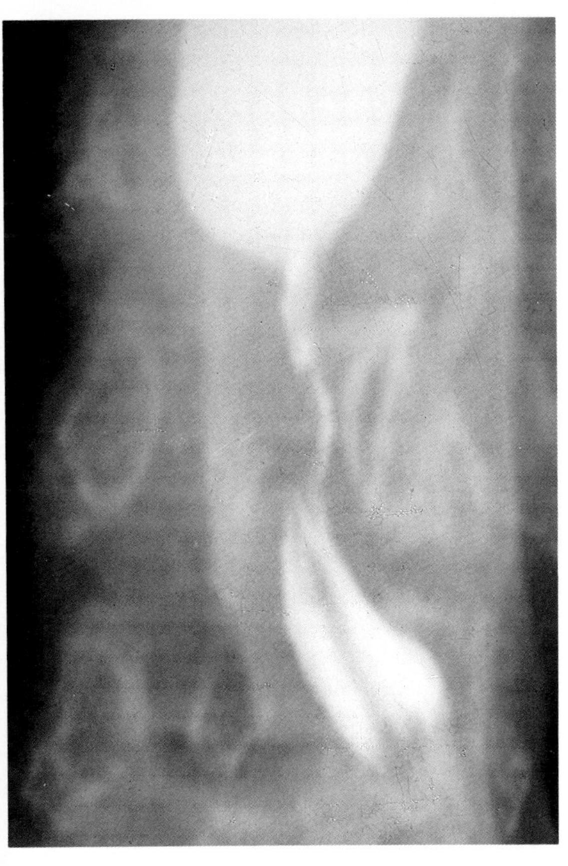

161

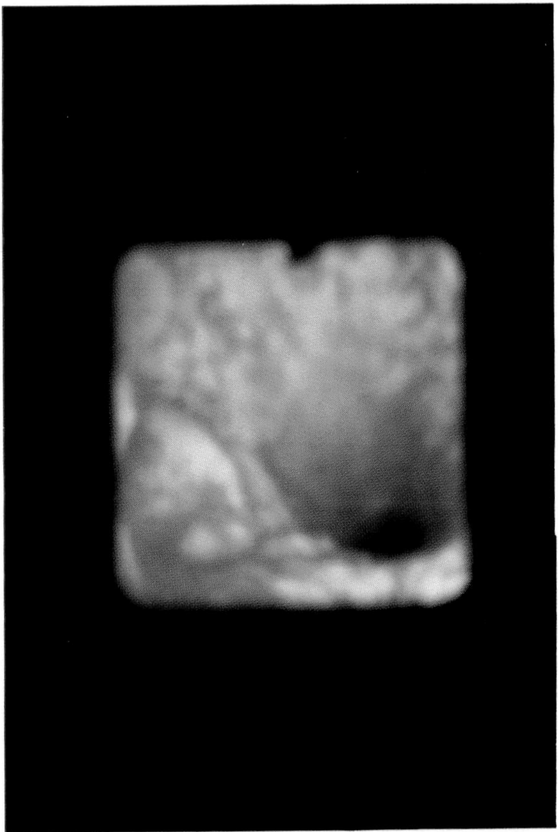

162

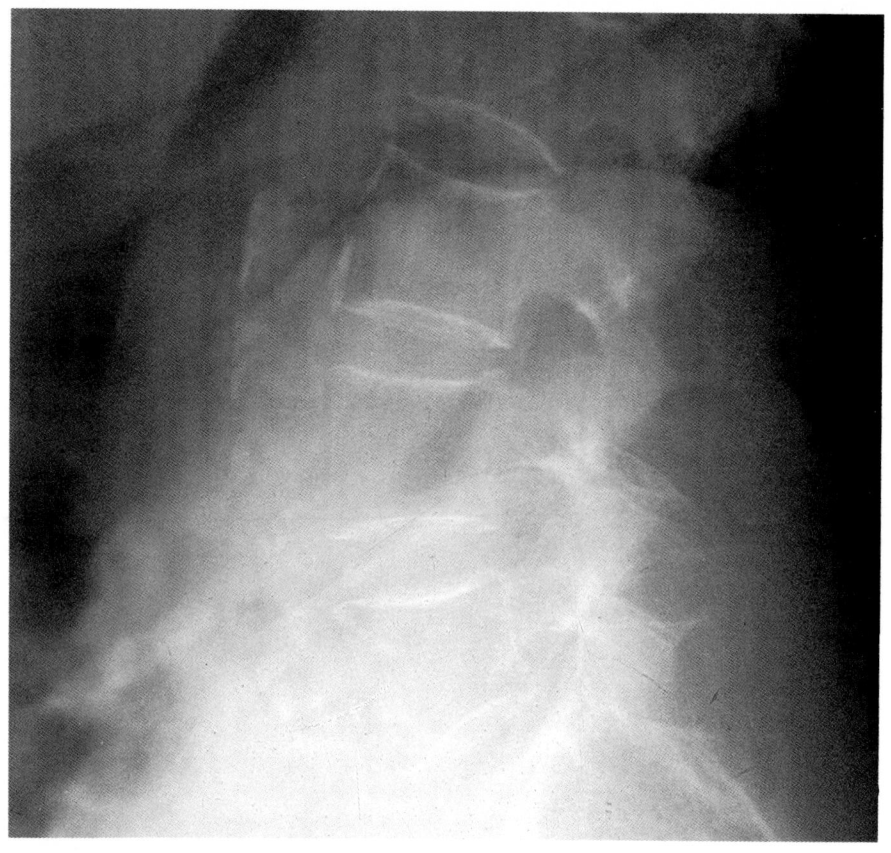

163

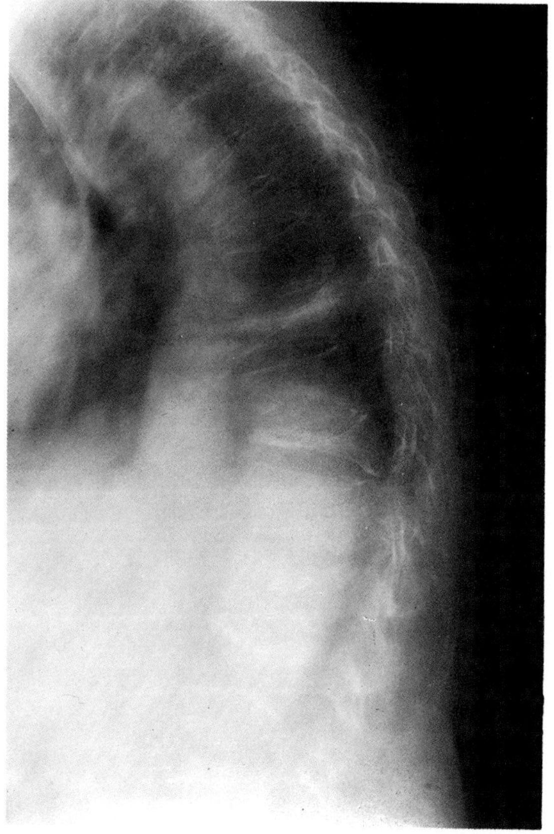

162 Osteoporotic spine. Biconcave vertebral bodies with reduced radiographic density. The trabecular bone is particularly affected. Note the calcification of abdominal aorta.

163 Osteoporotic spine. Increased translucency of the vertebral bodies with wedging and impaction fractures of the brittle midthoracic vertebrae.

This patient presented with severe backache spreading around to the front with weakness of the legs, kyphosis, and deteriorating mobility.

Osteoporosis

This is a common disorder of old age in which there is a reduced amount of bone per unit volume of bony tissue without any increase in osteoid.

Aetiology

1 Post-menopausal bone loss in females
2 Poor skeletal development of female
3 Prolonged negative calcium balance in some individuals. 8 per cent of UK population have insufficient dietary calcium intake
4 Nutritional factors – deficiencies of calcium, Vitamin D, Vitamin C, protein, and fluoride. Gastrectomy and malabsorption
5 Immobilisation
6 Hyperadrenocorticism
7 Hyperthyroidism
8 Acromegaly
9 Rheumatoid arthritis

Clinical features:

Usually asymptomatic
Backache caused by vertebral collapse
Fractured neck of the femur and Colles' fracture
Nerve-root compression
Increasing kyphoscoliosis and loss of height, marked transverse abdominal crease

Diagnosis

Normal serum calcium, phosphate and alkaline phosphatase
Xrays show reduced bone density (ghost-like bones), hollow vertebral bodies, biconcare (codfish) bodies, compression fracture of vertebrae and sometimes Schmorl's nodes
Bone biopsy with histological examination of bony tissue will indicate the degree of osteoporosis

164
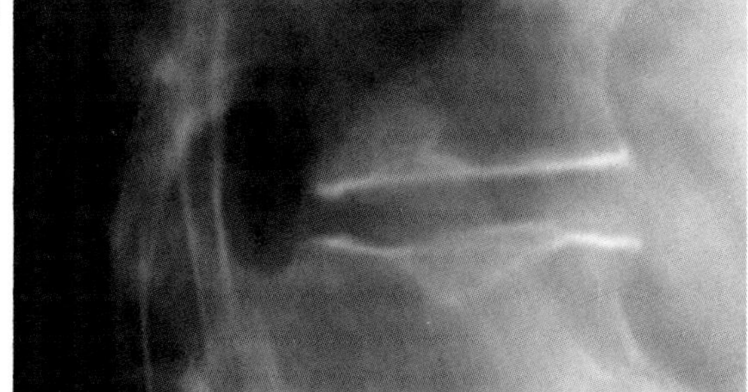

165
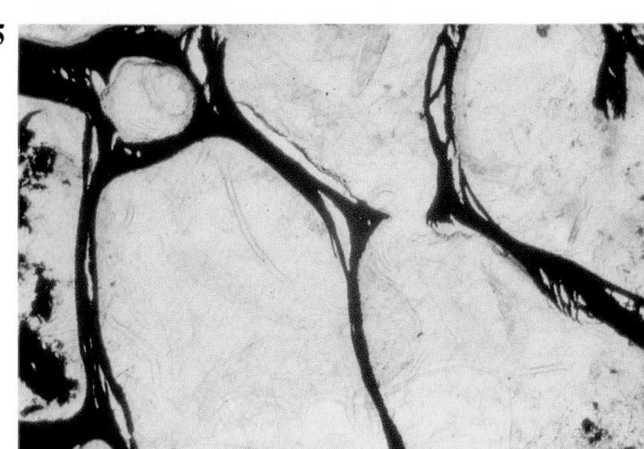

166
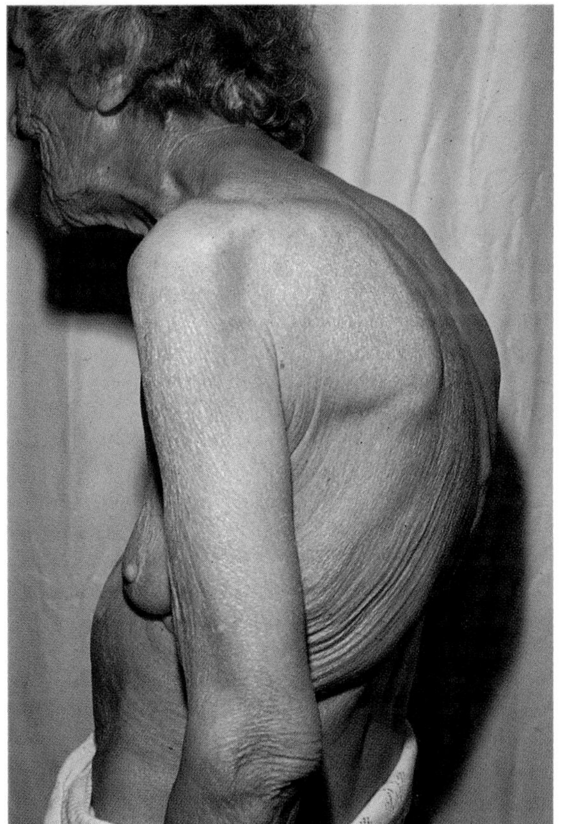

164 Schmorl's node. A sign of advanced spinal osteoporosis. There is herniation of the intervertebral disc into the body of the osteoporotic vertebra.

165 Osteoporosis. Bone histology showing reduction of both protein matrix and mineralisation.

166 Kyphosis. This elderly lady's condition was caused by a combination of spinal osteoporotic vertebral collapse and chronic degenerative changes in the vertebral column.

167

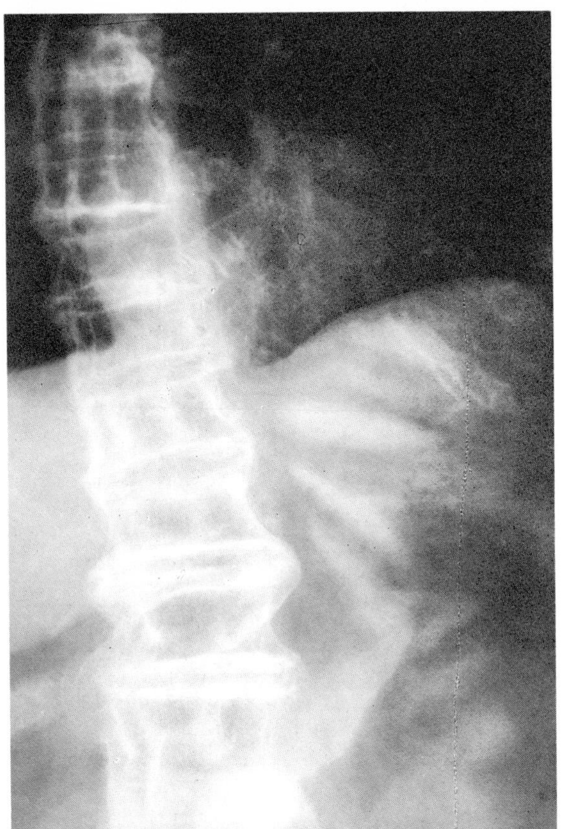

167 Spinal degenerative disease (osteoarthrosis). A common problem in old age and a frequent cause of chronic disability. Degenerative changes may extend throughout the whole of vertebral column and are particularly marked in apophyseal joints, the neurocentral joints, and the costovertebral joints. The pathology is further complicated by changes in the intervertebral discs. Spondylotic changes in the dorsolumbar spine produce backache. Intervertebral disc protrusion, with osteophytes, may give rise to symptoms of nerve-root compression.

168a and 168b Spinal scoliosis. This is a common radiological finding in the elderly and is usually associated with spinal osteoarthrosis.

168a

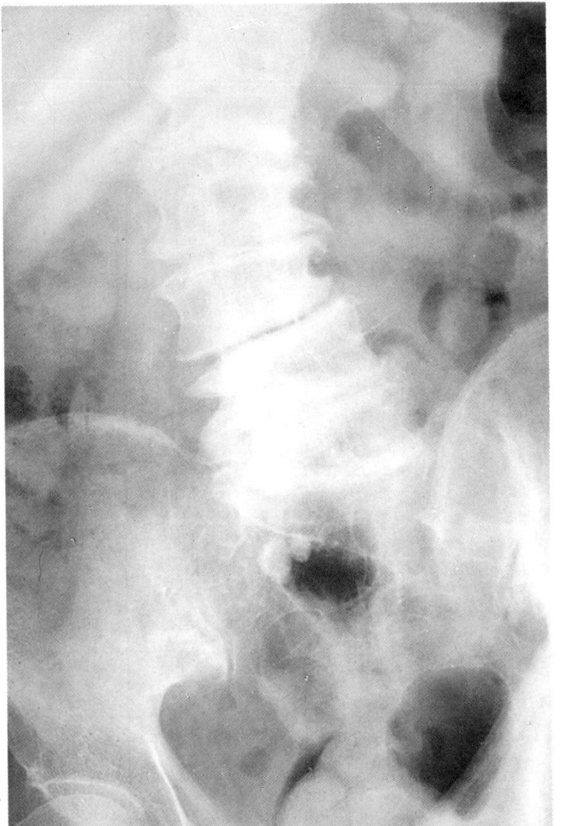

168b

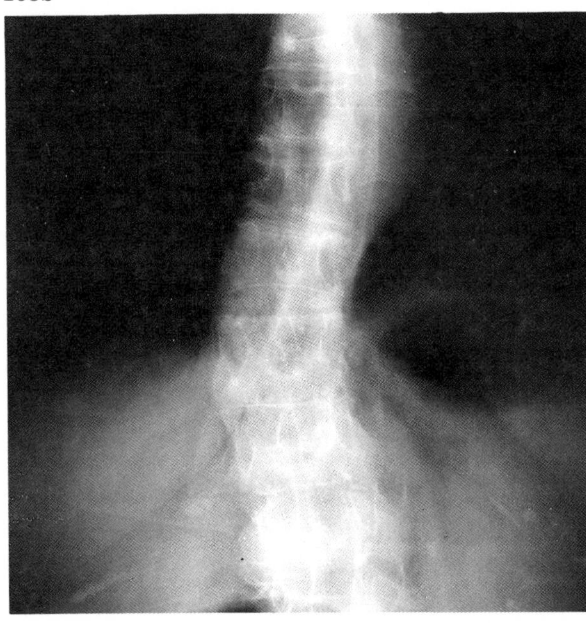

7 Disorders of the abdomen

169

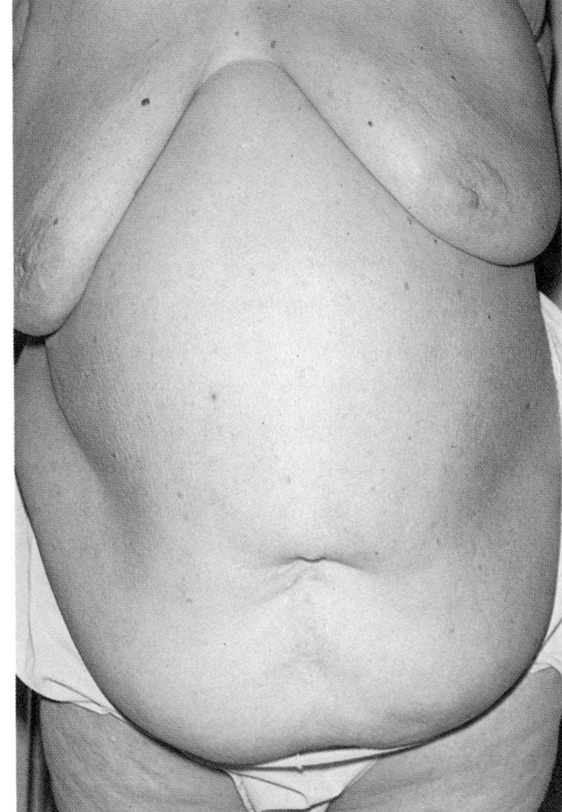

169 Obese abdomen. Fatty 'apron' of obesity in an elderly lady. She suffered from advanced osteoarthritis and hypertension.

170 Cachexia. Wasted abdomen of an 80-year-old man who had carcinoma of the colon with secondary spread. Note the slight generalised hyperpigmentation.

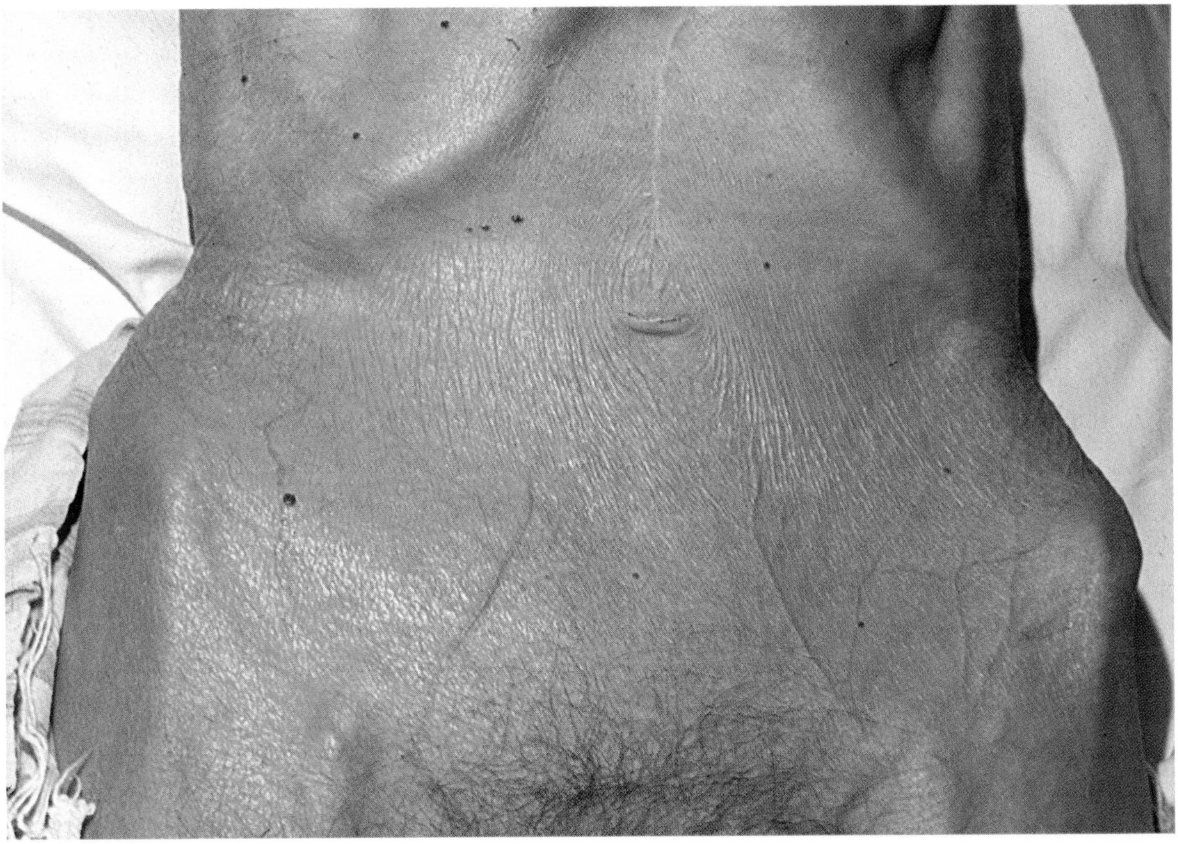

171

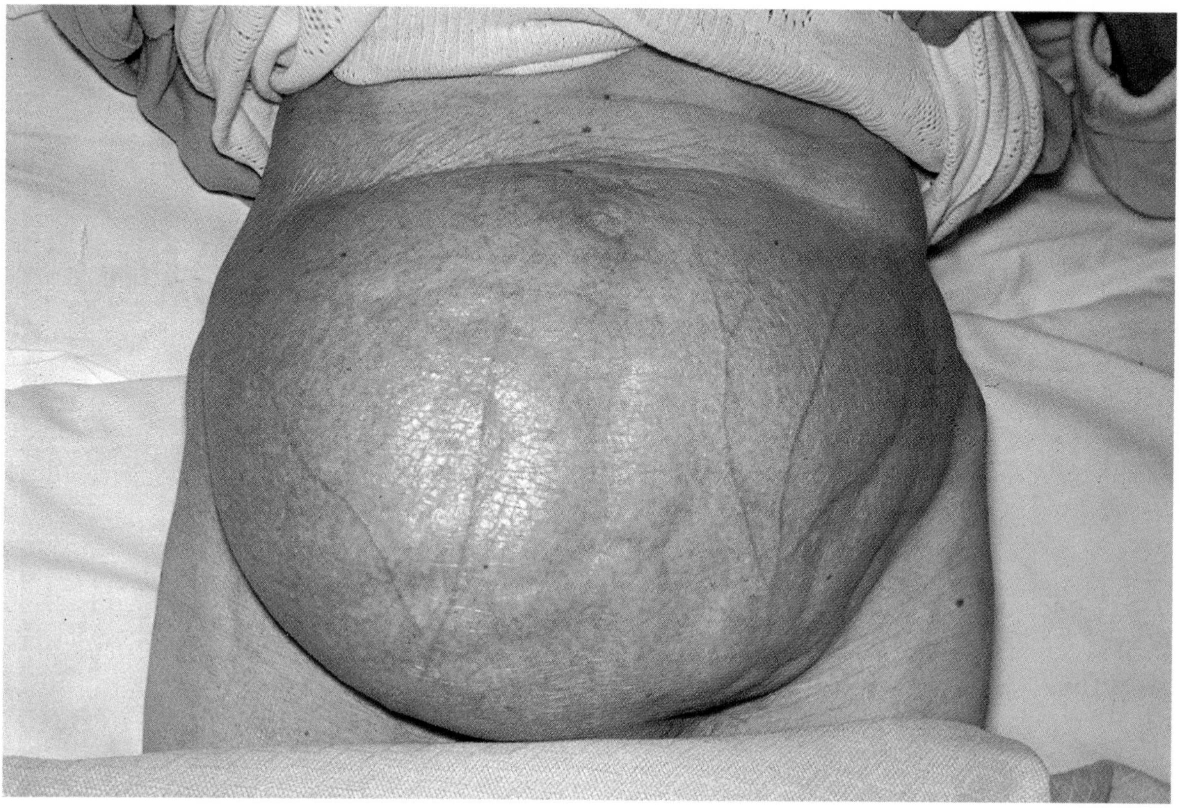

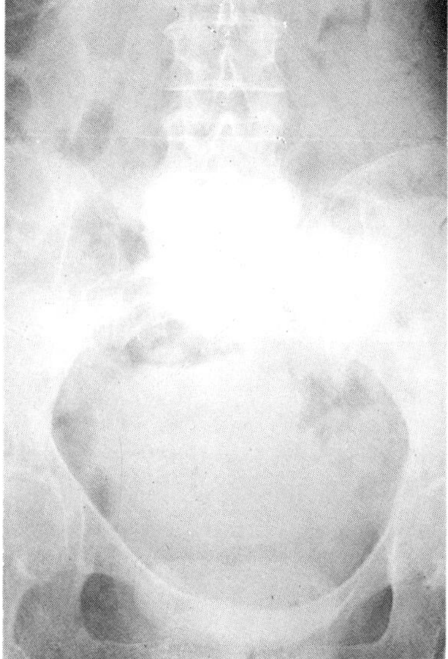

171 Severe constipation. Prominent bowel pattern caused by severe constipation. This Parkinsonian patient's bowels were impacted with faeces. Enemas were required to relieve the condition.

172 Constipation. Plain xray of the abdomen showing dense faecal shadows distending most of the colon and rectum.

Constipation in the elderly

Aetiology

1 Low dietary intake of fibre and roughage
2 Immobility and lack of exercise
3 Poor bowel habits
4 Lack of privacy and new environment
5 Drugs – codeine, antidepressants, laxative dependence, iron salts, anticholinergics
6 Colonic lesions – diverticular disease, cancer of colon, idiopathic megacolon, obstruction, spastic colon
7 Anal lesions – fissure, abscess, haemorrhoids
8 Metabolic and endocrine – myxoedema, hypokalemia, hypercalcemia, dehydration
9 CNS disorders – depression, Parkinsonism, autonomic neuropathy, cerebrovascular accidents, spinal cord lesions

Complications of constipation

Impaction and faecal incontinence
Urinary retention and overflow incontinence
Bowel obstruction
Agitation, irritability
Confusion

Faecal incontinence in the elderly

Causes

Constipation and impaction – overflow incontinence
Diverticular disease of colon
Rectal carcinoma
Laxative abuse
Antibiotics
Toxic confusion
Ischaemic colitis
Ulcerative colitis
Rectal prolapse
Cerebral cortex lesions
- CVAs
- Dementias
- Tumours

Spinal cord lesions
Cauda equina lesions

173

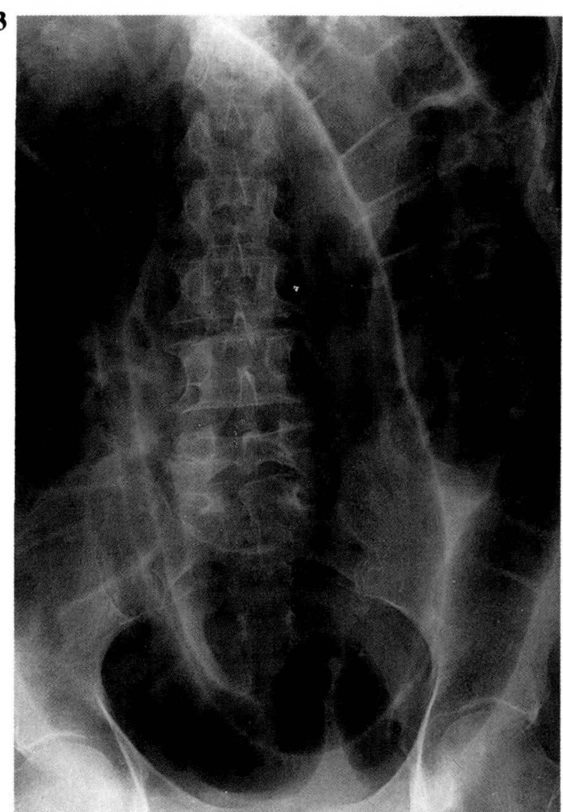

173 Megacolon. Plain xray of the abdomen showing megacolon in an elderly patient. In the elderly it is usually a complication of chronic constipation and cathartic colon syndrome and presents as gross tympanitic abdominal distension, sometimes associated with diarrhoea and faecal incontinence. Sigmoid volvulus is a further complication.

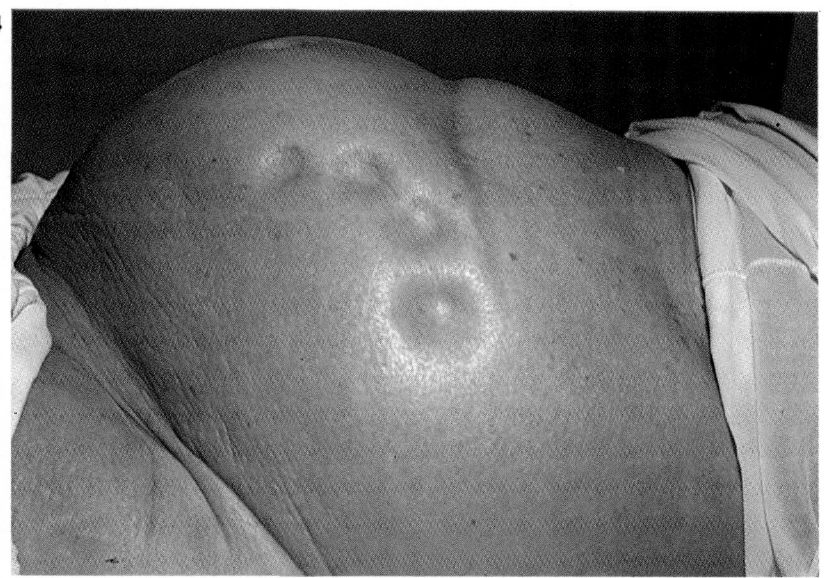

174 Oedema of the abdominal wall. Secondary to hypoalbuminaemia associated with nephrotic syndrome.

175
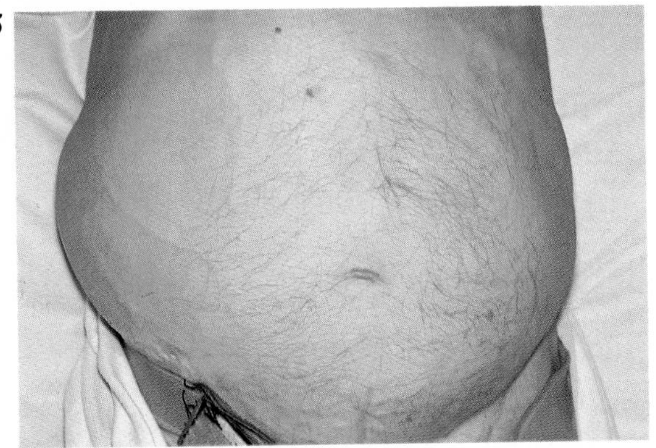

175 Ascites. Tense, distended abdomen caused by gross ascites. The patient had hepatic cirrhosis, with features of portal hypertension and hepato-cellular failure.

Common causes of hepatomegaly in the elderly

Congestive cardiac failure
Myeloproliferative disorders
Neoplastic especially metastasis
Biliary obstruction
Cirrhosis of the liver

176
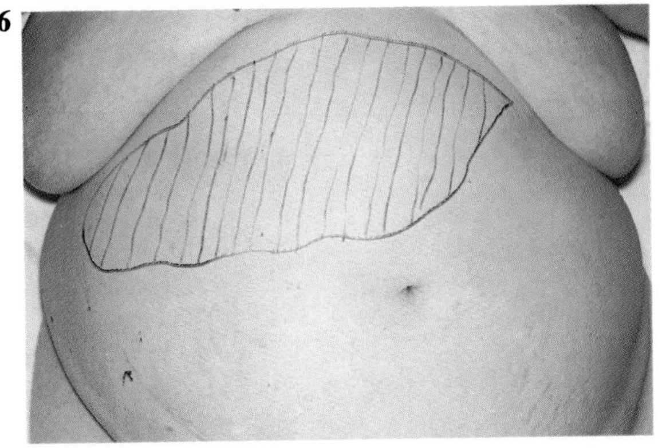

176 Hepatomegaly. Caused by hepatic metastases from carcinoma of the rectum. The liver is enlarged, hard, and painless with a nodular surface.

177
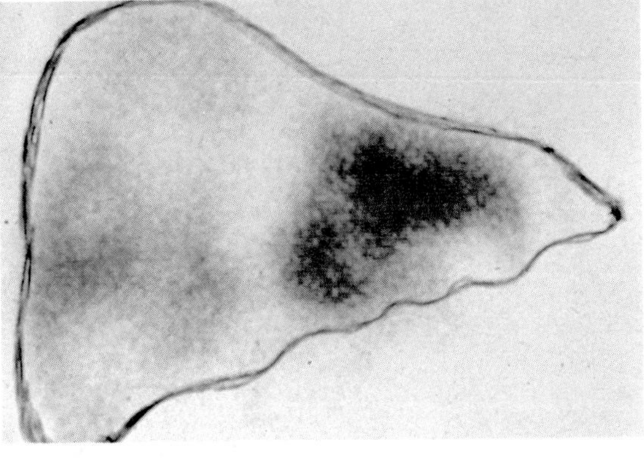

177 Liver scan. Multiple filling defects caused by secondary deposits.

178
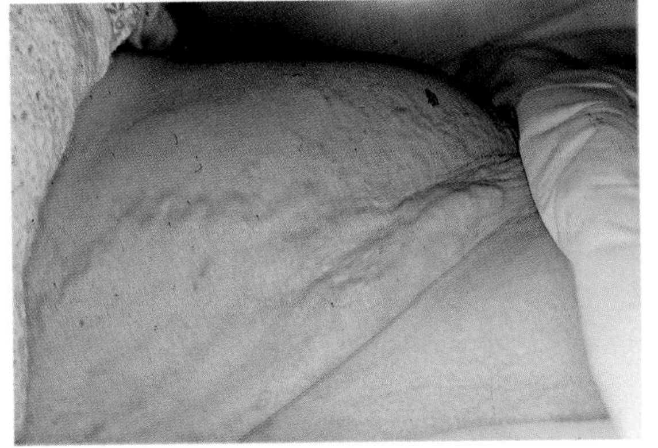

178 Caput medusae. Visible venous collateral circulation over the anterior abdominal wall in a patient with advanced cirrhosis of the liver.

79

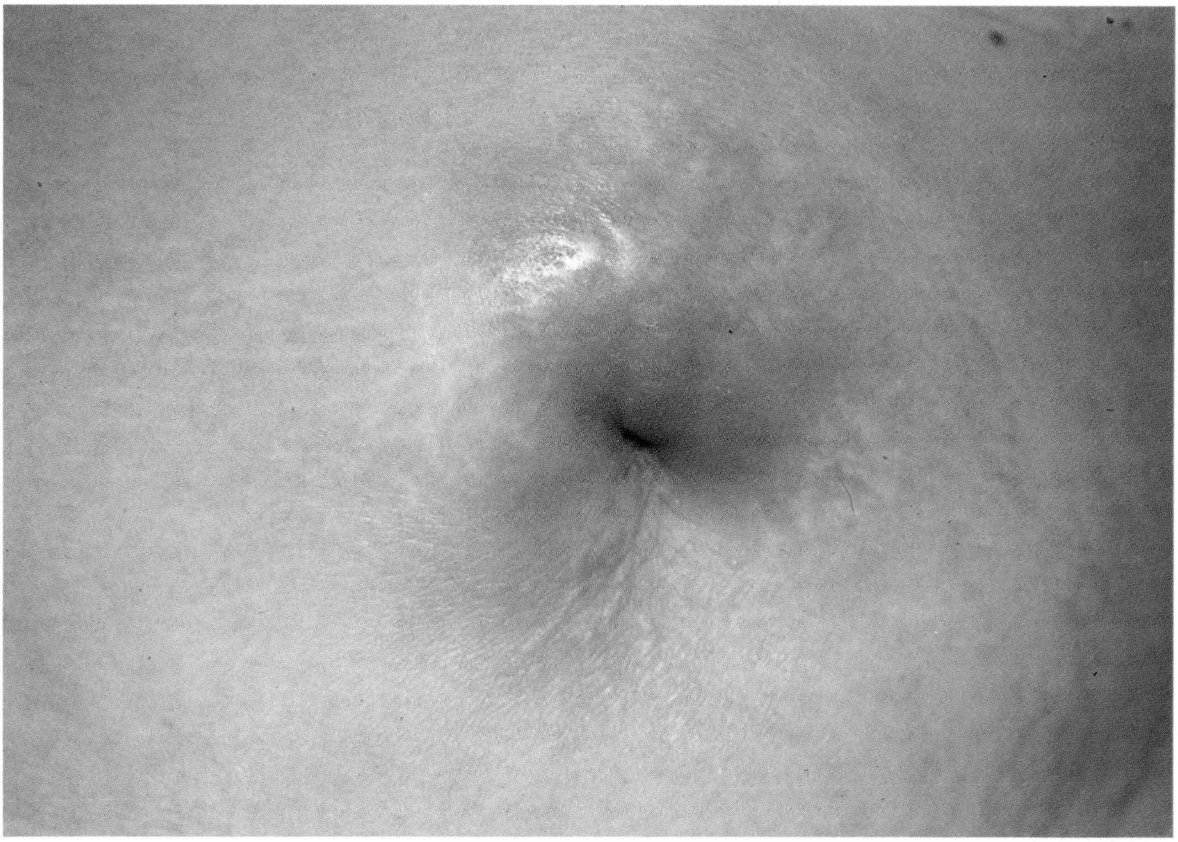

180

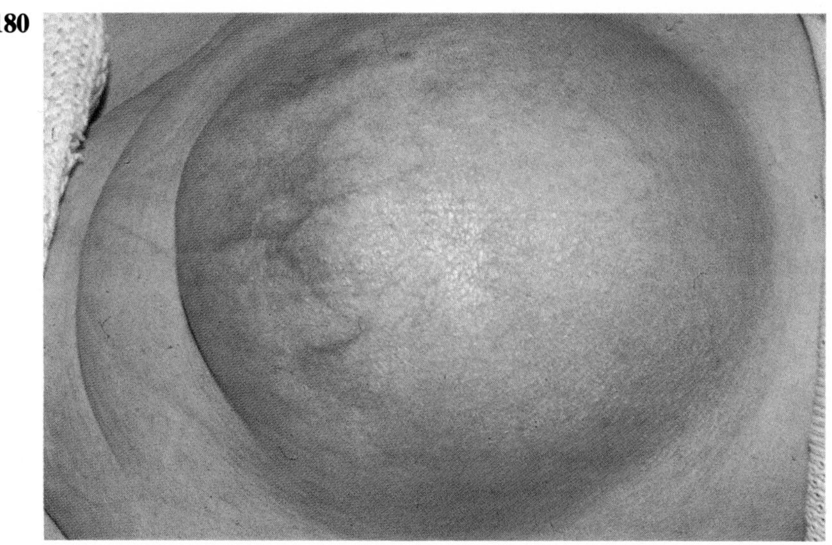

179 Umbilical infection. A result of self-neglect and poor hygiene.

180 Umbilical hernia. A common finding in old age. Usually symptomless.

181
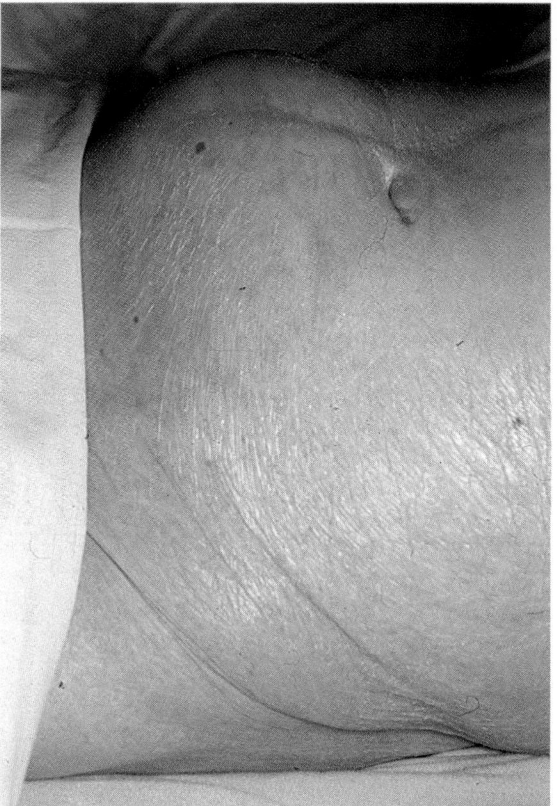

182
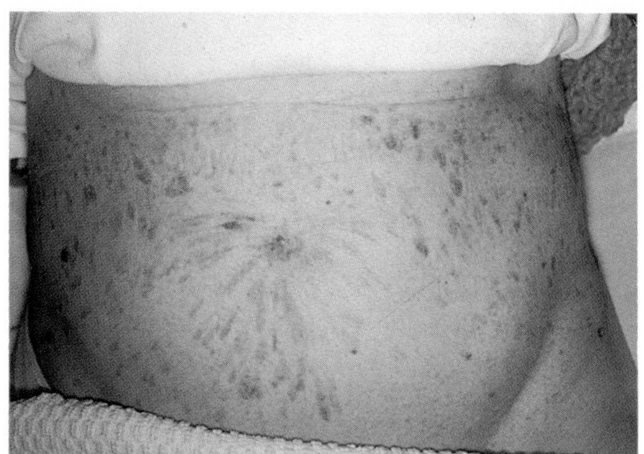

183
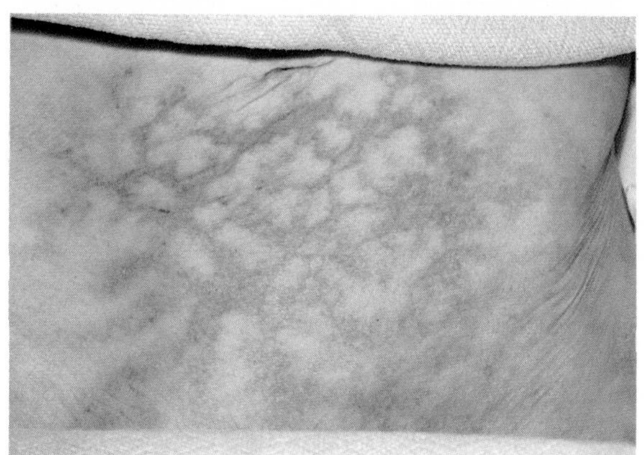

Common causes of urinary retention in old age

Abdominal operations
Prostatism
Faecal impaction
Pelvic tumours
Urethral stricture
Drugs – anticholinergics, diuretics
Anxiety and fear
Atonic neurogenic bladder
Spinal lesions

181 Urinary retention. Distended bladder in an elderly man who had prostatic hypertrophy and had developed urinary retention with overflow incontinence.

182 Seborrhoeic warts. These warts are benign lesions which become increasingly common with ageing. They appear as brownish macules on the head and trunk. Darkness and size tend to increase with advancing age.

183 Erythema ab igne on the anterior abdominal wall. This patient had recurrent abdominal pain caused by peptic ulcer disease. She used hotwater bottles to relieve her symptoms.

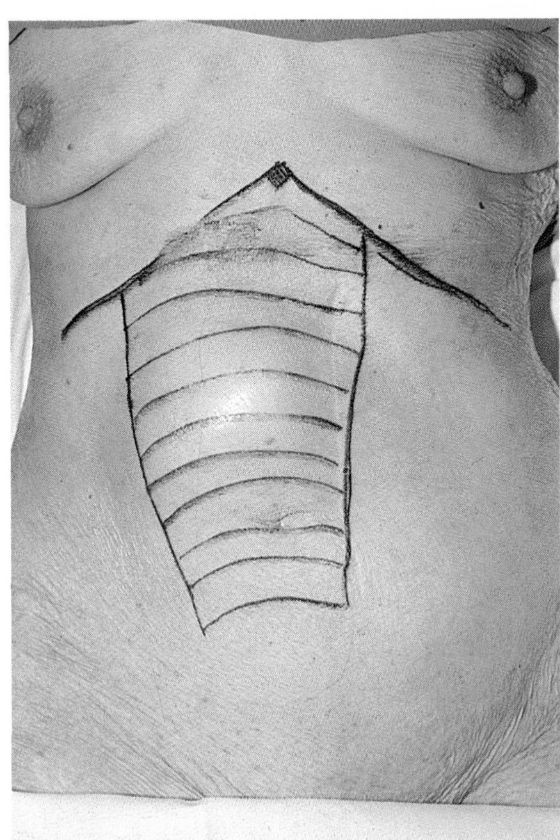

184a Aortic aneurysm presenting as a pulsatile abdominal mass. Nearly all aneurysms in the abdominal aorta are caused by atherosclerosis; most occur in men over 60 years of age. However, this patient is a female!

184b Aortic aneurysm. Calcified abdominal aortic aneurysm. May need to be differentiated from other causes of intra-abdominal calcification. The main complication is rupture of the aneurysm. Note spinal osteoporosis.

185 Calcified fibroid. A frequent cause of intra-abdominal calcification in elderly women. Usually benign and found incidentally.

186 Aortic aneurysm. Autopsy specimen showing a ruptured abdominal aortic aneurysm.

b

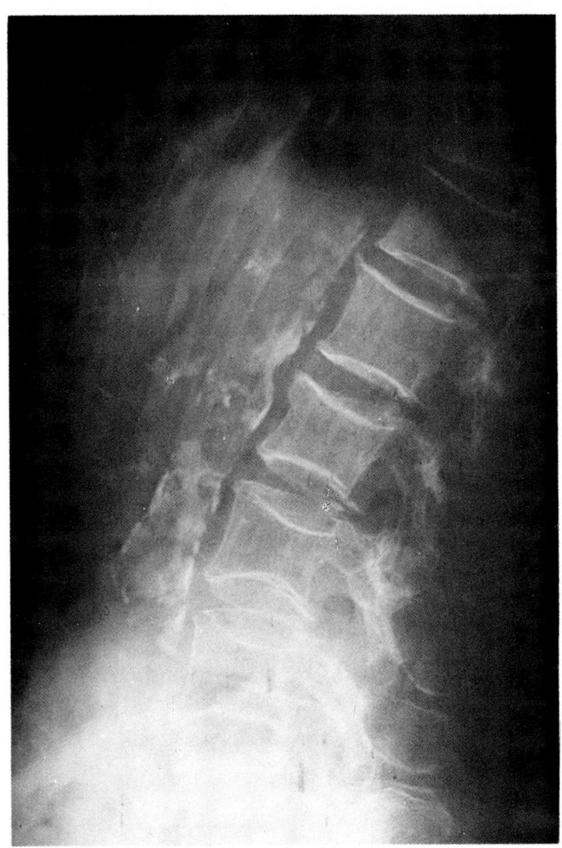

185

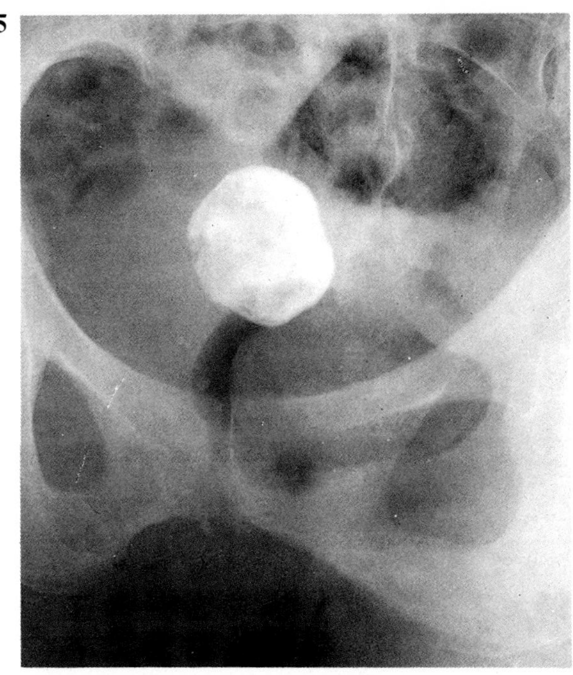

186

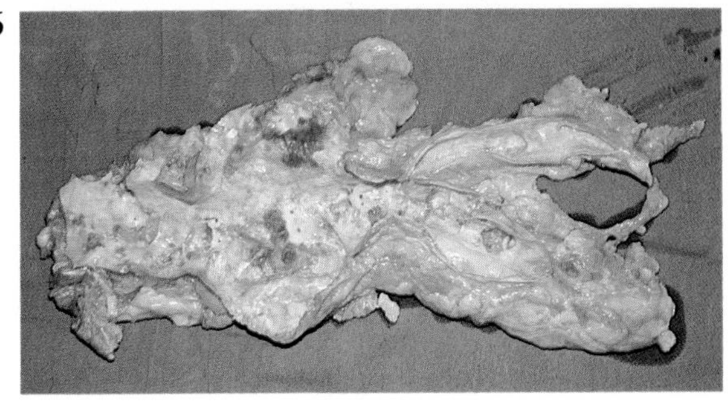

187

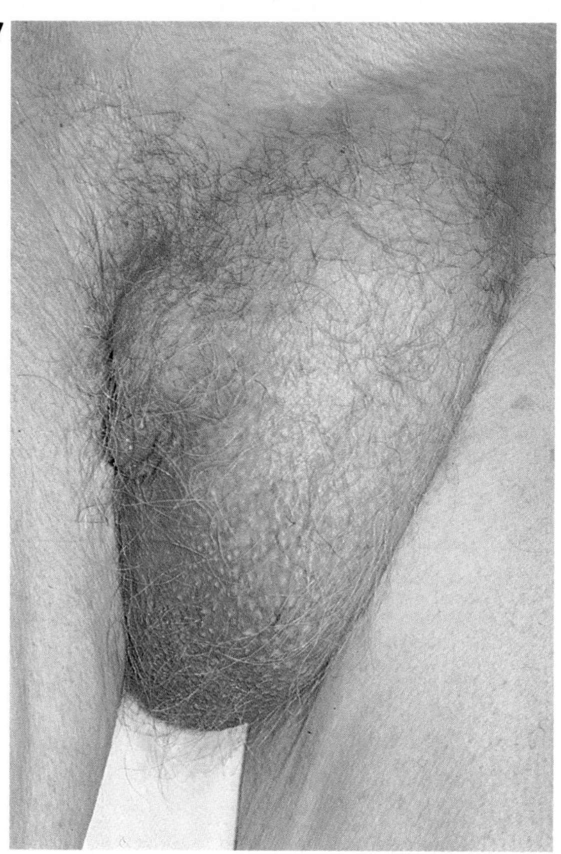

187 Scrotal hernia. A large scrotal hernia causing considerable discomfort. This elderly man refused surgical intervention.

188 Splenomegaly. Caused by chronic lymphatic leukaemia whose incidence rises with advancing age. Usually asymptomatic in the elderly.

189 and 190 Chronic lymphatic leukaemia. Bone-marrow section showing lymphocytic infiltration, with some focal pattern and paratrabecular sparing. (×*100*)

188

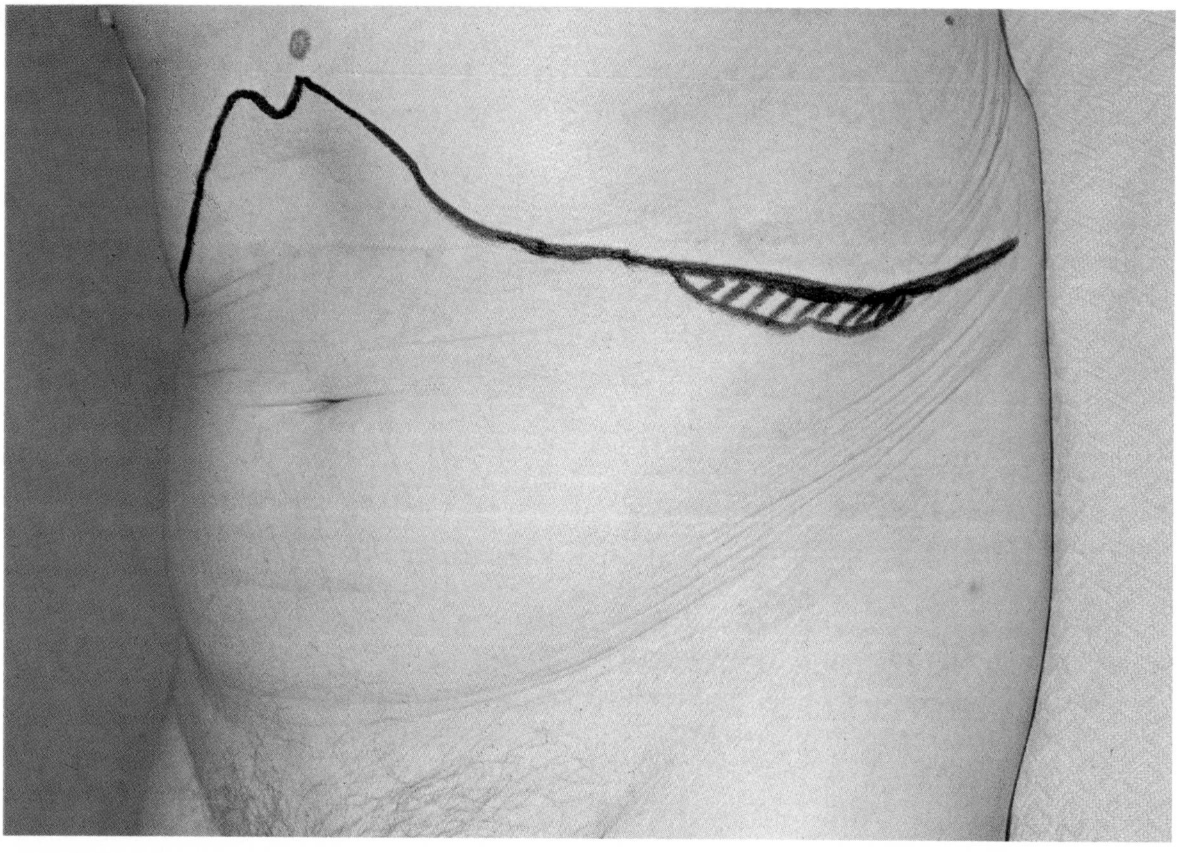

89

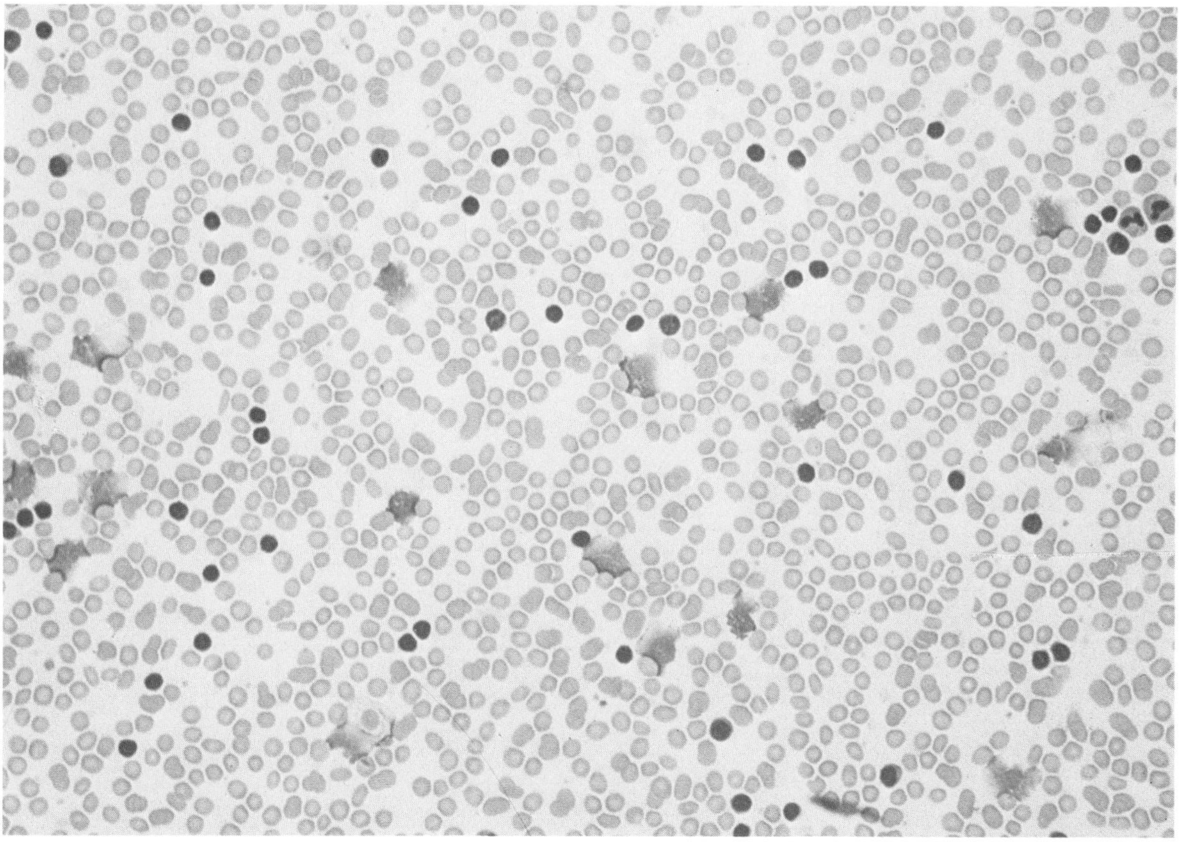

90

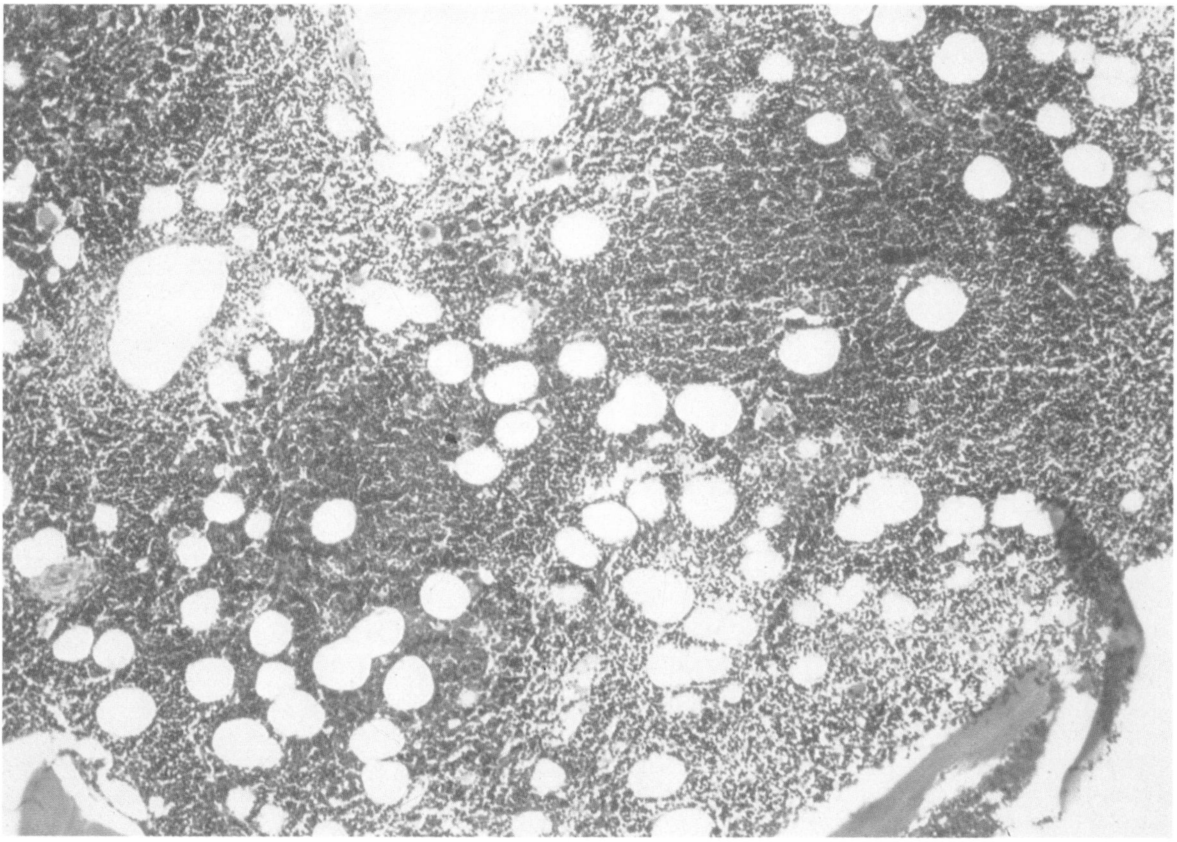

191 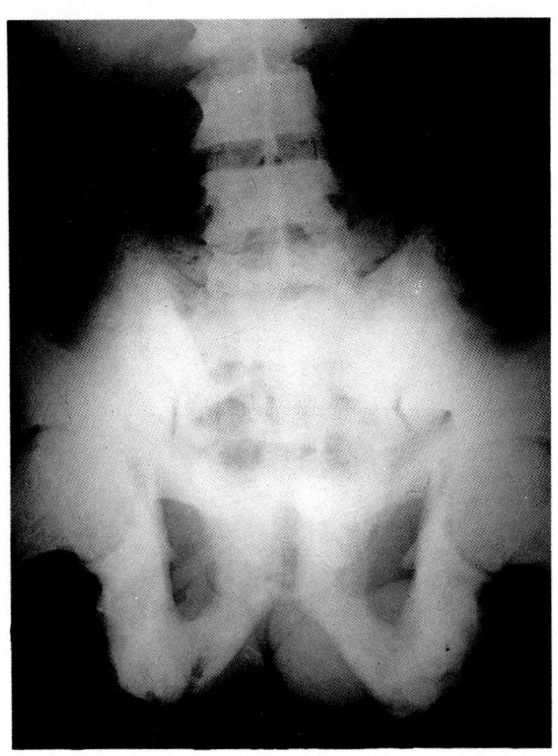

191 Bony metastases. Xray pelvis and lumbar spine showing areas of increased bone density due to secondary deposits from carcinoma of prostate: the most common malignancy of men over age 65 years. The incidence rises with age and is about 190 cases per 100,000 population per year.

192 Benign gastric ulcer. Endoscopic view of a benign gastric ulcer. In the elderly the symptoms may be less acute and the patient may present with weightloss, mild indigestion, and anaemia. The condition may be symptomless.

193 Malignant gastric ulcer. Endoscopic view of a malignant gastric ulcer. This is the third most common malignancy in old age, with an incidence of 110 cases per 100,000 per year.

192 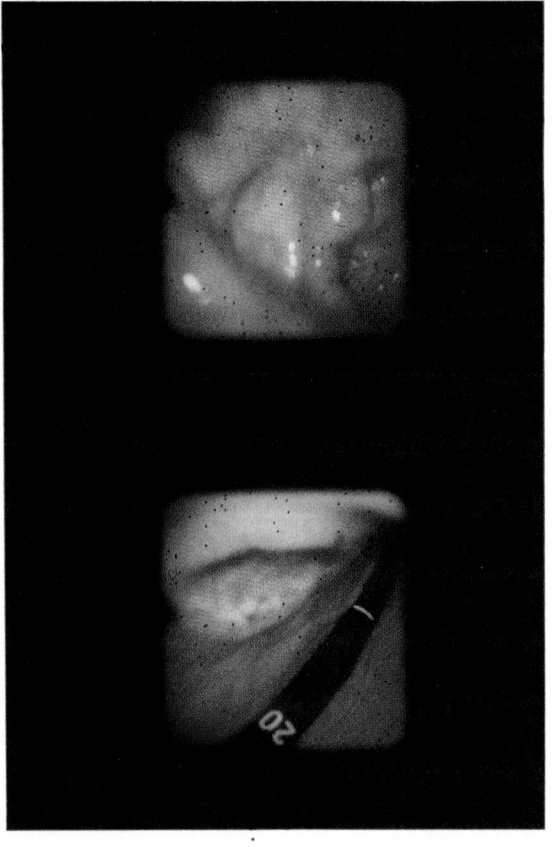

193 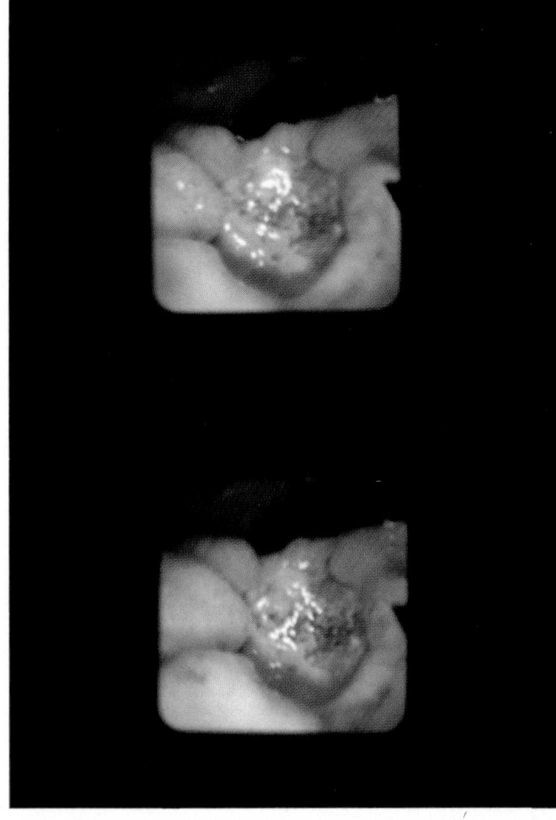

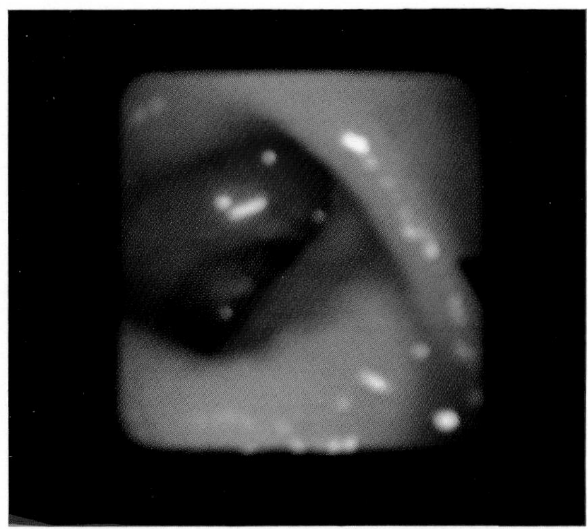

194 Duodenal ulcer. Ulcer in duodenal bulb seen through an endoscope.

195 Bleeding gastric ulcer. Endoscopic view shows clearly the haemorrhage from the ulcer.

196 Duodenal ulcer. Barium-meal xray showing an active duodenal ulcer. The patient had mild anaemia but no symptoms of pain or indigestion.

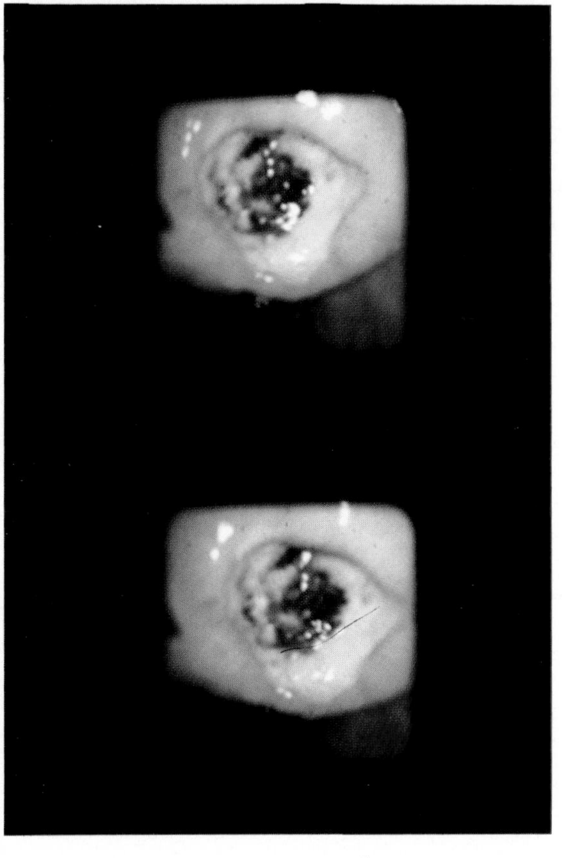

196

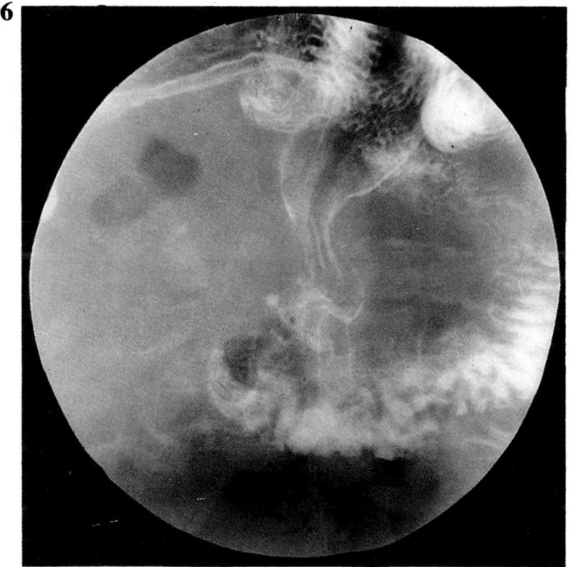

197

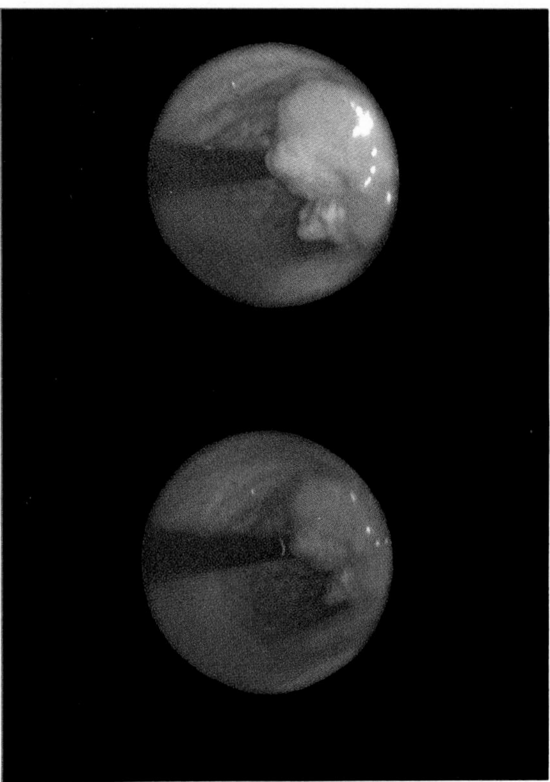

197 Polypoid carcinoma. Endoscopic view of polypoid carcinoma in gastric fundus.

Diverticular disease of the colon

Incidence

Diverticulosis can be demonstrated in up to 50 per cent of people over 80 years of age, by barium enema radiology

Aetiology

Several different factors play a part including lack of fibre in diet

Clinical features

Usually asymptomatic
Pain in left illiac fossa in 78 per cent
Constipation in 35 per cent
Diarrhoea in 19 per cent
Flatulence in 13 per cent
Rectal bleeding in 30 per cent
Nausea and loss of appetite

Complications

Diverticulitis
Haemorrhage
Abscess formation
Perforation – peritonitis, pericolic abscess, fistula formation into other viscera
Anaemia

198

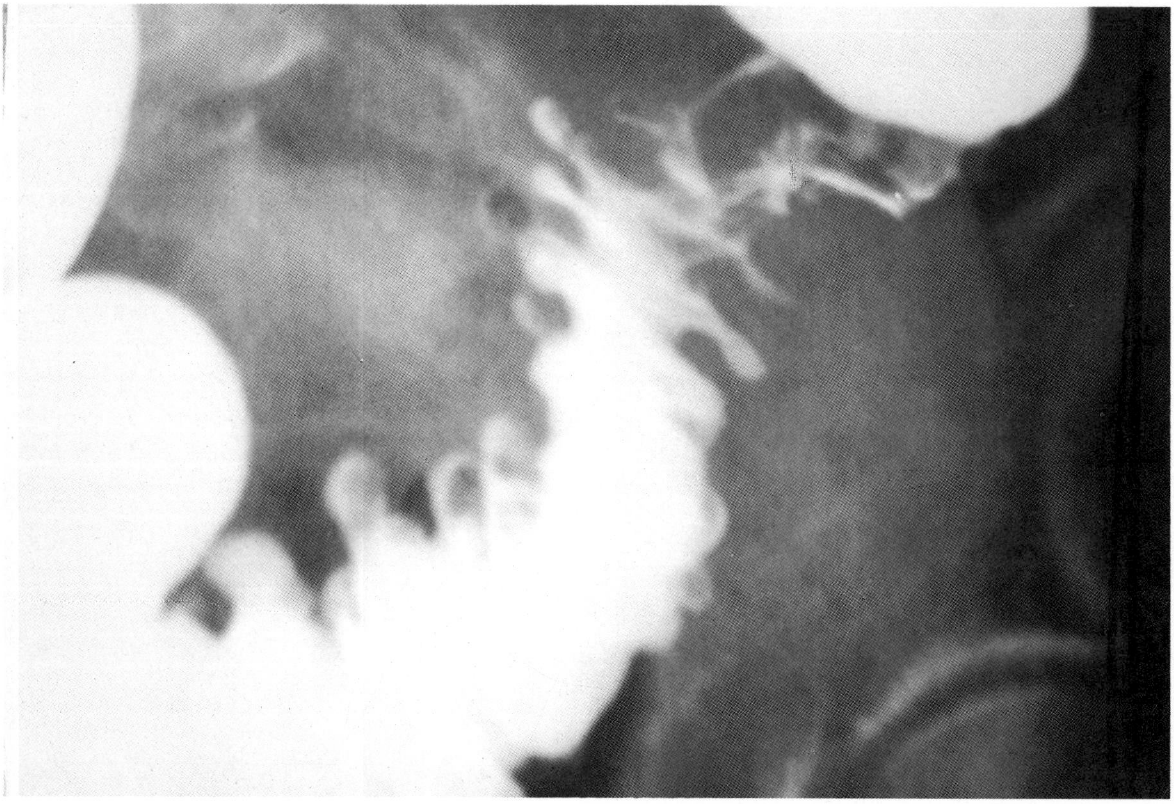

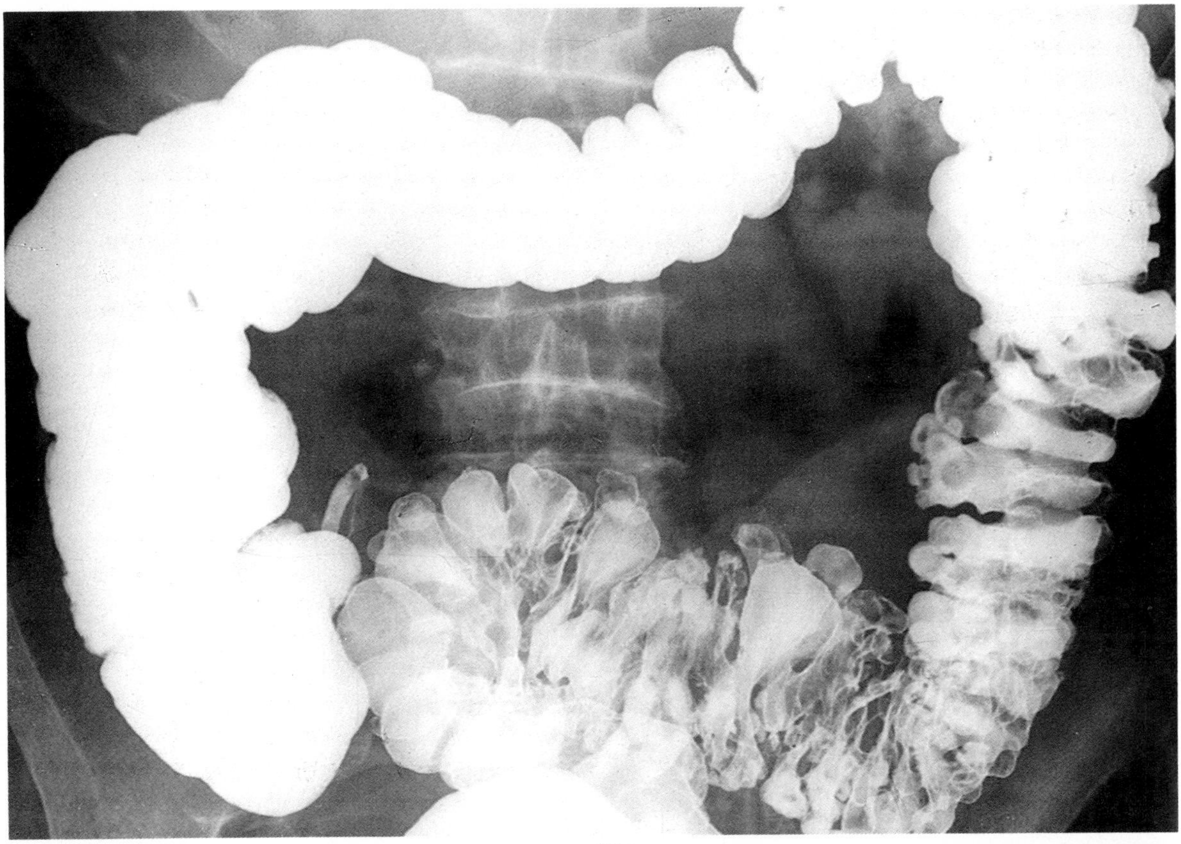

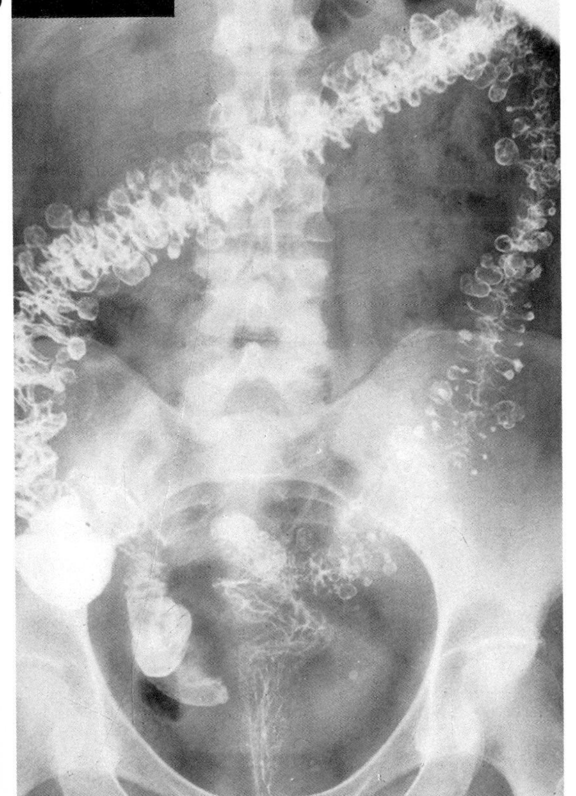

201

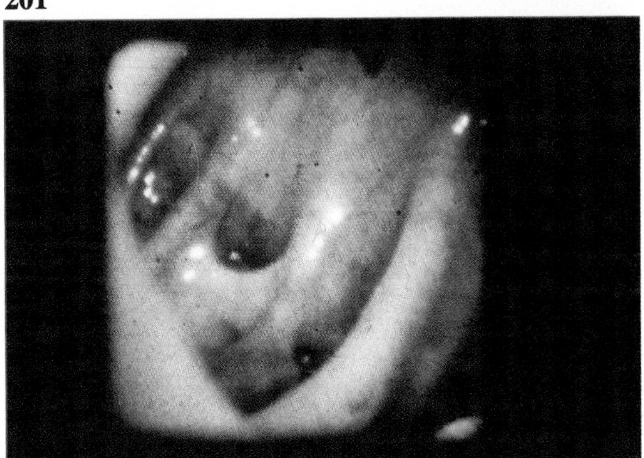

198 to 200 Diverticulosis. A frequent radiological finding in the elderly producing various large-bowel problems including constipation, diarrhoea, anaemia, and acute diverticulitis. However, it is mostly symptomless.

201 Diverticulosis. Colonoscopy showing the mouth of a diverticulum with some surrounding muscle spasm.

202 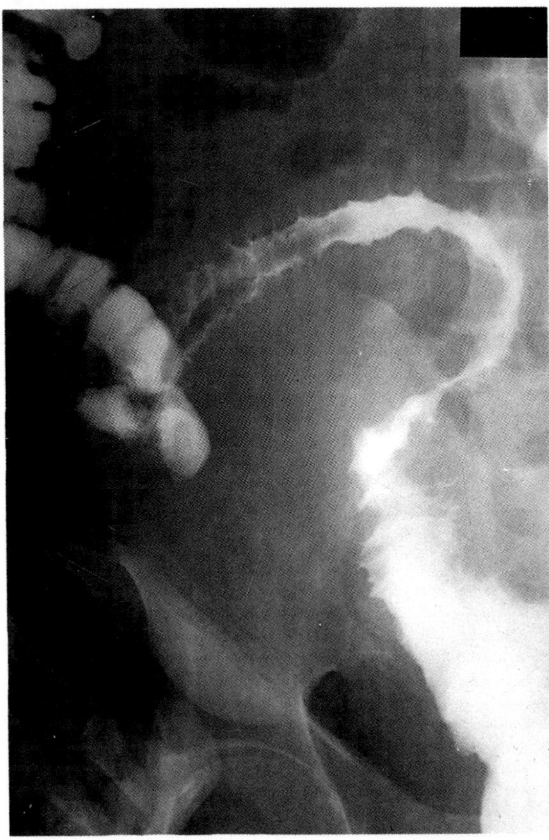

203a 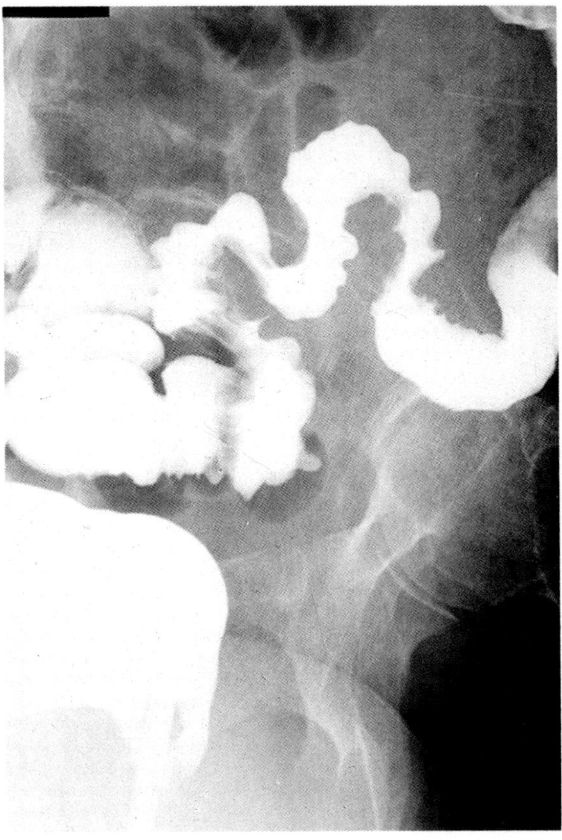

203b 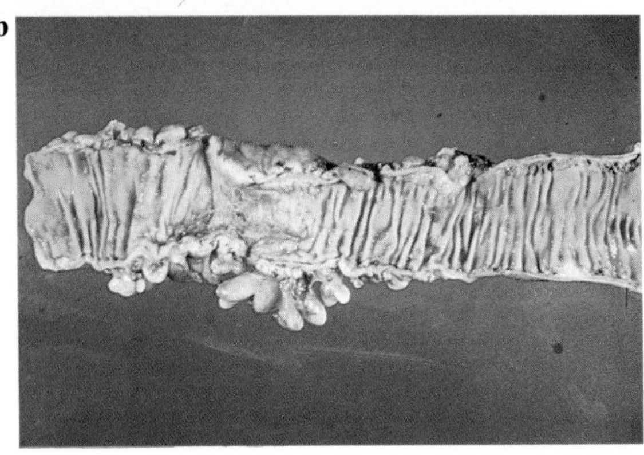

202 Ischaemic colitis. Typical radiological appearance in the region of splenic flexure. 'Saw-tooth' and 'thumb-printing' signs are clearly shown. These are caused by oedema of the bowel wall.

203a Ischaemic colitis. This barium enema xray shows both 'thumb-printing' and sacculation caused by the formation of pseudodiverticula.

203b Ischaemic colitis. Pathology specimen of the colon showing narrowed ischaemic segment.

Ischaemic colitis occurs in later life and the causative factors are atherosclerosis, congestive heart failure, use of Digitalis, and haemorrhage caused by bleeding from a duodenal ulcer.

The clinical presentation may be acute or chronic and consists of abdominal pain and diarrhoea, which may be bloodstained. In some cases, an ischaemic area causes bowel constriction which results in obstruction.

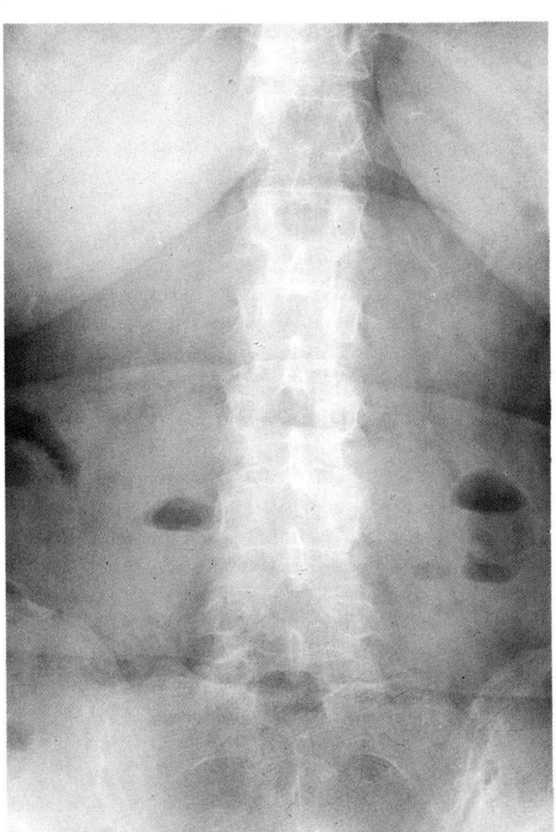

204 Intestinal obstruction. Plain xray of the abdomen (erect) showing multiple fluid levels in a case of intestinal obstruction. This elderly patient was found to have a carcinoma of the colon.

205 Carcinoma of the colon. Colonoscopy showing a neoplasm which may present with recurrent diarrhoea, weightloss, and anaemia. Carcinoma of the colon is the most common form of malignancy in old age.

206 Ulcerative colitis. Colonoscopy. The mucosa is red and inflamed and bleeds easily on contact. This disease is uncommon in old age.

205

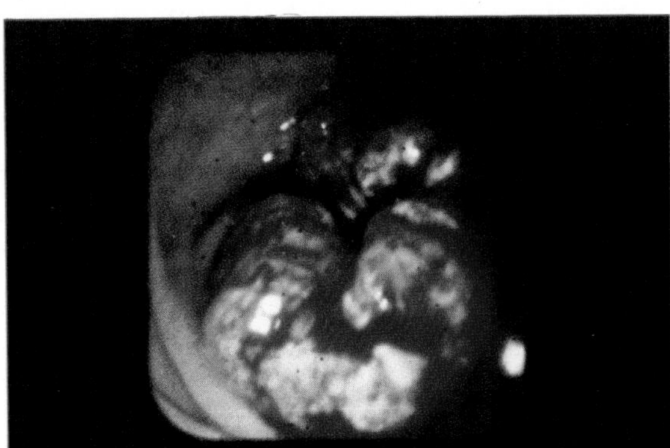

206

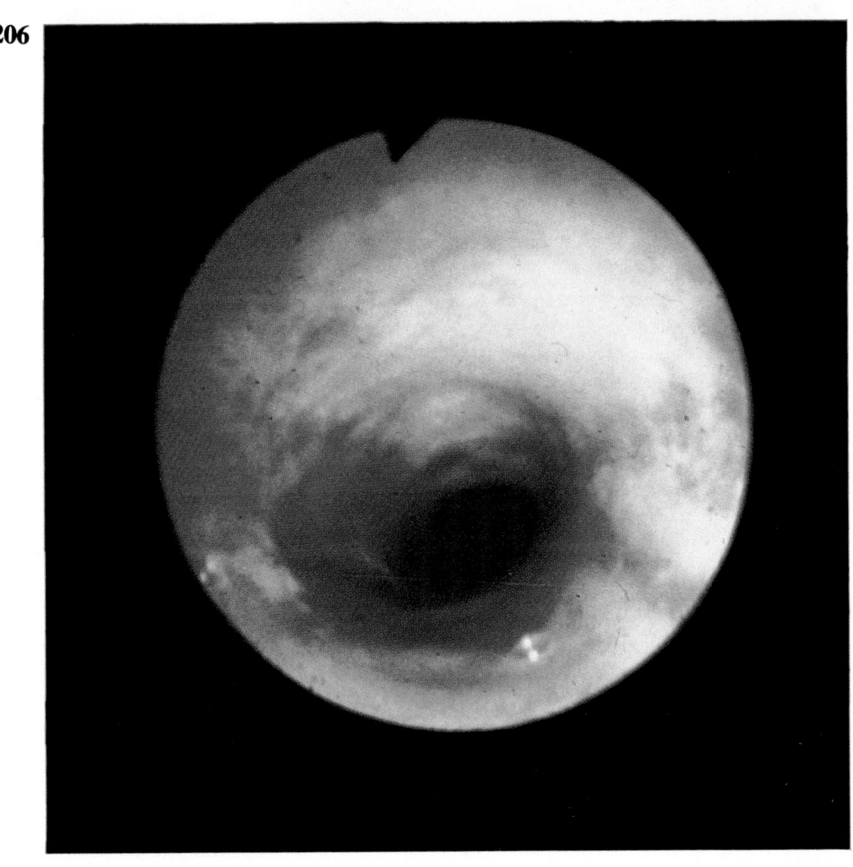

Incontinence of urine

It is estimated that there are about 140,000 elderly people in the United Kingdom who suffer from incontinence. Precipitating factors are a combination of restricted mobility, distant or awkward toilet, and increased frequency or urgency.

Incontinence of urine may be caused by lesions at four different anatomical levels:

1 The muscles of the pelvic diaphragm
2 The urethra
3 The bladder
4 The brain, spinal cord, and autonomic nerves controlling micturition.

Weakness of the pelvic diaphragm leads to 'genuine-stress incontinence' – called 'genuine' to distinguish it from pseudo-stress incontinence in patients with detrusor instability. In this latter case coughing or moving may fire off a bladder contraction because of an unstable bladder.

Disorders of the urethra include atrophic urethritis in females in association with atrophic vaginitis (to be treated with oestrogens) and obstruction as a result of constipation or prostatic enlargement.

Diseases of the bladder include cystitis and, rarely, tumours or calculi.

Disorders in the central nervous system depend on whether they involve the reflex arc of micturition (through 2nd, 3rd or 4th sacral segments of the spinal cord), in which case it will be of a 'lower motor neurone' type or the spinal cord above the sacral segments, brainstem or cerebral cortex, in which case it will be of a 'upper-motor neurone' type. The first is often called a neurogenic atonic bladder and the second a neurogenic reflex or uninhibited bladder. Full diagnosis requires cystometry.

Urinary incontinence can also be classified as follows:

A Transient urinary incontinence – reversible

Infective – urinary tract infection

Retention with overflow – faecal impaction, anticholinergic drugs

Increased diuresis – diuretics, diabetes mellitus

Toxic confusional states, oversedation and psychological

207

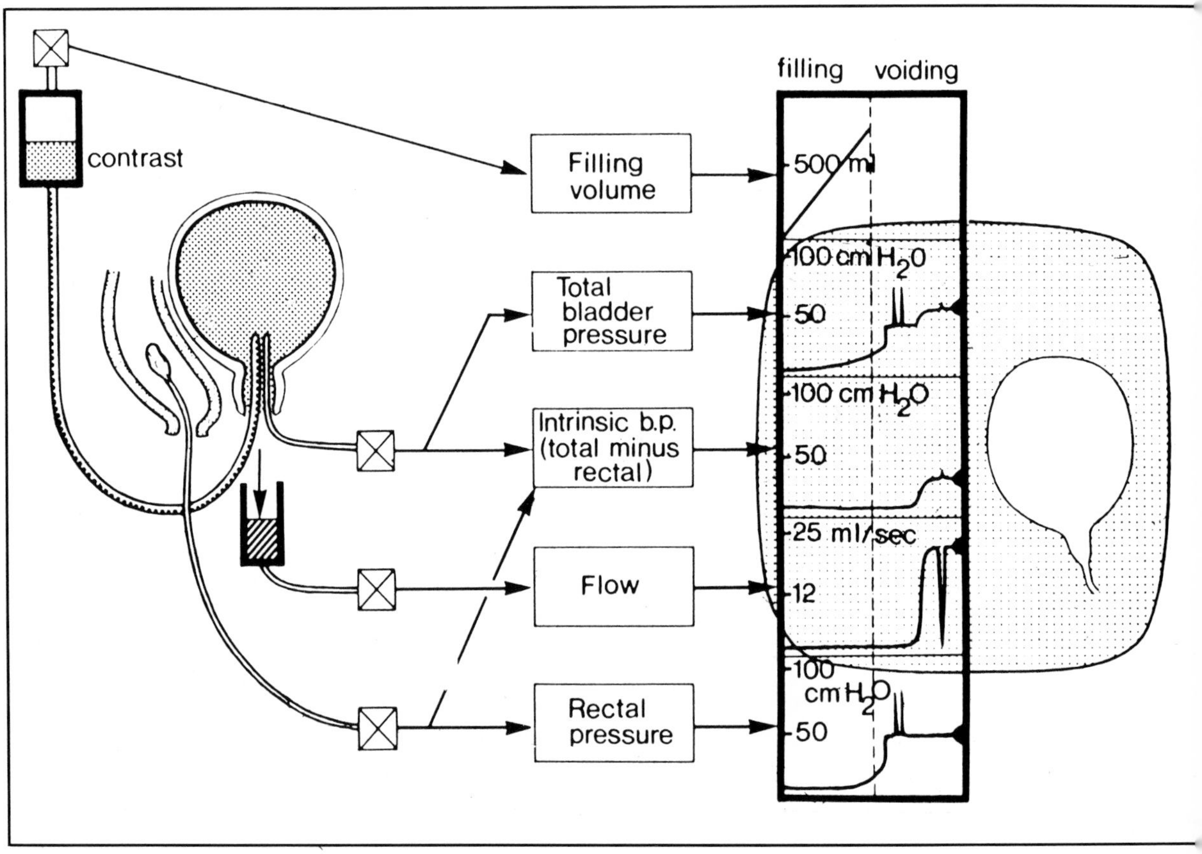

B Established urinary incontinence

Uninhibited neurogenic bladder – dementias, cerebrovascular accidents, parietal and frontal lobe lesions
Reflex neurogenic bladder – paraplegia
Retention with overflow – tabes, diabetes, prostatism
Autonomous bladder – cauda equine lesions

207 Cystometry. Diagrammatic representation of equipment for simultaneous cystometry and cystourethrography, with video-tape recording as first described by Bates and his colleagues in the *British Journal of Urology,* 1970. The equipment shown includes a reservoir which fills the bladder with radio-opaque fluid, and a second line from the bladder through a transducer which records intravesical pressure. To distinguish intrinsic bladder contractions from those that are transmitted from the abdominal cavity, a second pressure recording line is taken from the rectum, and by subtracting this pressure from that of the bladder, the pure bladder muscle contraction is shown as 'subtracted' pressure. This sophisticated system also allows the recording of the degree of filling, the degree of emptying, and a simultaneous picture of the shape of the bladder and urethra taken by xray.

208

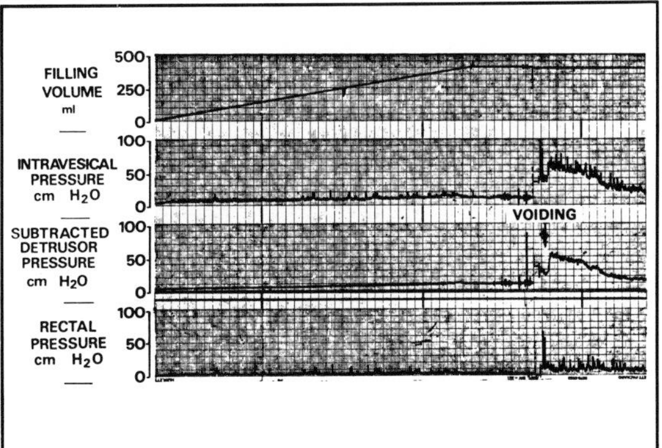

208 Normal cystometrogram. Bladder filling up to 450ml of fluid with no intrinsic contractions occurring until the patient attempts to void.

209

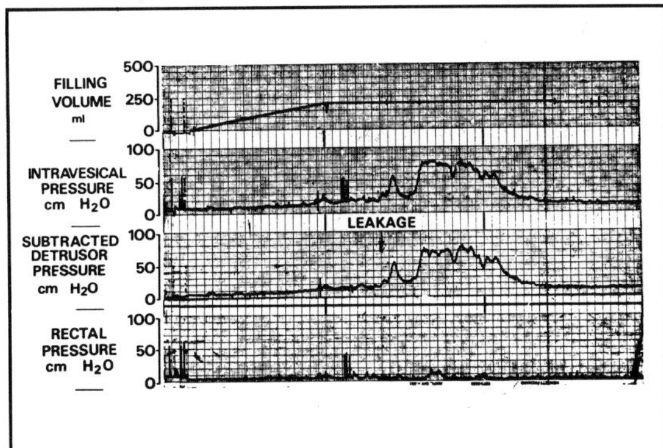

209 Uninhibited neurogenic bladder. In this cystometrogram tracing the bladder contractions occur at 250ml filling, followed by a series of contractions associated with leakage.

Cystography

Changes which may be demonstrated in the bladder by cystography are associated either with bladder outlet obstruction (for example, enlargement of the prostate) or with functional outlet obstruction in the uninhibited or reflex neurogenic bladder in which intrinsic bladder contractions occur against a closed outlet. The findings which may then be seen include:
(These three xrays are all of females and such findings are not uncommon in aged incontinent women.)

210

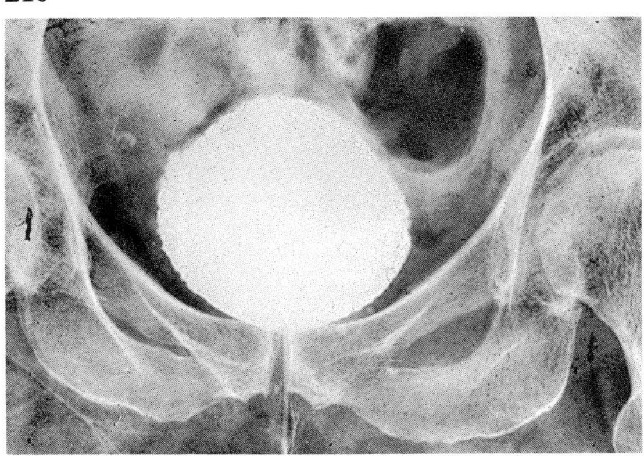

210 Trabeculation.

211

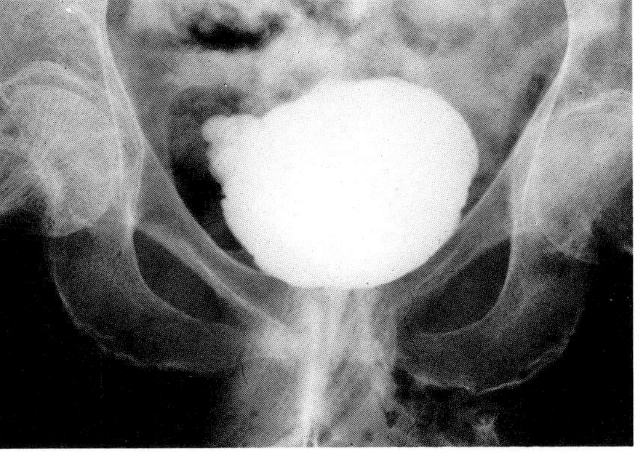

211 Formation of cellules or pseudodiverticula.

212

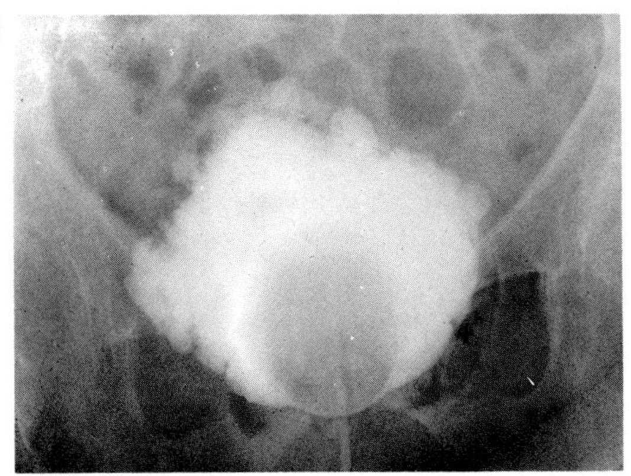

212 Formation of diverticula.

213 Bisected female bladder showing trabeculation and cellule formation.

214 Monilial infection. Severe monilial infection in an aged incontinent woman with poor hygiene and obesity.

215 Caruncle. This is a granulomatous and ulcerating lesion, presumably the end stage of a urethrocele. This anatomical abnormality is seen frequently in elderly incontinent women.

213

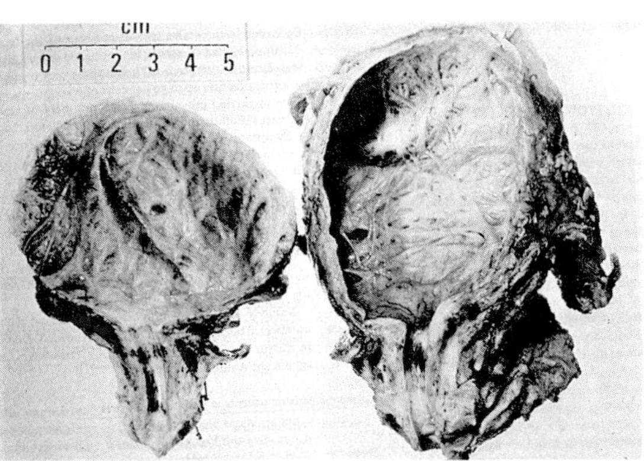

214

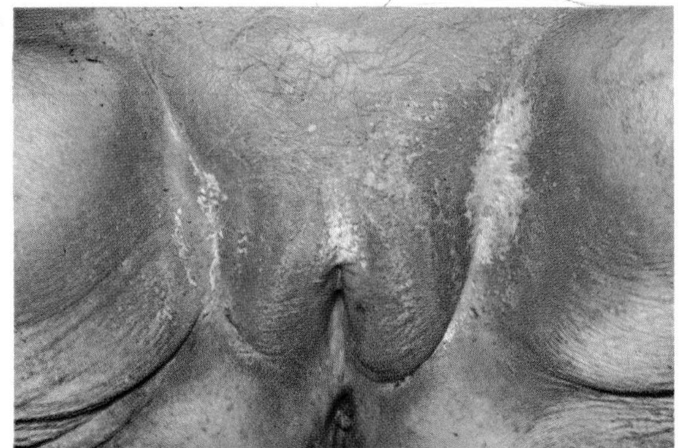

215

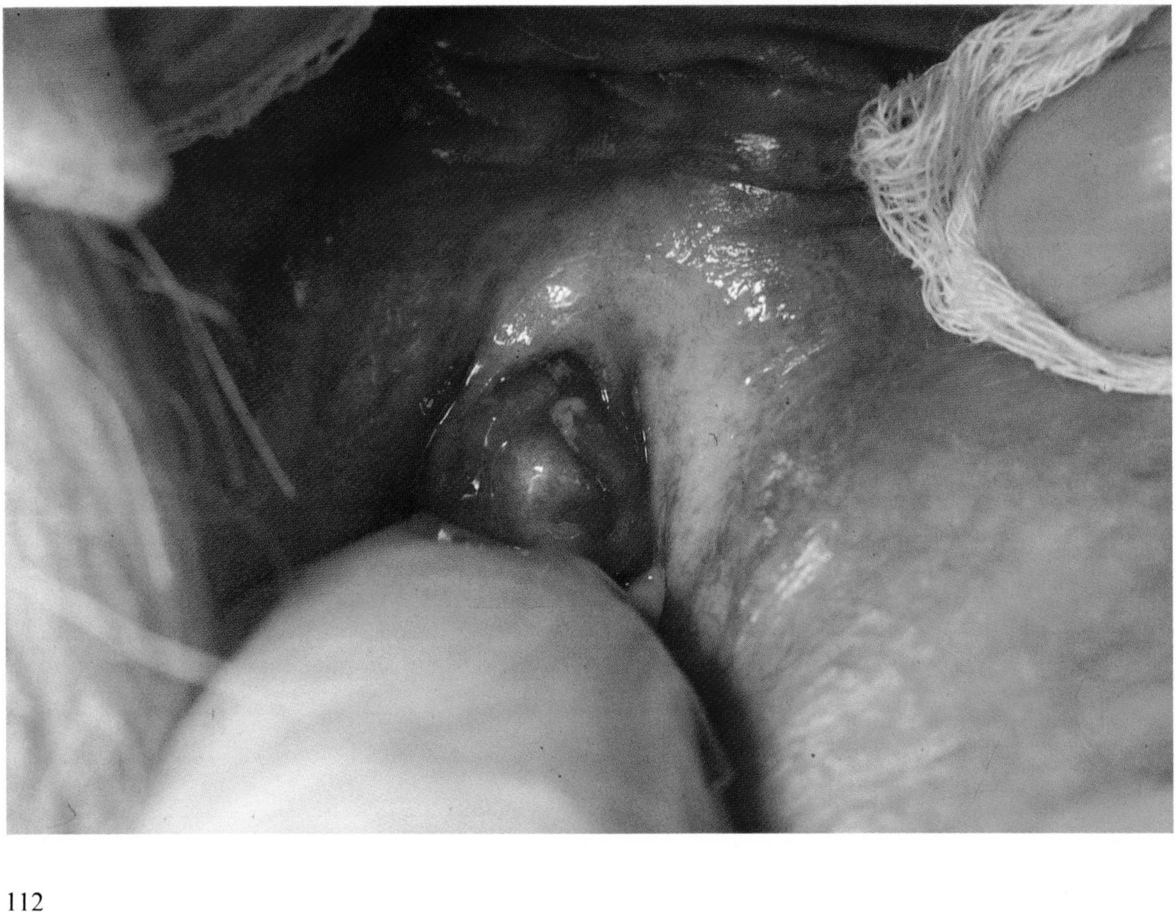

216

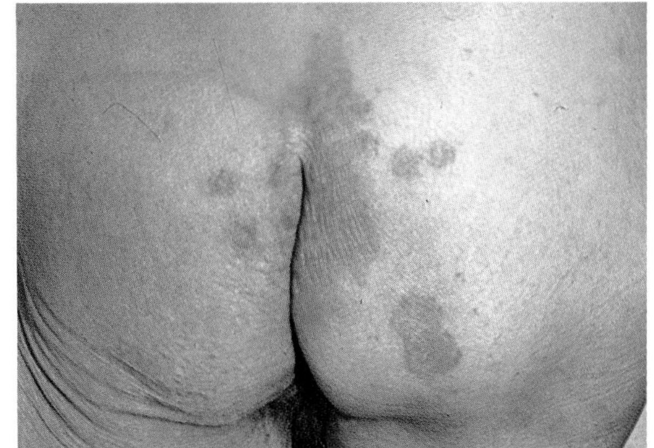

216 Rash caused by urinary incontinence. Early stages. Contributory factors consist of immobility, ill-health, pressure, and lack of nursing care.

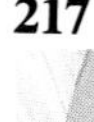

217

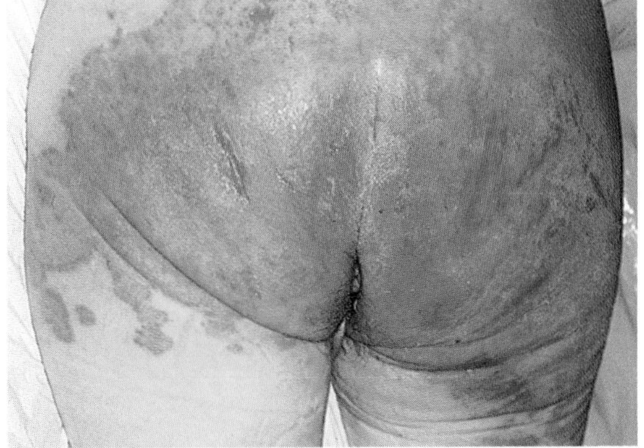

217 Rash caused by urinary incontinence. Advanced stages with cellulitis, excoriation, and a serious risk of a pressure sore.

218a Slight urethral prolapse. There is minimal prolapse of the urethral mucosa. This is a fairly common condition in elderly women, probably associated with age changes affecting the supporting tissues of the urethra, and a frequent cause of incontinence.

218b Uterovaginal prolapse. A more advanced case. Vaginal atrophy, weakness of vaginal walls, and ageing skeletal muscle can cause this condition which can result in urinary incontinence.

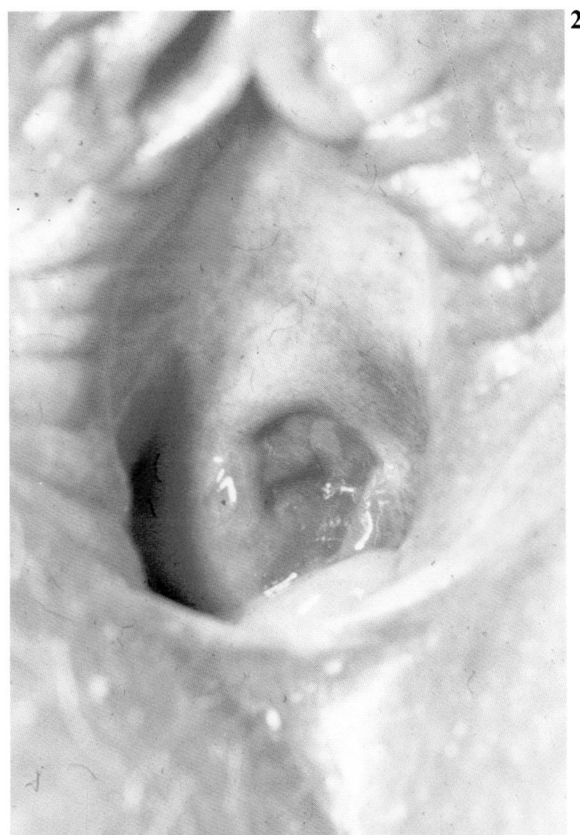

218b

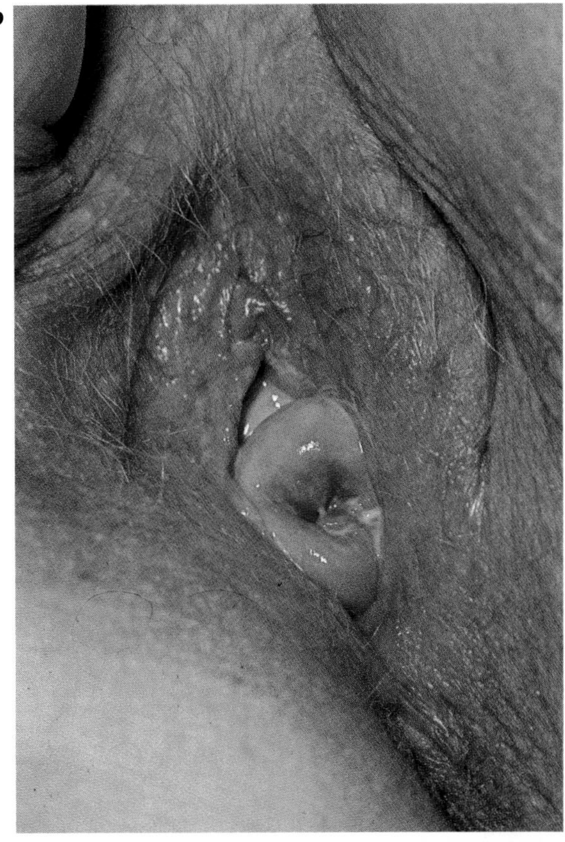

8 Disorders of the upper limbs

219 and 220 Wasting of small muscles of hand. This is caused by a lesion involving the lower brachial plexus (8th cervical and 1st thoracic roots). There is paralysis and wasting of the small muscles of the hand. The second picture is of a patient who had bilateral incomplete cervical ribs causing bilateral brachial plexus compression.

220a Thenar eminence wasting. This patient has mild wasting of hand muscles, especially of thenar eminence. He was found to have motor-neurone disease.

220b Claw-hand deformity. Wasting of small muscles of the hand with 'claw hand' deformity caused by ulnar-nerve palsy.

219

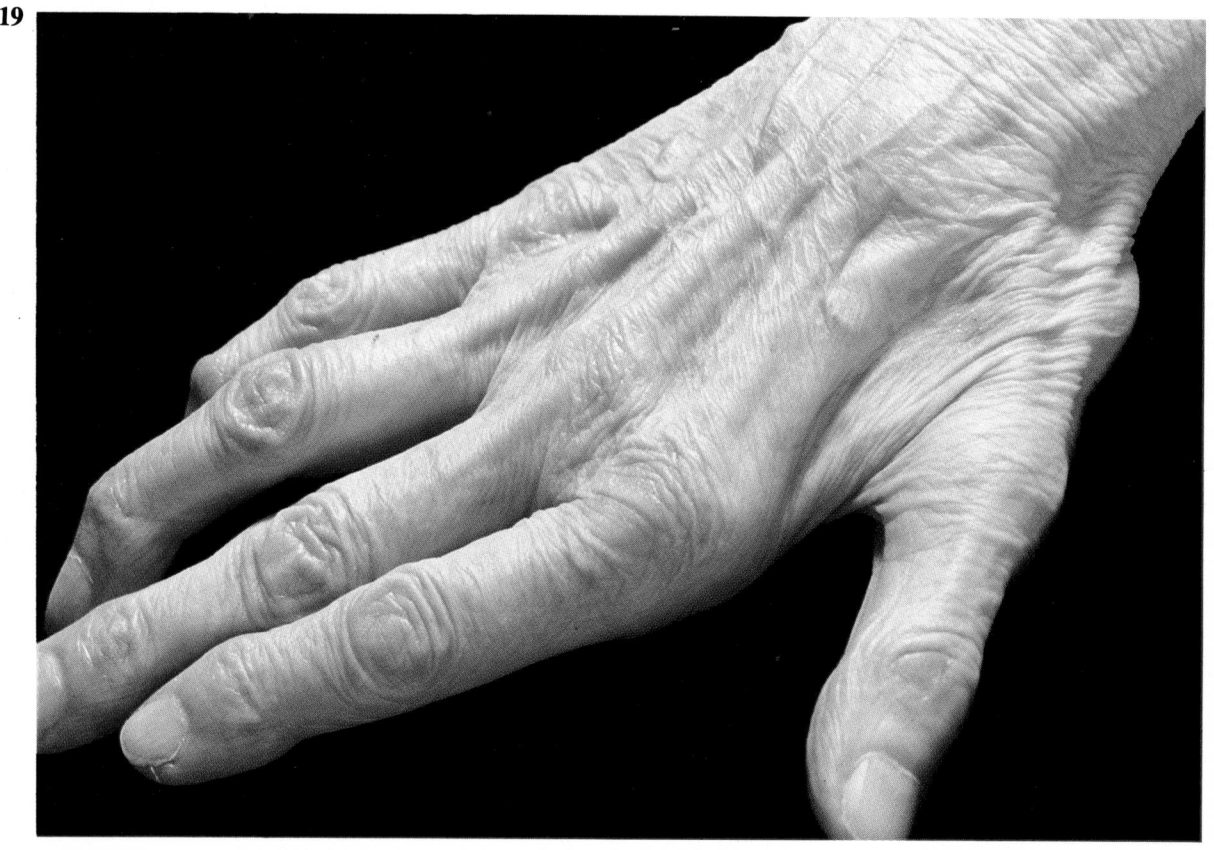

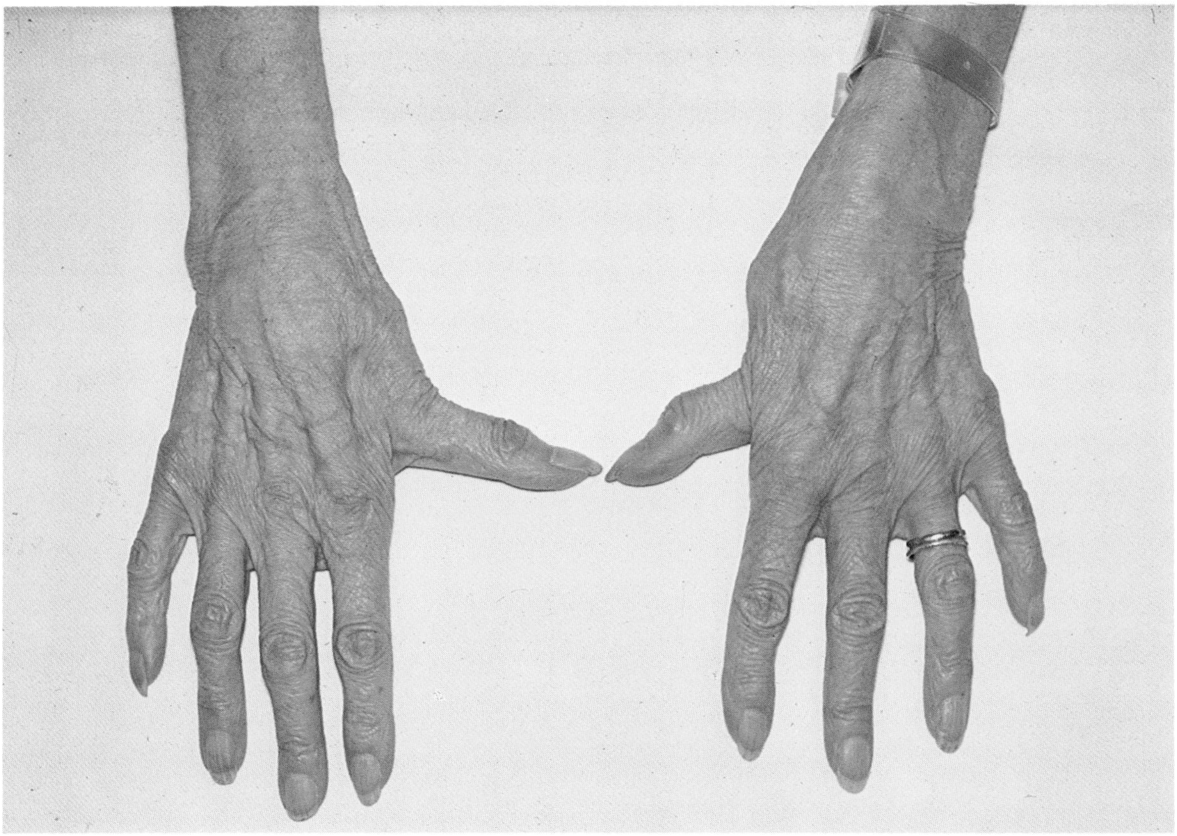

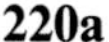

220a

Causes of wasting of small muscles of the hand

1 *Cord lesions*
  Tumour, e.g. meningioma
  Motor neurone disease
  Cord compression
  Trauma
  Vascular lesions
  Syringomyelia
2 *Root lesions*
  Cervical spondylosis
  Neurofibroma
3 *Brachial plexus lesions*
  Cervical rib
  Pancoast's tumour
  Scalenus anterior syndrome
4 *Nerve lesions*
  Carpal tunnel syndrome (median nerve)
  Ulnar nerve lesion
  Polyneuropathy
5 *Miscellaneous*
  Shoulder-hand syndrome
  Arthritis – e.g. RA
  Disuse atrophy, e.g. paralysis

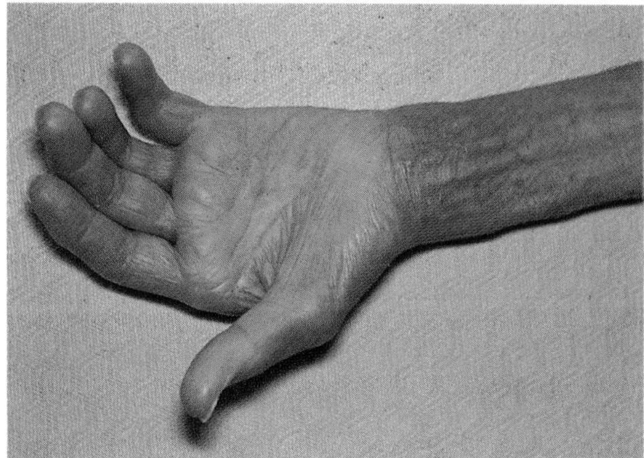

220b

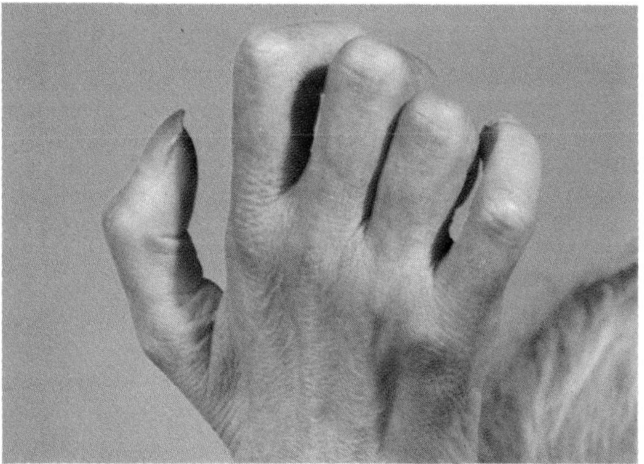

221

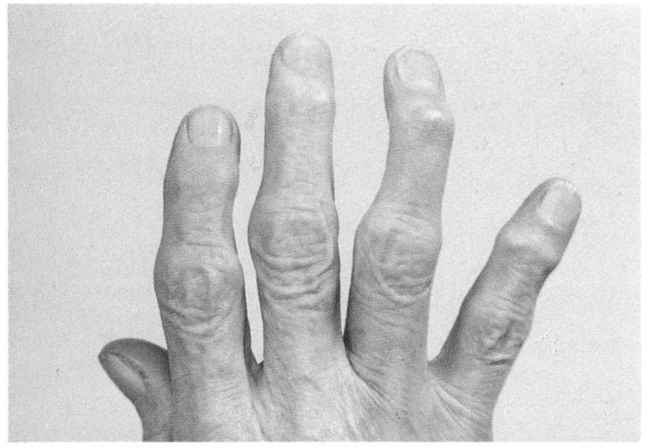

221 Osteoarthritis. Primary generalised osteoarthrosis showing both Heberden's and Bouchard's nodes.

222

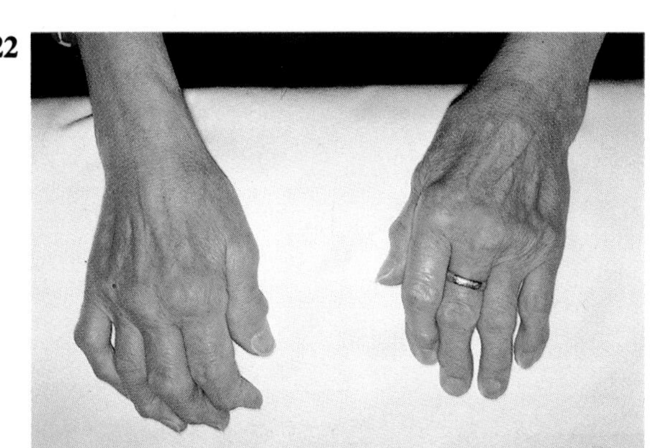

222 Osteoarthritis. Common destructive arthropathy in the elderly. In this case the distal interphalangeal joints, the carpometacarpal joints of thumbs and the proximal interphalangeal joints show changes of osteoarthritis. Note the associated wasting of the small muscles of the hands.

223a

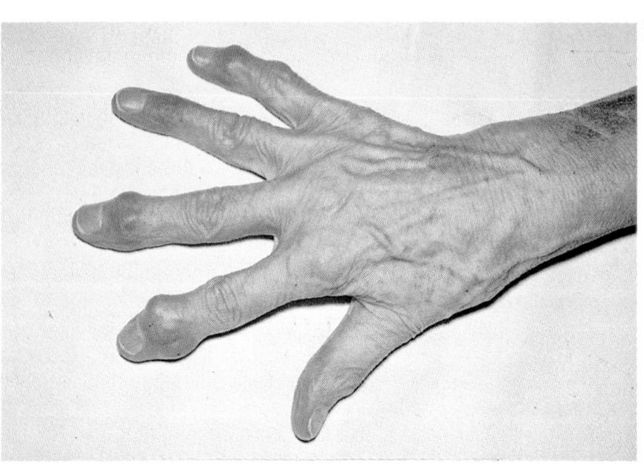

223b

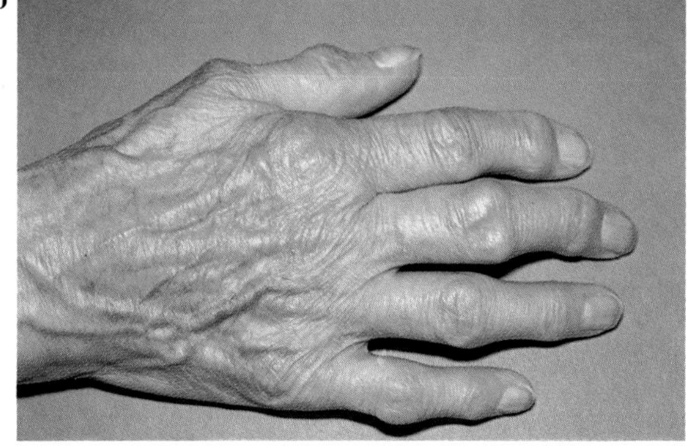

224a

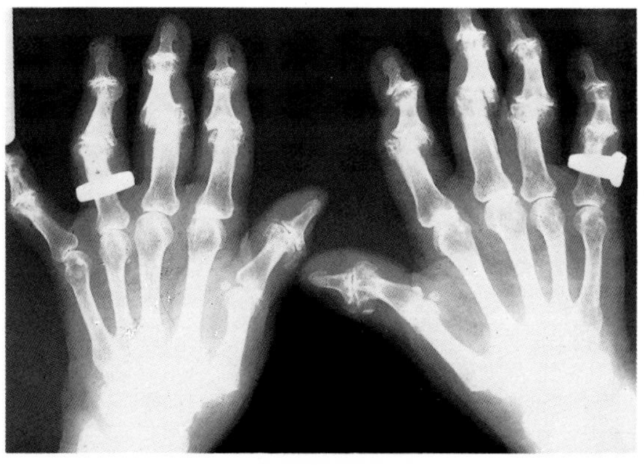

223a Heberden's nodes. Bony swellings in the distal interphalangeal joints; a typical feature of longstanding osteoarthritis. Women are affected much more frequently than men.

223b Bouchard's nodes. Also a feature of osteoarthritis. They are similar to Heberden's nodes but occur in the proximal interphalangeal joints.

224a Osteoarthritis. Xray of hands showing an advanced case of osteoarthritis. There is bony overgrowth and loss of joint space in distal interphalangeal and proximal interphalangeal joints.

224b

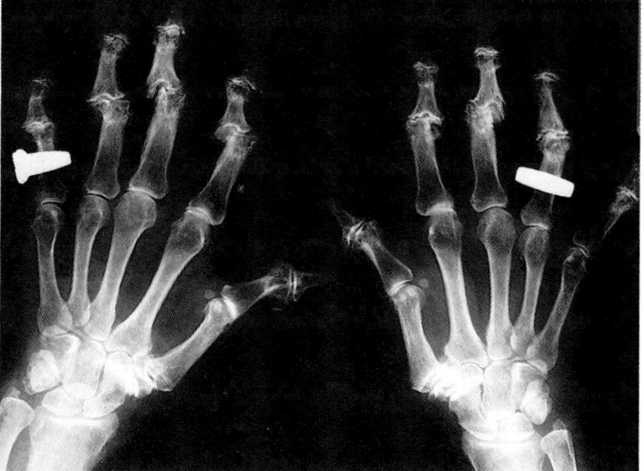

224b Osteoarthritis. Another xray of moderately advanced case of osteoarthritis showing typical changes in DIP and PIP joints.

Osteoarthritis in old age

Osteoarthritis is a chronic degenerative joint disease. Radiological surveys have indicated an incidence in old age of over 80 per cent. It affects the spine, hips, knees and less frequently the joints of the upper limbs. It is more common in obese, relatively immobile people.

The disease is usually primary but secondary osteoarthritis can occur with congenital anatomical abnormalities of joints, trauma and mechanical problems, crystal deposition disease, avascular necrosis, septic arthritis, and often recurrent haemarthrosis in haemophiliacs.

Symptoms

Pain in one or more joints, worst towards the evening and increased by particular activity. Eighty per cent of patients have morning stiffness. Other symptoms are immobility associated obesity, depression, falls and insomnia.

Signs

Knee – bony swelling, effusions, tenderness, crepitus, painful limitation of movement, and Baker's cyst.
DIP joints – bony swelling and deformity and Heberden's nodes.
Chronic stages – slowly progressive course with exacerbation and remissions. Joints develop painful restriction of movement, sometimes with deformity such as hip flexion, knee valgus or laxity. There are no extra-articular manifestations.

Xray features

Loss of joint space, sclerosis of adjacent bone, marginal osteophytes, and subarticular cysts.

Laboratory tests

No specific diagnostic test. ESR is normal and latex test is negative. Synovial fluid is clear, viscous, and non-inflammatory.

Rheumatoid arthritis in old age

There are three main groups:
1st Group – those patients who carry their rheumatoid arthritis with them into old age
2nd Group – those who have fresh joint damage in later years
3rd Group – those who have symptoms of rheumatoid arthritis for the first time in old age.

Features of rheumatoid arthritis appearing for the first time in old age:

The male : female ratio is altered.
In old age – male : female ratio 1 : 25
In younger age groups – 1 : 5
Distribution of joint involvement is similar but synovitis of ankles and wrists of less frequent in older age. Involvement of the hip also tends to be less frequent in elderly males.
Radiological changes tend to be more severe but there is relatively less deformity. Response to gold therapy is better in the elderly.
Systemic features such as weightloss, lymphadenopathy, splenomegaly, and prolonged morning stiffness are of less intensity.
Onset tends to be abrupt.
Nodules slightly less frequent.
Anaemia common and ESR is usually high.
Osteoporosis is frequent.
Rheumatoid factor tests tend to show high titres.
Rheumatoid arteritis is rare.

Complications of rheumatoid disease

1 *Chronic Ill Health*
Weightloss, depression, pressure sores, immobility, constipation, social isolation.
2 *Locomotor*
Deformity, joint subluxations, tendon rupture, nerve compression (carpal tunnel syndrome), cervical subluxation, Baker's synovial cyst, rupture of synovial sac, cricoarytenoid arthritis, arthritis of auditory occicles, osteoporosis, muscle atrophy.
3 *Cardiopulmonary*
Pleural effusion, pulmonary nodules, fibrosing alveolitis, Caplan's syndrome with pneumoconiosis, pericarditis.
4 *Ocular*
Scleritis, uveitis, Sjogren's syndrome, scleromalacia perforans.
5 *Arteritis*
Raynaud's phenomenon, leg ulcers, mesenteric ischaemia.
6 *Miscellaneous*
Peripheral and autonomic neuropathy, amyloidosis, Felty's syndrome and complications of drug therapy.

225

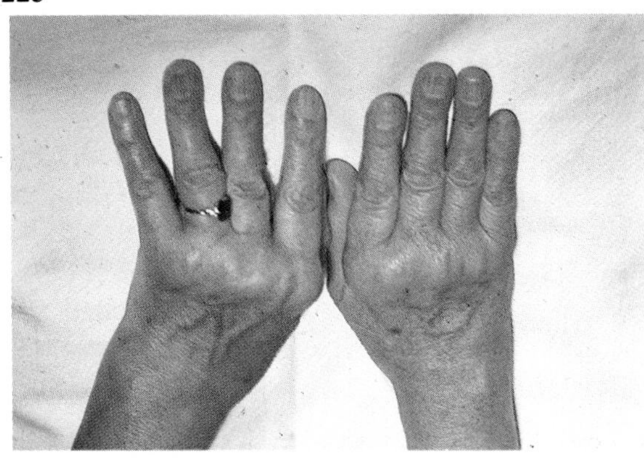

225 Rheumatoid arthritis. Changes of rheumatoid arthritis in the hand of an elderly lady. There is considerable destruction of the proximal interphalangeal and metacarpophalangeal joints. The rheumatoid disease had started in middle age and was still active with pain, anaemia and high ESR.

226 Severe rheumatoid arthritis. Chronic burnt out rheumatoid disease. All the joints, including wrists, are affected and there is gross deformity with shortening and subluxation and complete loss of function.

226

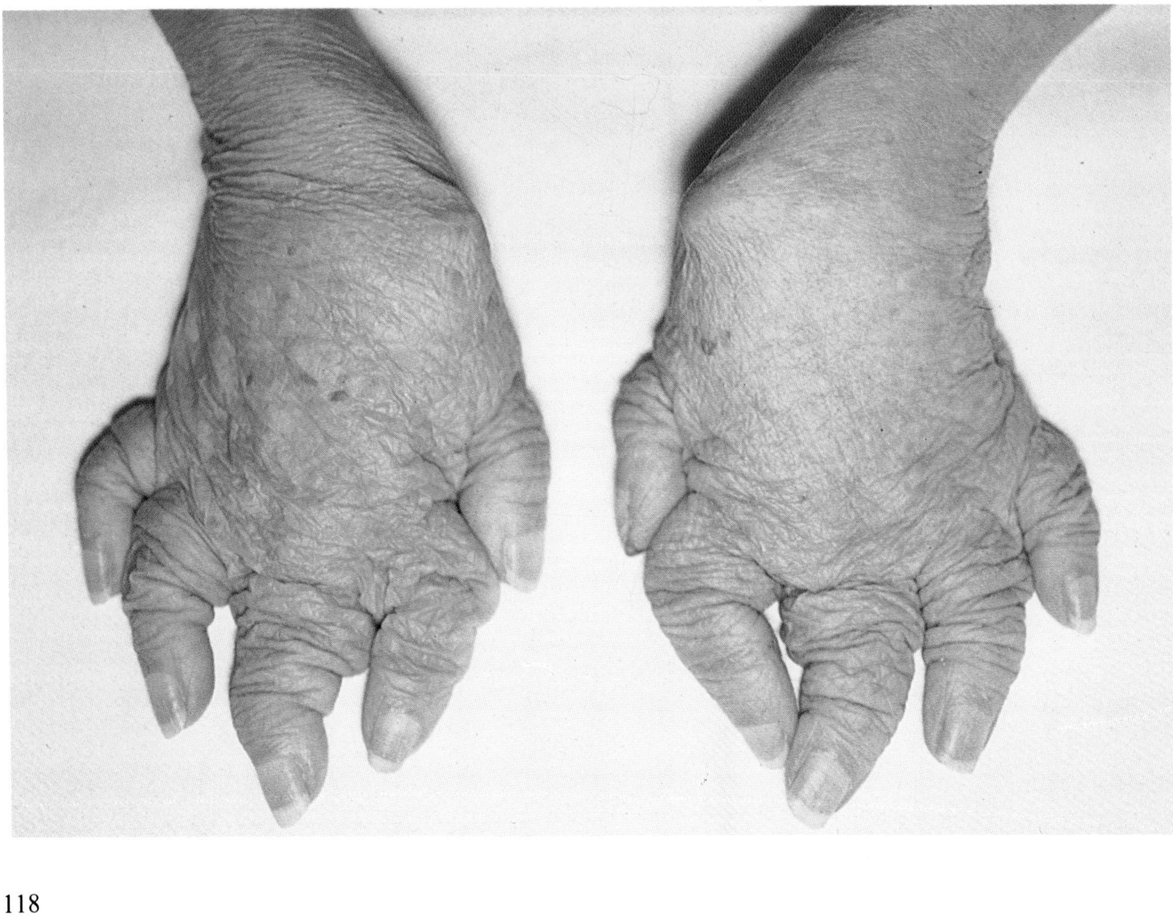

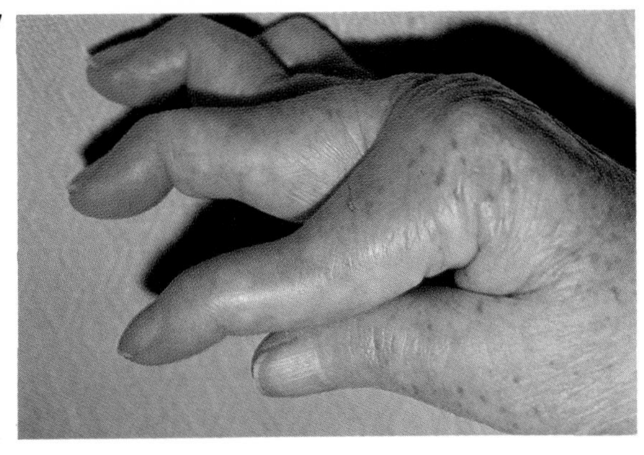

227 Swan-neck deformity. Hyperextension at proximal interphalangeal joint caused by rheumatoid disease producing the classic swan-neck deformity.

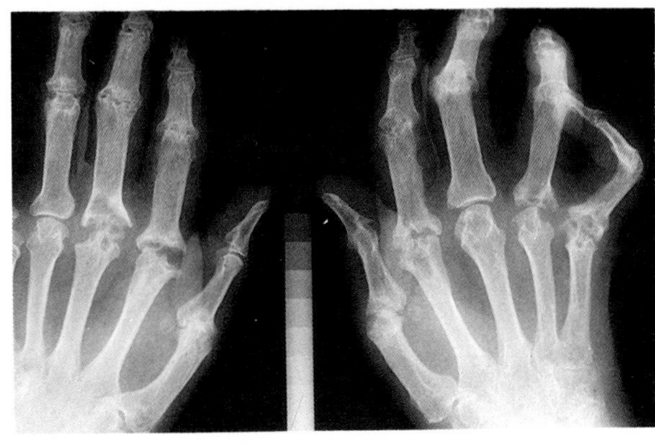

228 Rheumatoid arthritis. Xray of the hands of an elderly patient showing extensive joint destruction. There are marked erosions in metacarpophalangeal and proximal interphalangeal joints. Also osteoarthritic changes in the distal interphalangeal joints.

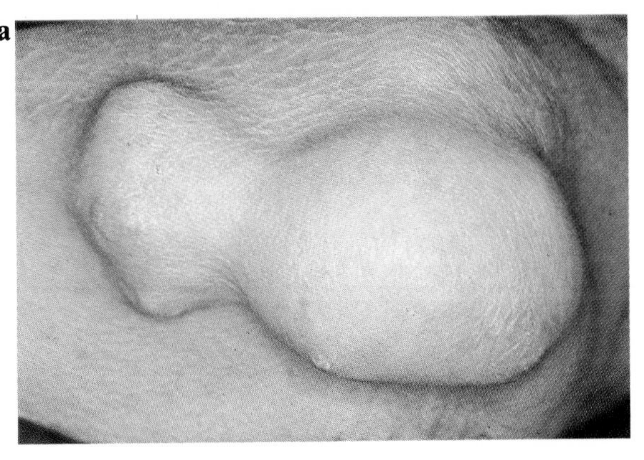

229a Rheumatoid nodule. A periarticular soft-tissue swelling occurring below the elbow on the extensor surface. Nodules are thought to form around an area of vasculitis. They may become necrotic and ulcerate.

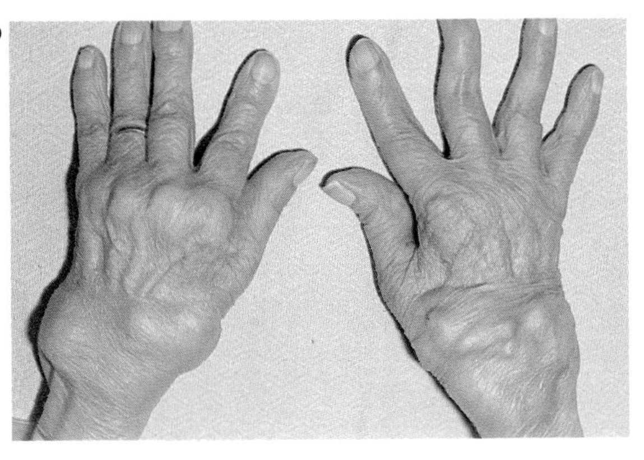

229b Rheumatoid arthritis. A case of advanced rheumatoid arthritis in an elderly lady – involving mainly the wrists and surrounding soft tissues.

230

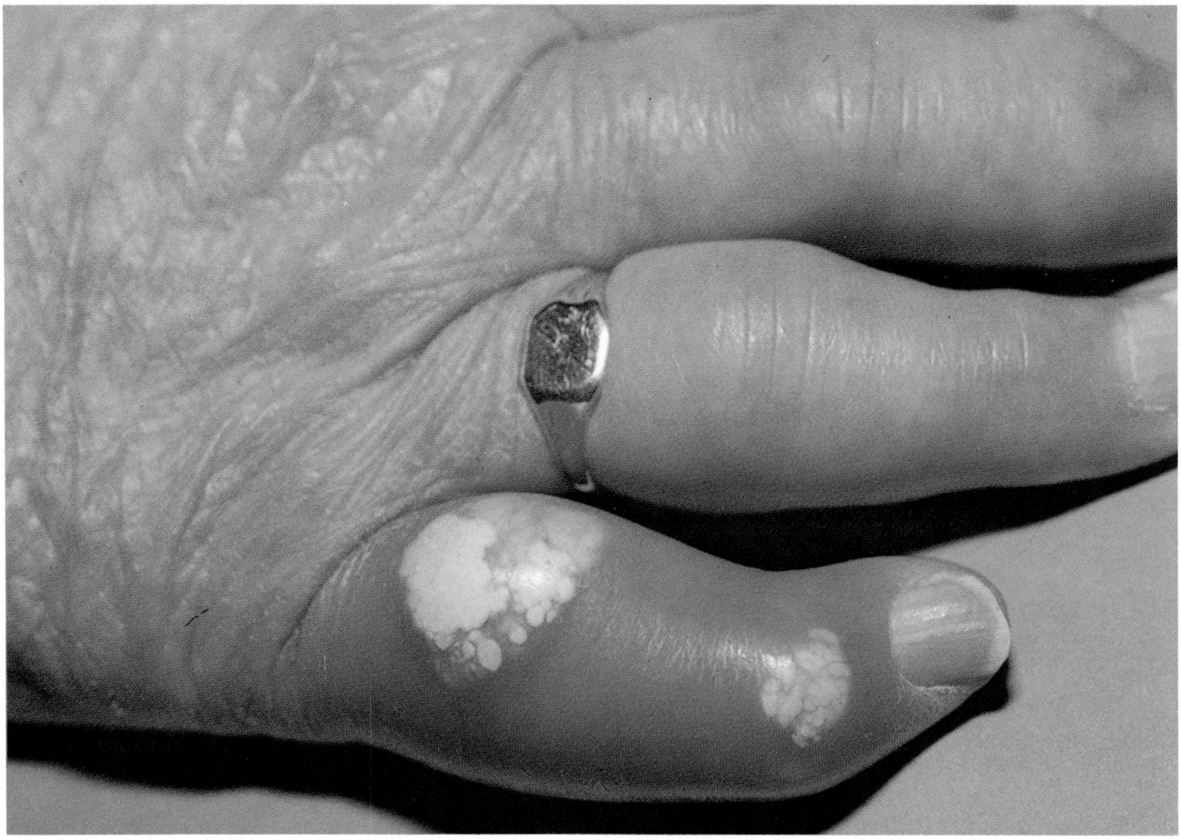

231

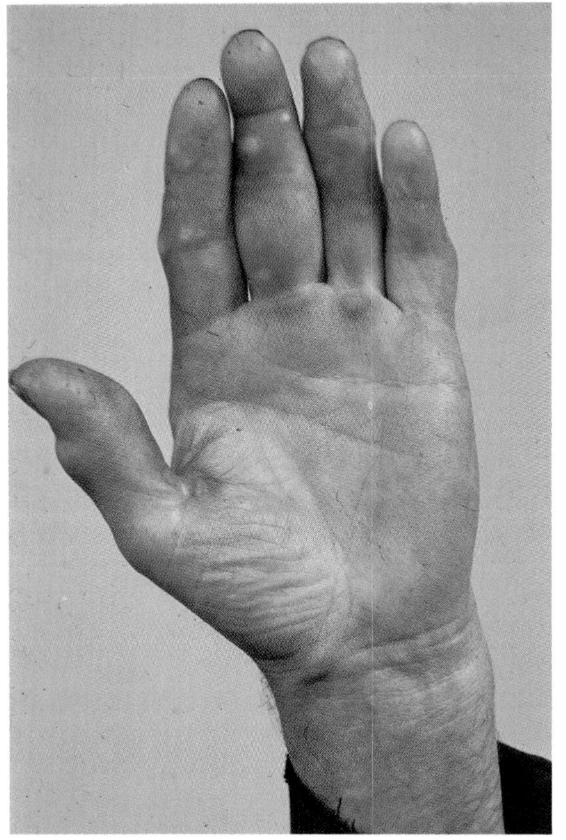

232

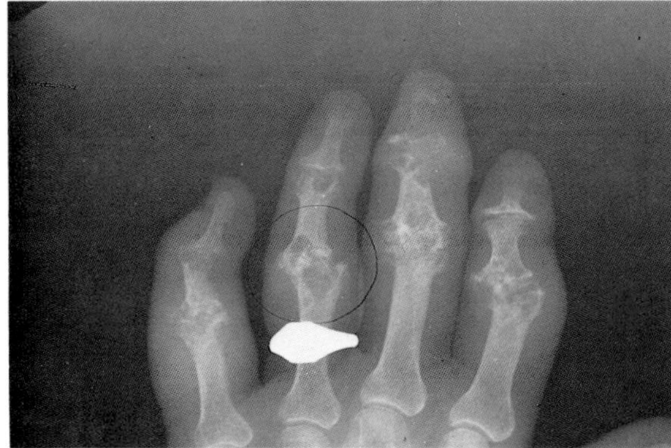

230 Tophaceous gout. This elderly lady had a longstanding history of 'rheumatism' and gout was only diagnosed when tophi appeared on the fingers. The feet were not involved but the serum uric acid level was elevated. She responded rapidly to appropriate therapy.

231 Tophaceous gout. Gouty tophi seen on the palmar surface of the fingers.

232 Gout: hand xray. Note the destructive changes in proximal interphalangeal and distal interphalangeal joints with punched-out radio-lucent areas in the bones.

233

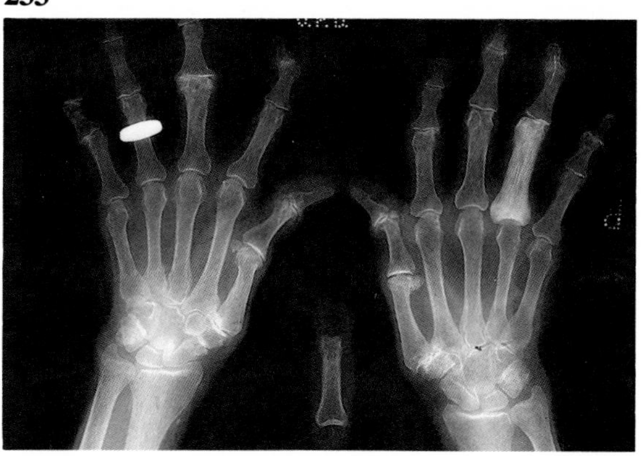

233 Paget's disease. Xray of the hands showing Paget's disease of the right 4th proximal phalanx. Note the increased density and thickening of the bone.

234a

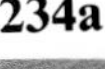

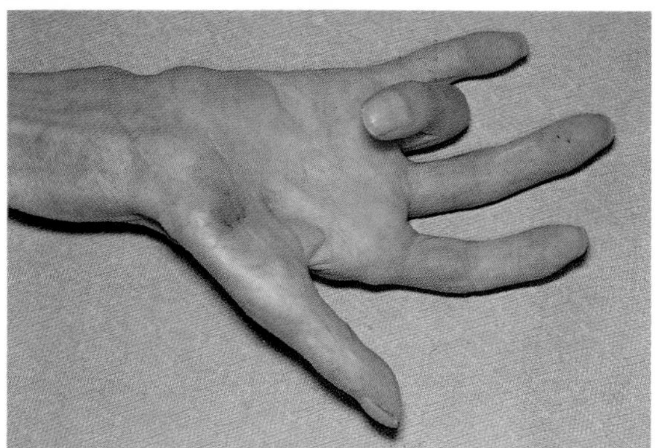

234a Dupuytren's contracture. Painless flexion contracture affecting the ring finger first and then involving the other fingers. It is caused by progressive fibrosis of the palmar fascia. About 25 per cent of people over 60 years of age have some thickening of the palmar fascia. Some cases are familial. There is an increased incidence in patients with alcoholic liver disease and epilepsy. Note the incidental wasting of the thenar eminence.

234b Dupuytren's contracture. In this case there is almost symmetrical involvement of both hands.

b

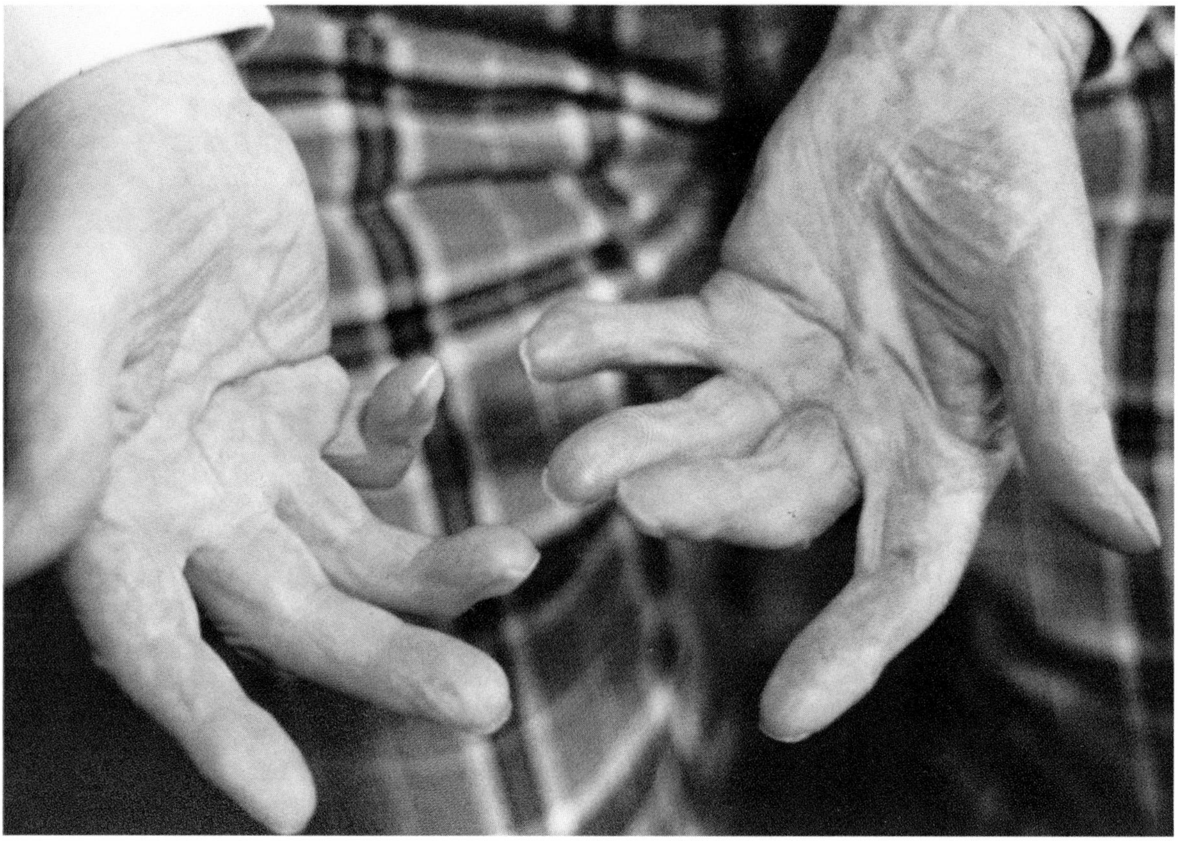

235

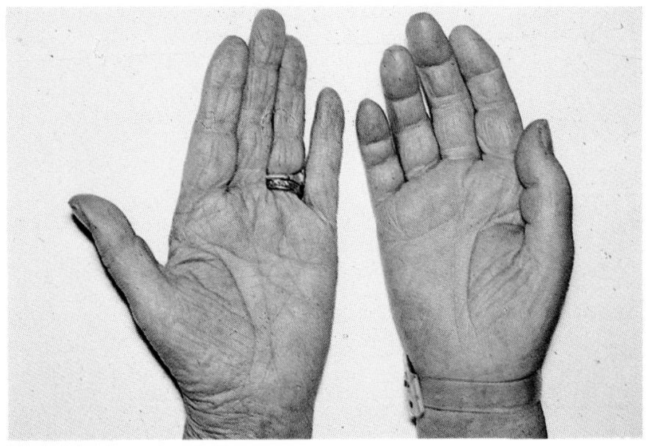

235 Hemiplegic oedema. Right-hand showing non-pitting oedema caused by disuse and autonomic changes associated with hemiplegia.

236

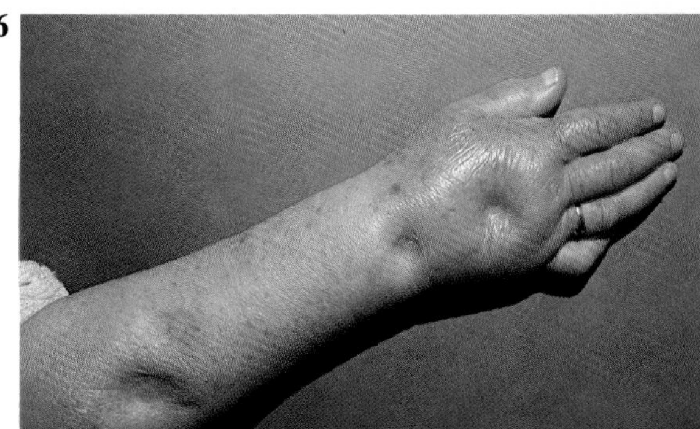

236 Oedema. This elderly lady had gross pitting oedema of the arms and hands (also legs) caused by hypoalbuminaemia resulting from a protein losing enteropathy.

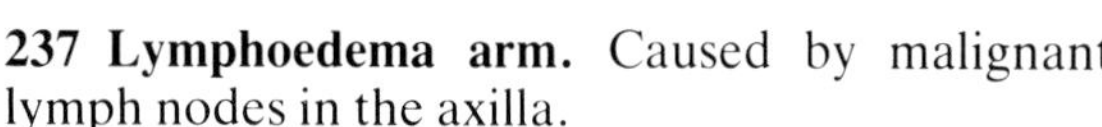

237 Lymphoedema arm. Caused by malignant lymph nodes in the axilla.

This patient was found to have carcinoma of the breast. Note the artificial right leg.

237

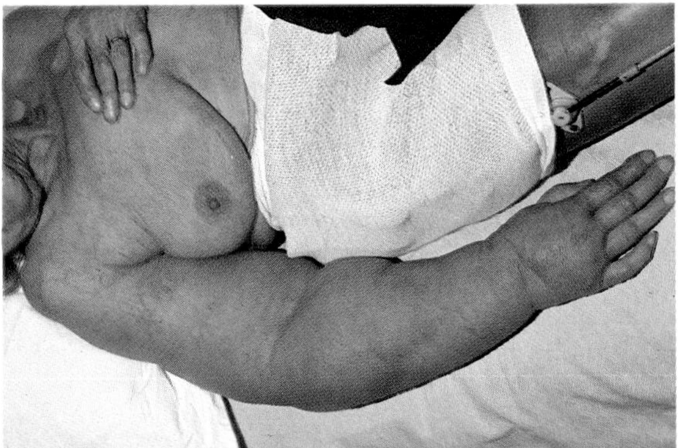

238a

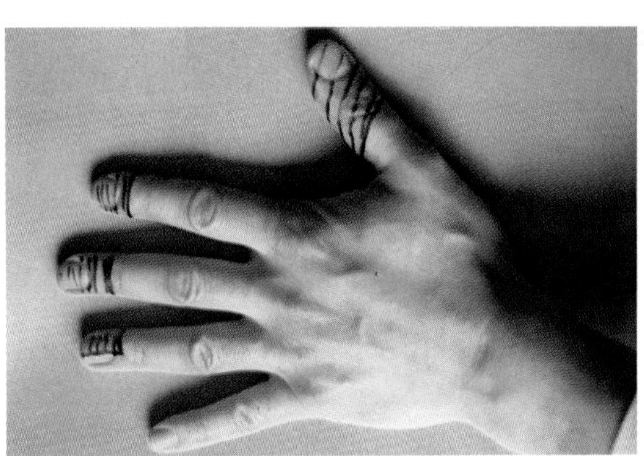

238b

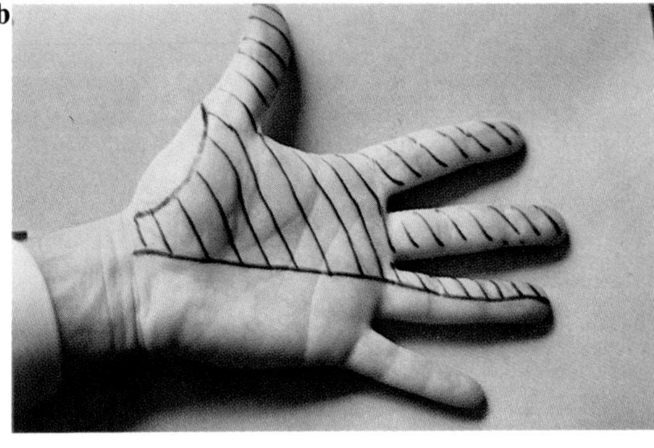

238 Carpal tunnel syndrome. Pictures (a and b) showing areas of sensory impairment as a result of a median-nerve lesion at the wrist. The median nerve also innervates the pronators of the forearm, long finger flexors, and abductor and opponens muscles of the thumb. Myxoedema is a frequent cause of carpal tunnel syndrome in older patients.

239

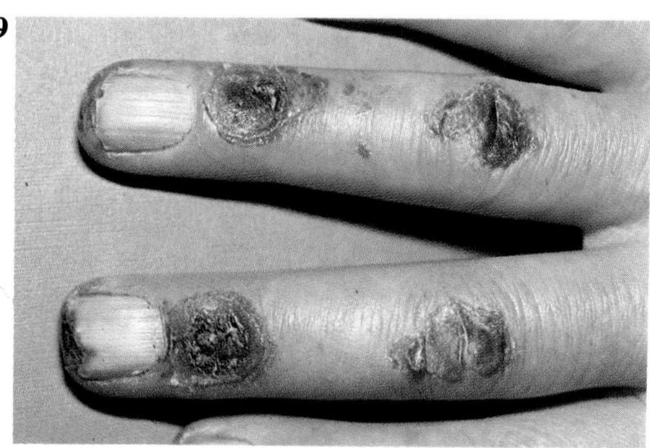

240

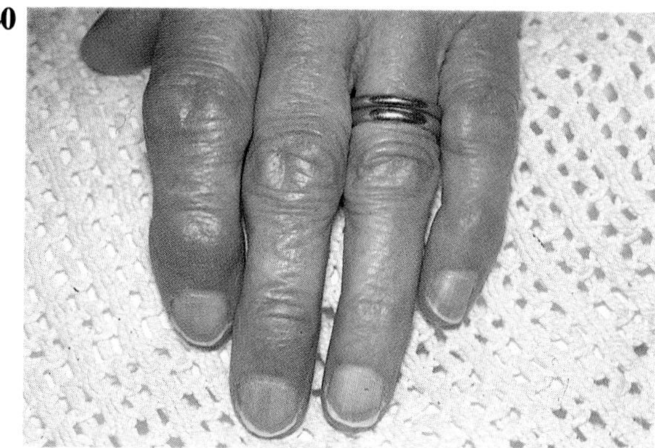

239 Burns. This elderly man had recurrent burns on the fingers. Examination of the central nervous system revealed sensori-motor neuropathy caused by cervical spine disease.

240 Peripheral cyanosis. Note the bluish discolouration of fingers and nails. The cyanosis in this case was of central origin and caused by corpulmonale.

241

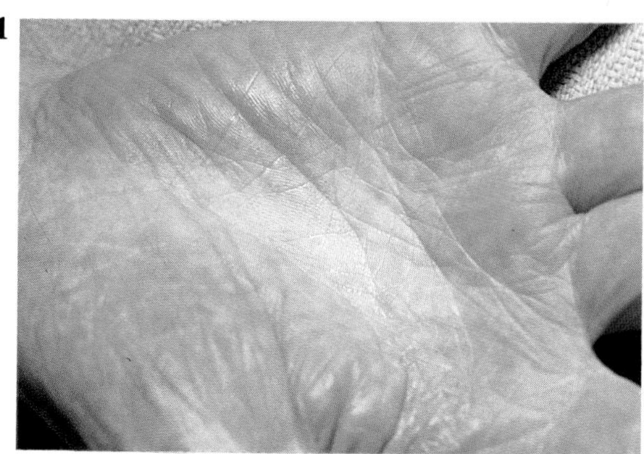

241 Palmer erythema. A peripheral ring of erythema around the palmar surface of the hand is a frequent finding in the elderly. It is usually 'innocent' but other causes are liver disease, polycythaemia, and thyrotoxicosis.

242

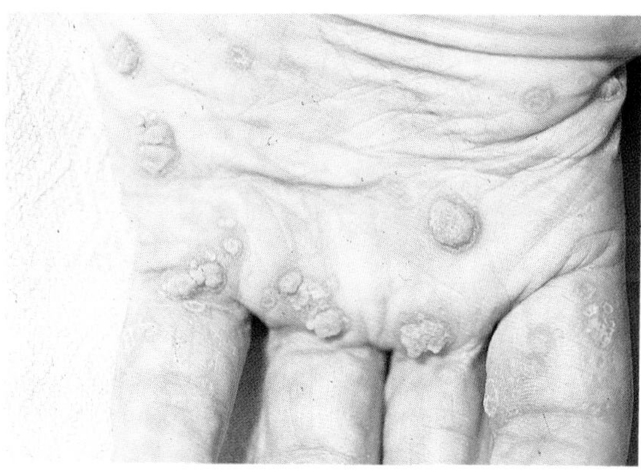

242 Palmer warts. These are deep, painful, flat lesions covered by a thick layer of cornified epithelium and occurring on the palms and soles. They are caused by a virus and are occasionally seen in the elderly.

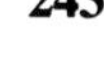

243

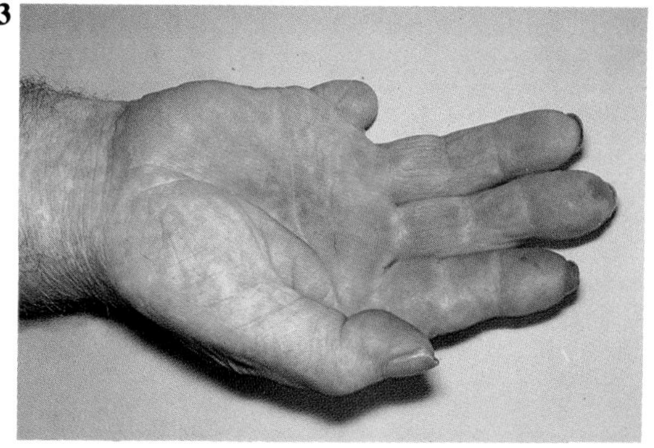

243 Faecal staining of the hands. This elderly patient was grossly confused and disorientated. He had chronic brain failure and was found to have faecal impaction. His hands and clothes were smeared with faeces because he had been attempting manual disimpaction.

244

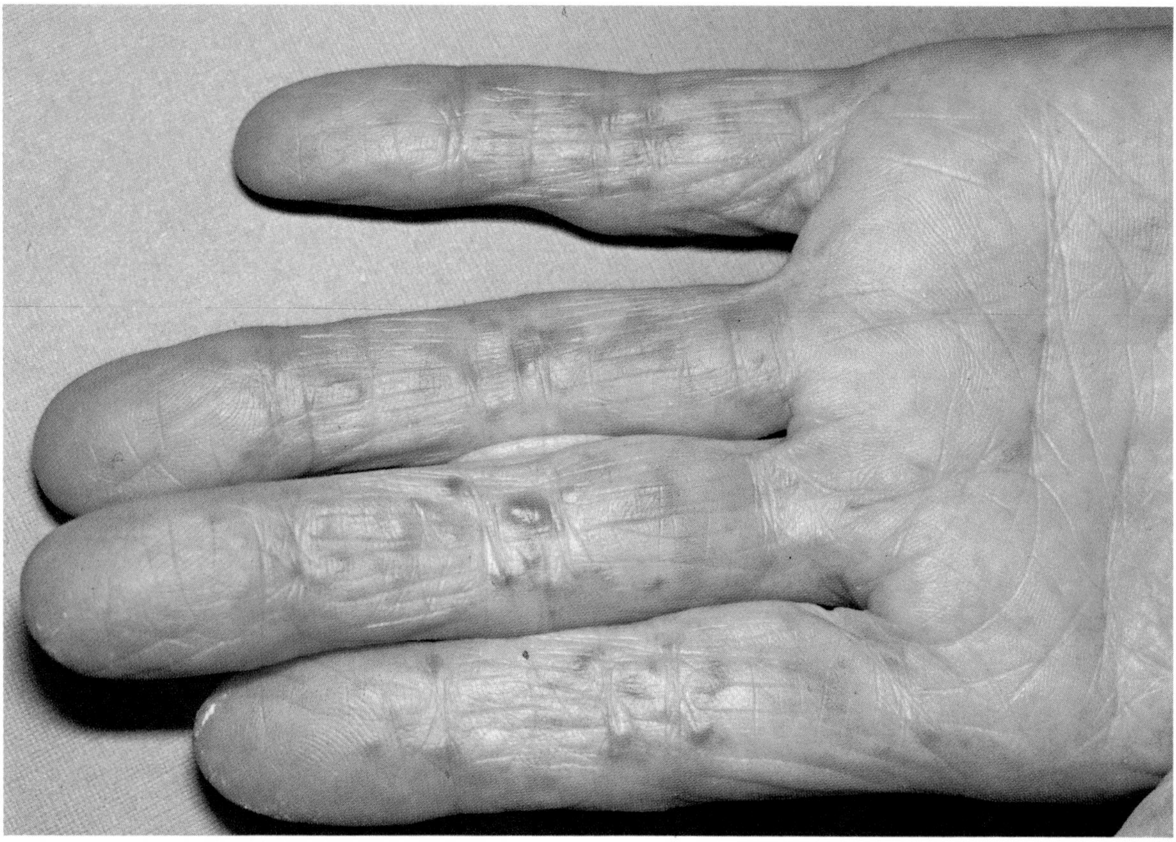

245

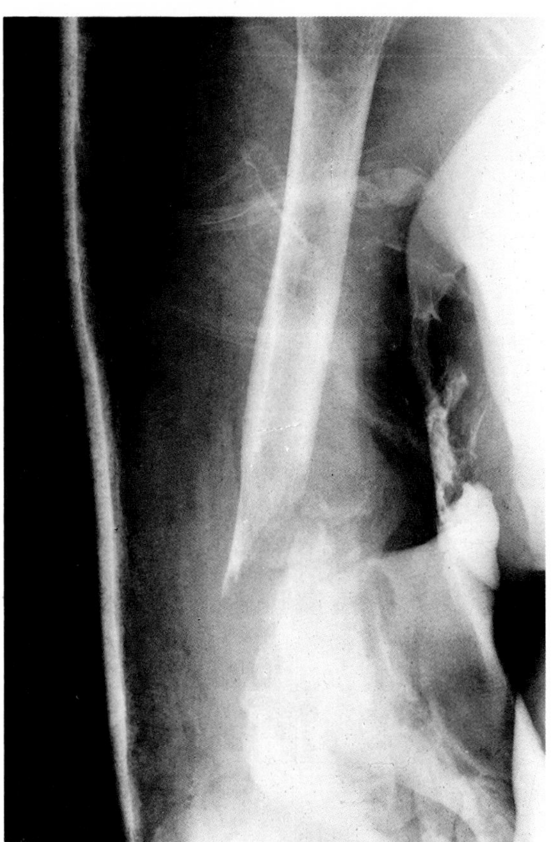

244 Finger varicosities. Dilated veins occur on the palmar aspects of the fingers in over 50 per cent of people over 70 years of age. There is no known relation with any venous abnormalities elsewhere in the body and the finding has no clinical significance.

245 Pathological fracture. Xray of the humerus showing a pathological fracture caused by secondary deposits from carcinoma of the colon. Note the destruction and sclerosis of bone around the fracture.

Elderly patients with osteoporosis, osteomalacia, Paget's disease, and bony metastasis are more prone to fractures.

246

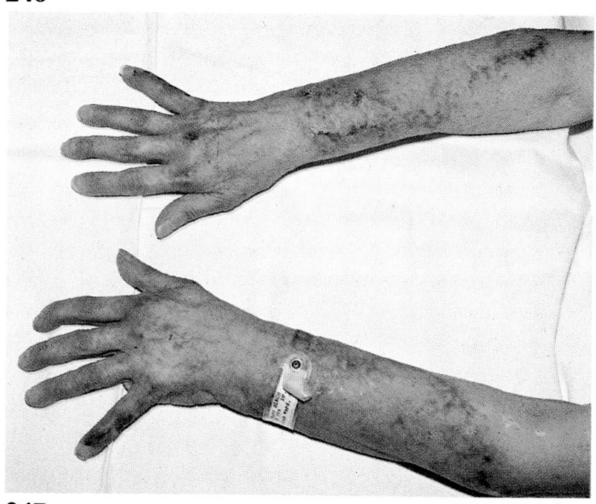

246 Cryoglobulinaemia. Purpuric spots and sores on the forearms, which appeared recurrently with exposure to cold and initially thought to be senile purpura. Investigations revealed the presence of cryoglobulinaemia with macroglobulins.

247

247 Raynaud's phenomenon. Note the finger-tip ischaemia and necrosis. This elderly female patient had severe cervical spondylosis.

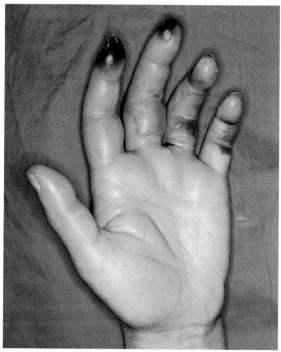

Raynaud's phenomenon

Paroxysmal digital ischaemia usually accompanied by pallor, cyanosis and followed by erythema.

Causes

1 Reflex vasoconstriction
   - Raynaud's disease
   - Cervical spondylosis
   - Shoulder-hand syndrome
   - Use of vibrating machinery

2 Arterial occlusion
   - Thoracic outlet syndrome
   - Arteriosclerosis
   - Embolus
   - Buerger's disease

3 Collagen diseases
   - Systemic sclerosis
   - Polyarteritis
   - Systemic lupus erythematosis
   - Rheumatoid arthritis

4 Increased blood agglutination
   - Cold agglutinins
   - Dysproteinaemias
   - Polycythaemia, leukaemia

5 Miscellaneous
   - Cold injury – frostbite
   - Toxins – ergot, tobacco
   - B-blocker drugs
   - Amyloidosis
   - Myxoedema

248

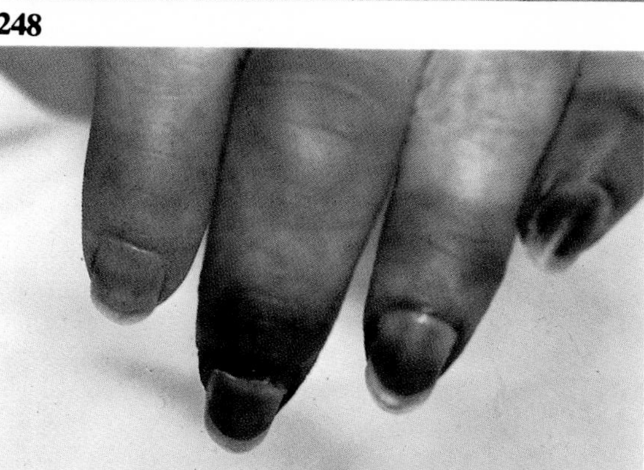

248 Vasculitis. Severe ischaemia of the fingers caused by polyarteritis nodosa.

249

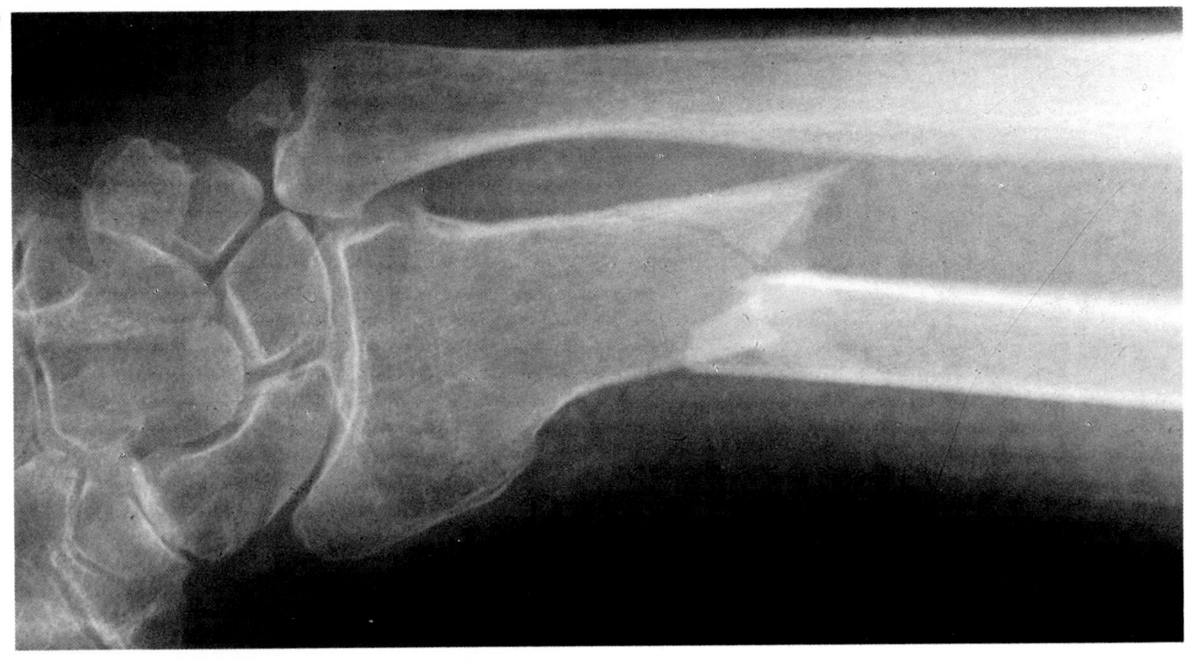

249 Fractured wrist. Common orthopaedic problem in the elderly. May result with slight trauma and cause considerable disability.

250

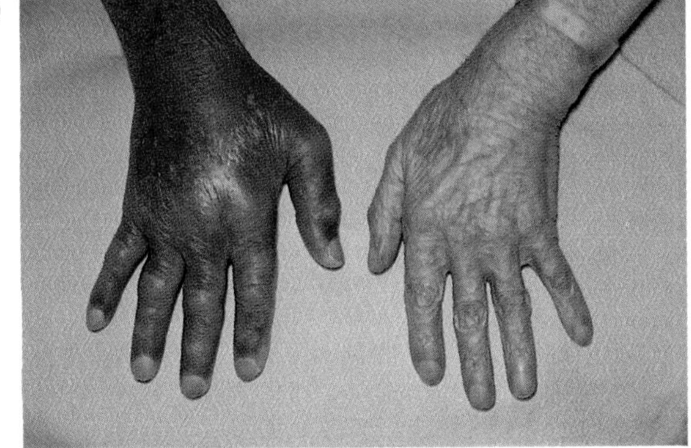

250 Ecchymosis. Severe ecchymosis of the right-hand in an 82-year-old widower who had a tendency to bruise excessively. Investigations revealed the presence of hypovitaminosis-C plus anaemia and painful joints. Leukocyte ascorbic acid levels were below normal.

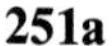

251a

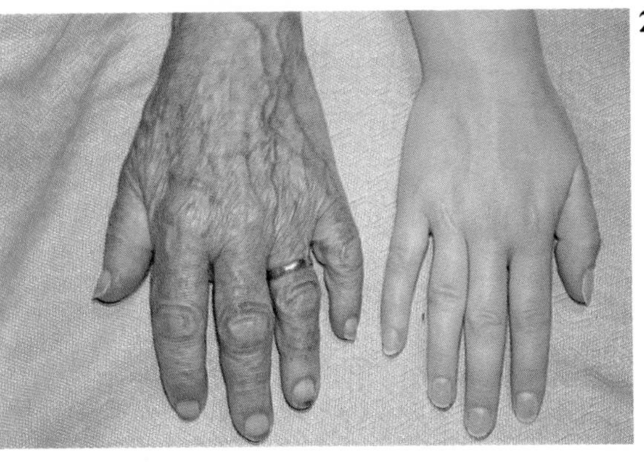

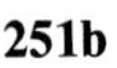

251b

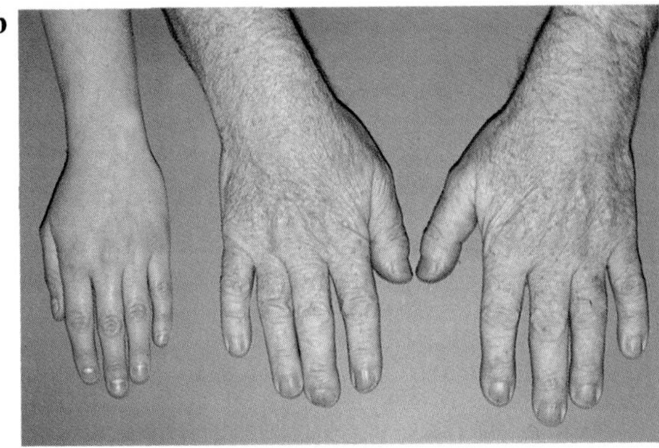

251a and b Acromegaly. Acromegalic hands compared with normal hands. Note the enlargement; the ends of the digits are square.

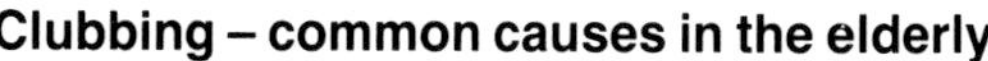

Clubbing – common causes in the elderly

1 Thoracic
  Carcinoma lung
  Chronic pulmonary suppuration
  Fibrosing alveolitis
  Mediastinal tumours
2 Cardiovascular
  Bacterial endocarditis
3 Extrathoracic
  Cirrhosis of liver
  Ulcerative colitis
  Pyelonephritis

252 Acromegaly. Xray showing generalised bony enlargement and tufting of the terminal phalanges.

253 Bronchiectasis. Note the clubbing of the fingers.

254 and 255 Koilonychia. Early and severe. Such nail changes may occur with anaemia, but sometimes they are quite 'innocent' in the elderly.

256 Psoriasis. Psoriatic changes in the nails. The patient also had extensive skin disease and arthropathy.

252

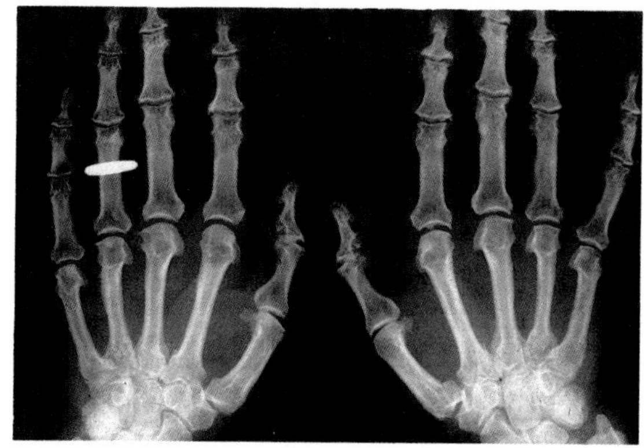

253

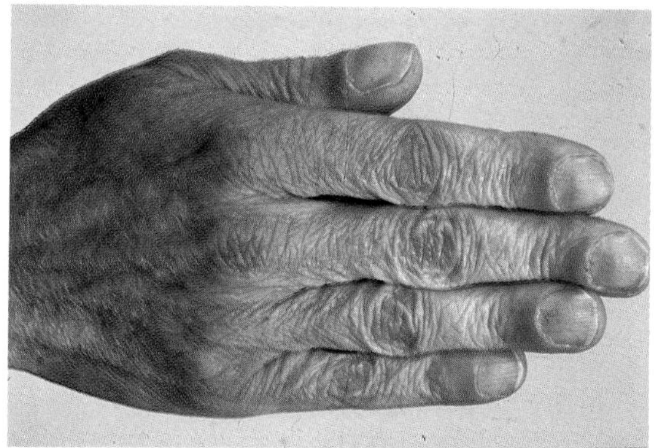

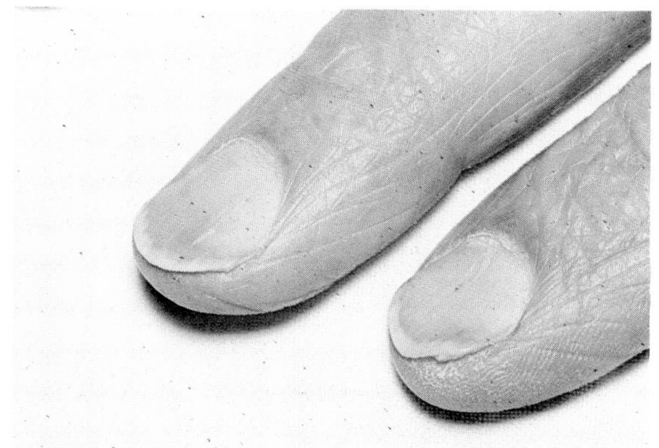

255

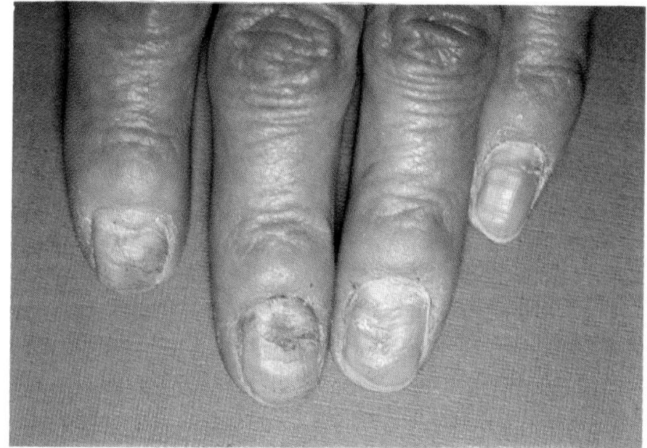

256

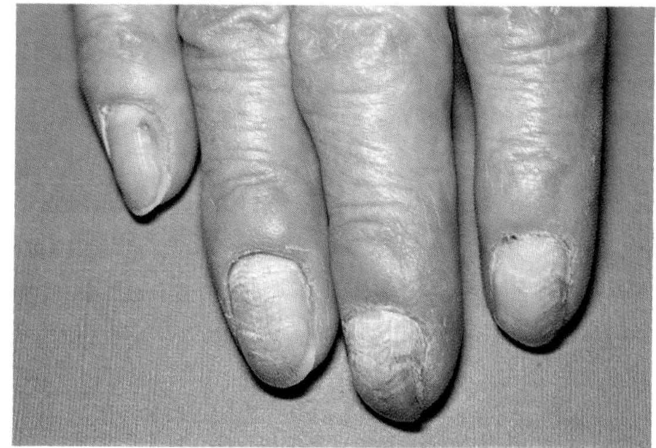

257 White nails. Note the marked pallor of the nail-bed caused by hypoalbuminaemia secondary to chronic liver cirrhosis. Occasionally three distinct zones are visible – white, pinkish and opaque – this pattern is called 'neopolitan' nails and is said to occur with collagen degeneration and osteoporosis in the very old.

258 Frozen shoulder. Right side. The patient is unable to abduct the arm at the shoulder joint, which is painful and stiff. It is caused by adhesive capsulitis, which is a common complication of hemiplegia.

259a Supraspinatus tendonitis. A form of frozen shoulder. Note the calcification in the supraspinatus tendon.

259b Adhesive capsulitis of the shoulder.

Shoulder-hand syndrome

Occurs in association with:

1 Myocardial infarction
2 Hemiplegia
3 Pulmonary lesions
4 Epilepsy
5 Cervical spine lesions
6 Herpes zoster
7 Brain tumour
8 Paniculitis
9 Vasculitis
10 Trauma

Causes of painful and stiff shoulder

Shoulder-hand syndrome
Adhesive capsulitis
Supraspinatuus tendinitis

257

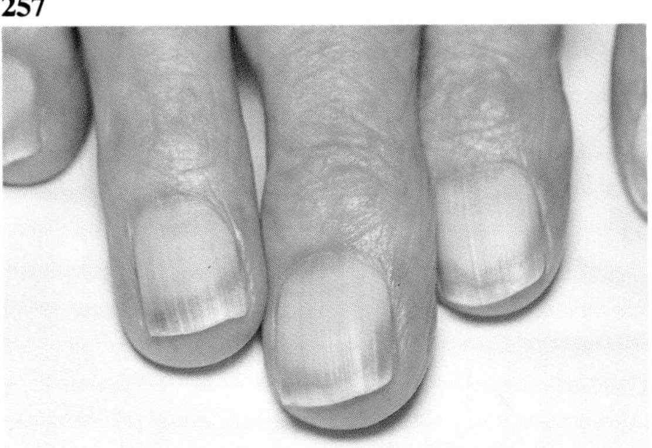

258

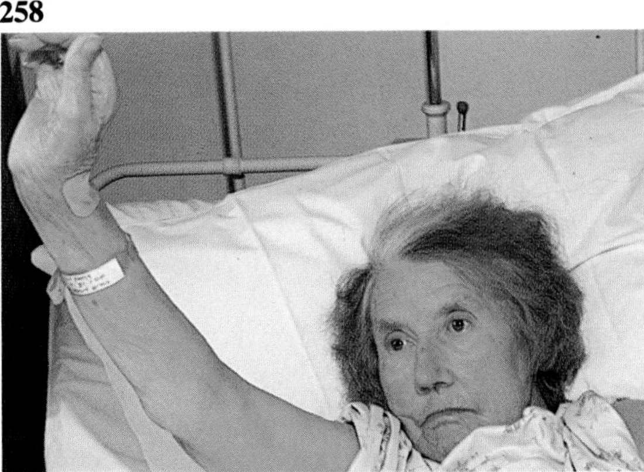

259a

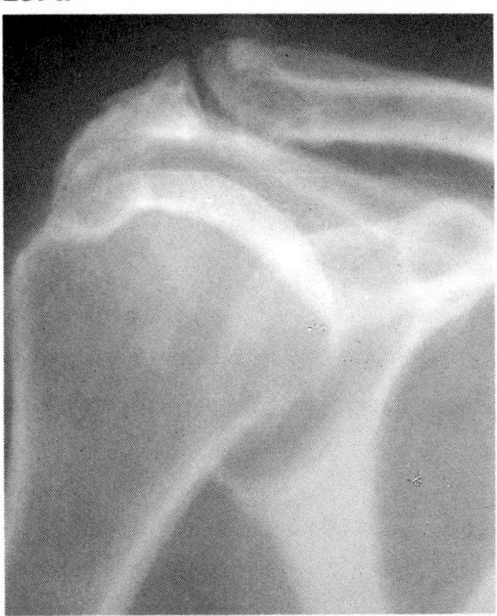

259b

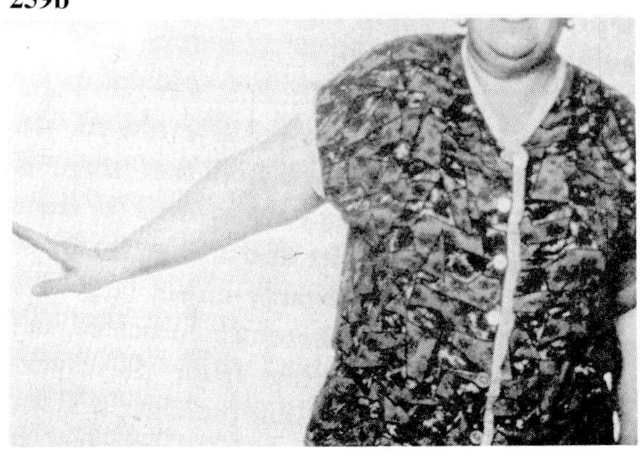

9 Disorders of the lower limbs

260 Wasting. Carcinomatous wasting of the legs with involvement of all muscle groups. This 76-year-old patient was found to have carcinoma of the stomach.

260

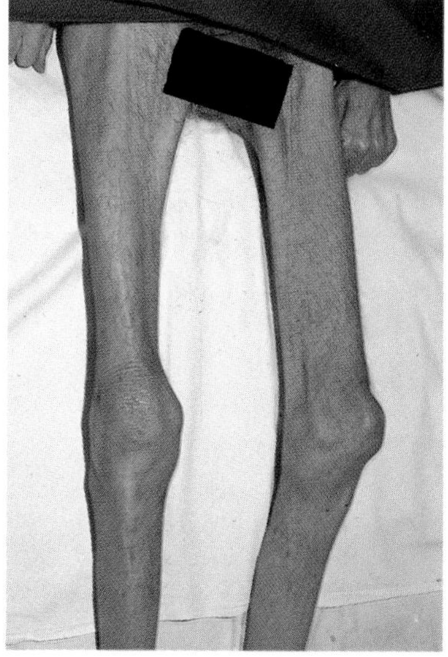

261

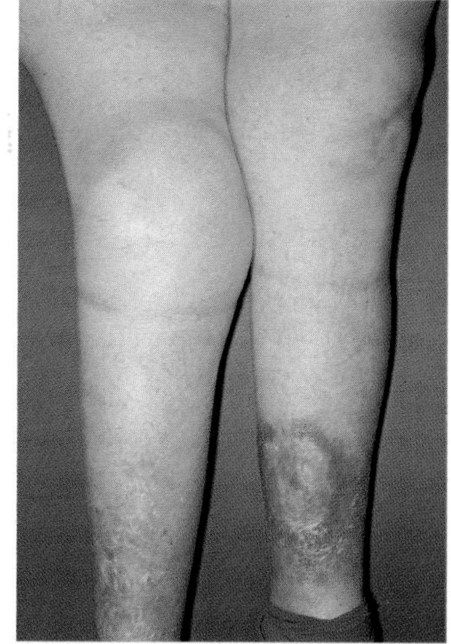

262

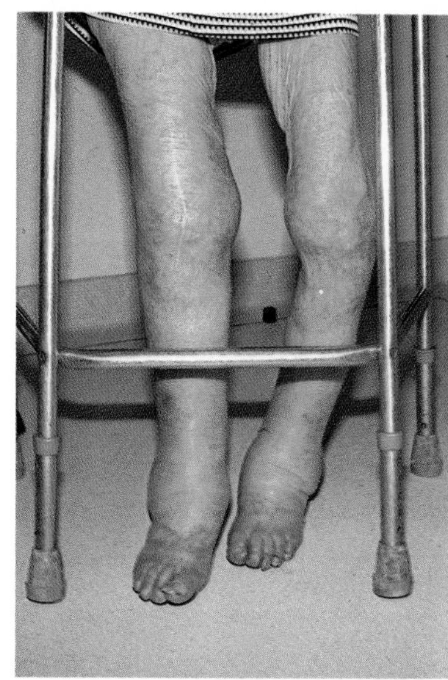

263

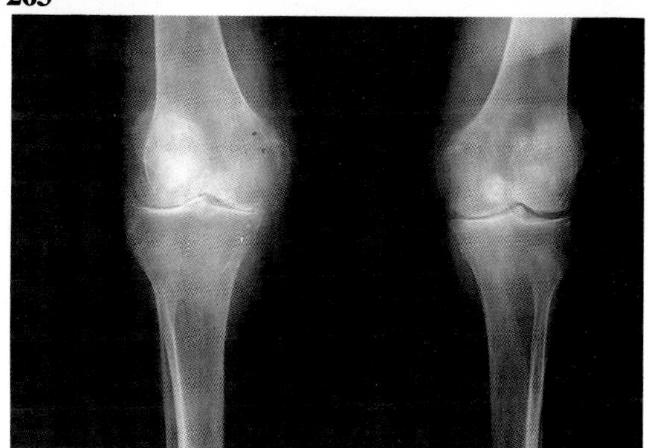

261 Osteoarthritis of the knees. Both knees are affected by the arthritis with pain, swelling, deformity, and reduced mobility. The left leg is shorter than the right as a result of arthritic destruction of the left hip joint.

262 Osteoarthritis of the knees. Advanced osteoarthritis affecting both the knees. The left knee shows secondary genu varus with joint instability and subluxation. Note the associated muscle atrophy about the knees, with postural oedema of the ankles. Note the arthrodesis.

263 Osteoarthritis. Xray of the knees showing loss of joint space and subchondral bony sclerosis.

264

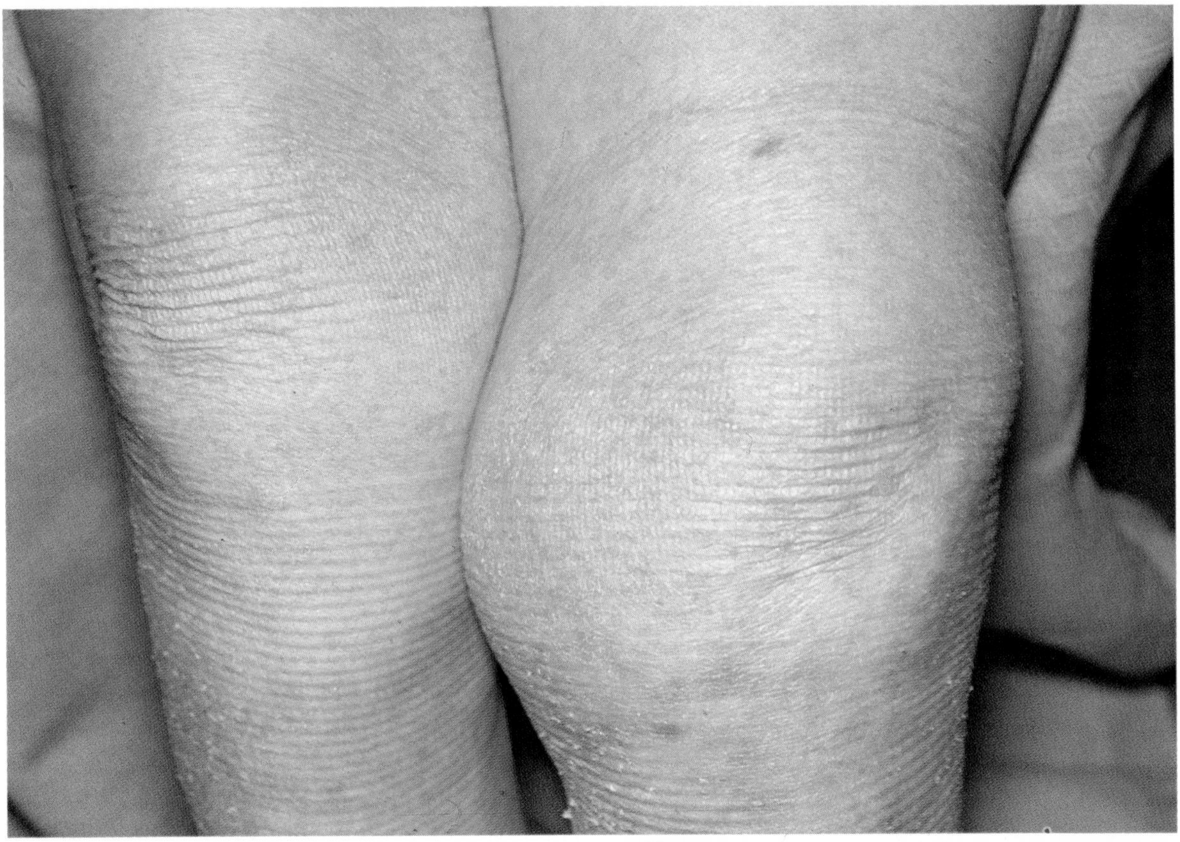

264 Pseudogout. Painful swelling of the left knee joint. Xrays revealed the presence of chondrocalcinosis. Aspiration of fluid from the knee showed typical birefringent microcrystals of calcium pyrophosphate dihydrate. The patient also had maturity onset diabetes mellitus and hypertension.

265

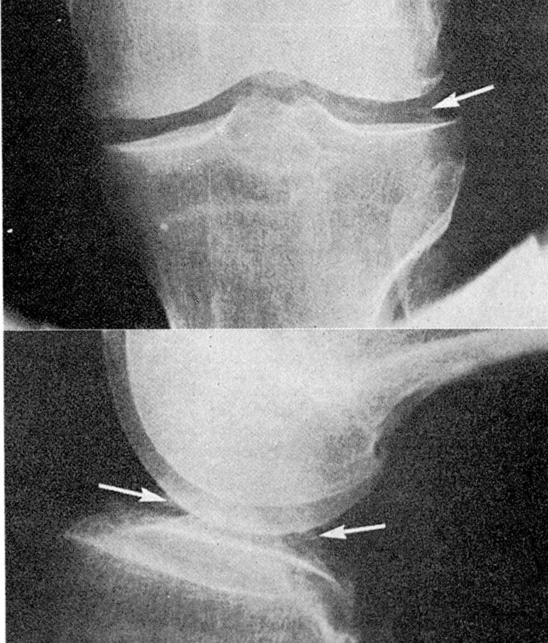

265 Pseudogout. Anteroposterior and lateral xrays of the knee showing typical linear deposits of CPPD in the menisci and articular cartilage, with degenerative changes indistinguishable from osteoarthritis.

Calcium pyrophosphate arthropathy

Associated conditions:

Osteoarthritis
Chronic renal failure
Hyperuricaemia
Hyperparathyroidism
Paget's disease of the bone
Diabetes mellitus
Hypertension
Haemochromatosis
Acromegaly

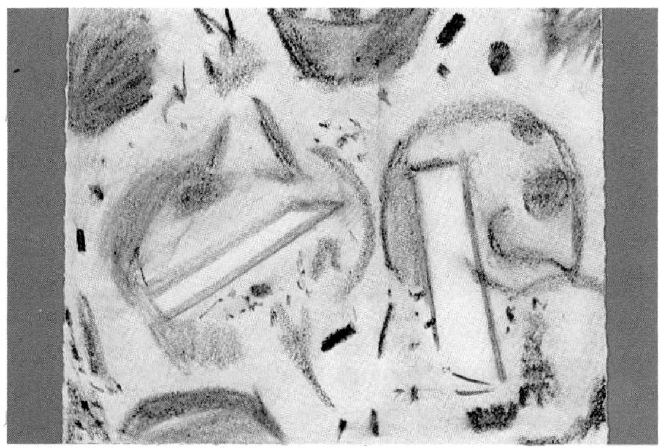

267

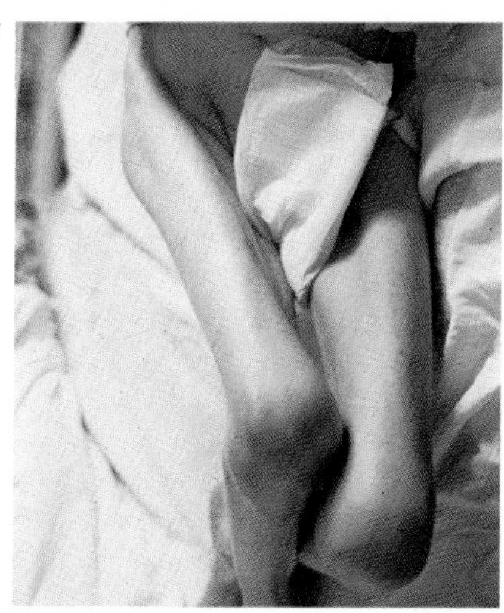

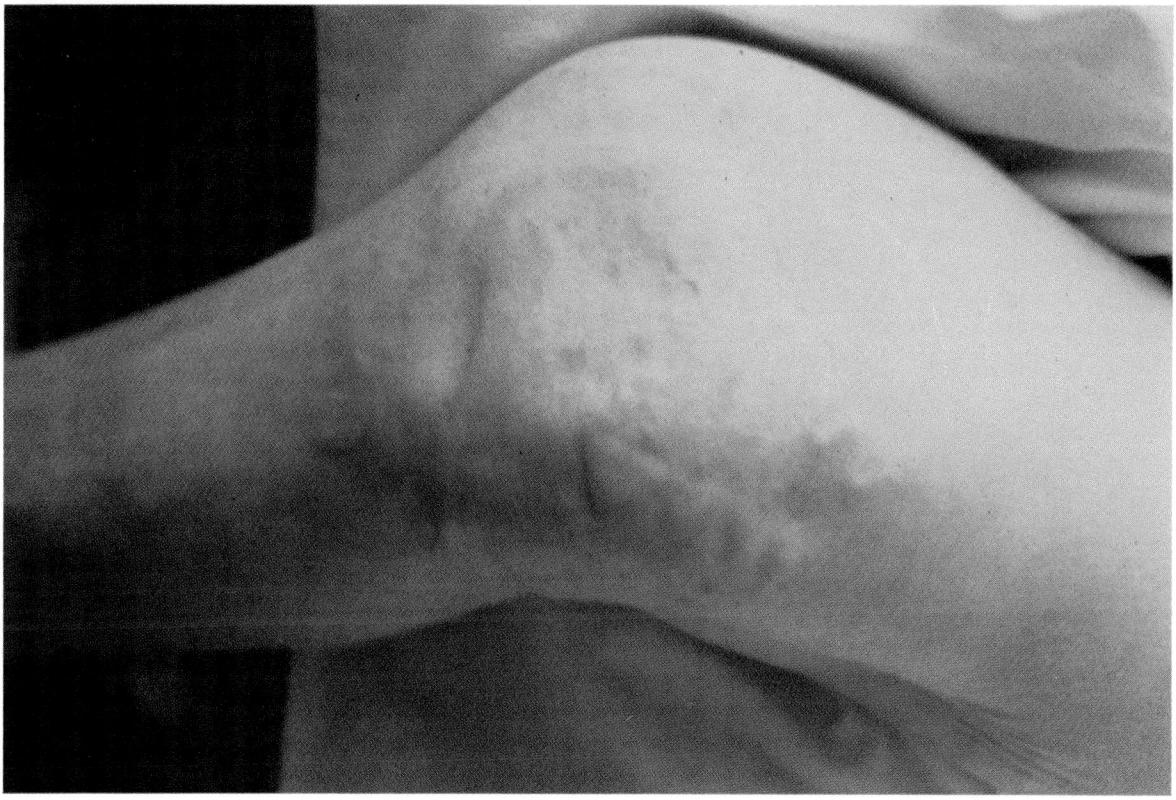

266 Chondrocalcinosis (diagramatic). Calcium pyrophosphate dihydrate crystals seen in the leukocytes show positive birefringence under polarized microscope.

267 Quadriceps wasting. Marked wasting of the quadriceps muscles caused by immobility and bilateral cerebrovascular disease. Such cases may go on to develop contractures.

268 Knee-joint effusion in a case of chronic degenerative joint disease.

269

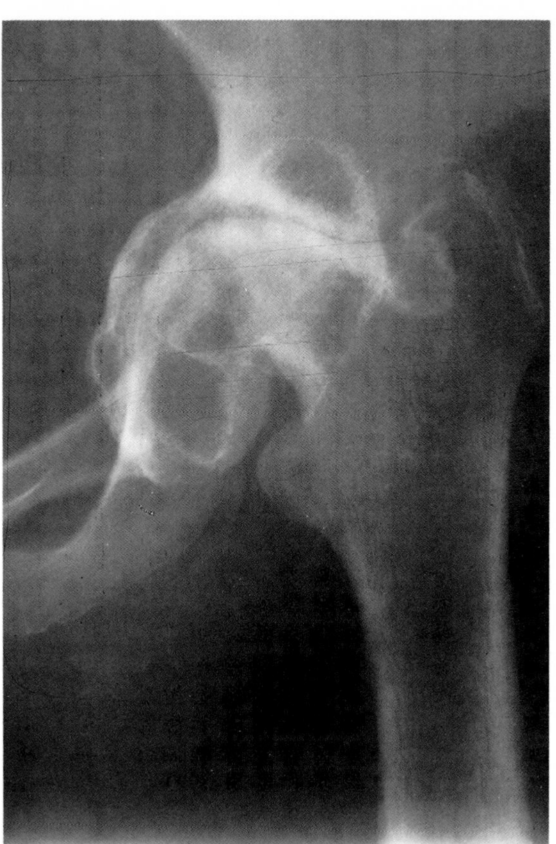

Fractures in the elderly

Aetiology

Falls or sudden mechanical stress plus:
- Osteoporosis
- Osteomalacia
- Paget's disease
- Bony metastasis

Types

Femur – commonest type of fracture in the elderly: Subcapital or pertrochanteric
- Humerus – usually impacted
- Colles' fracture
- Pelvic fracture
- Rib fracture
- Pathological fractures
- Compression fractures of vertebrae in osteoporosis

269 and 270 Osteoarthritis of the hip joint. Note the almost complete loss of articular cartilage with flattening of the femoral head and small cystic areas in the head and neck of the femur. Subchondral bone has areas of sclerosis and protrusio acetabuli is developing.

270

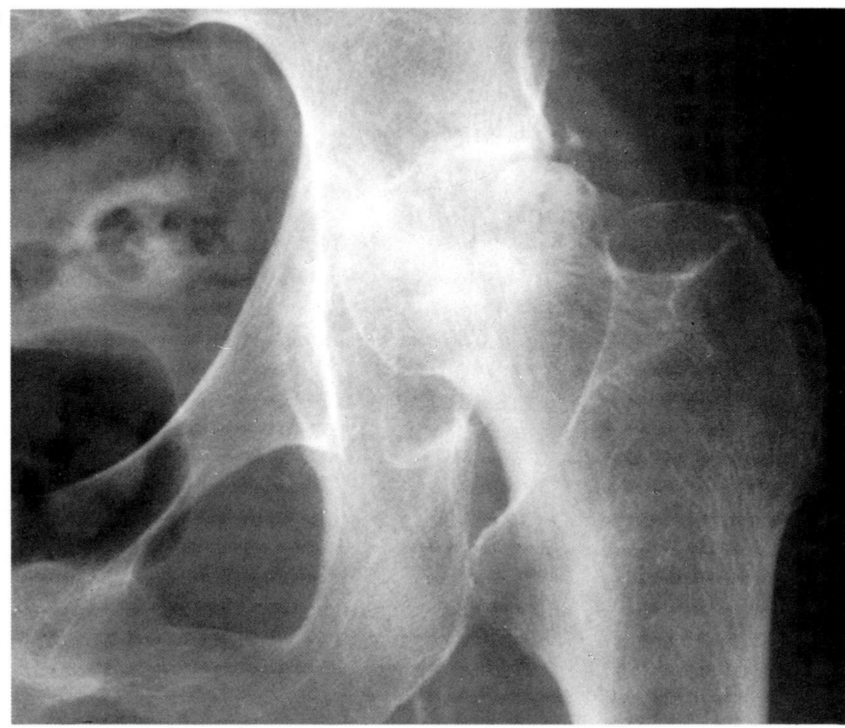

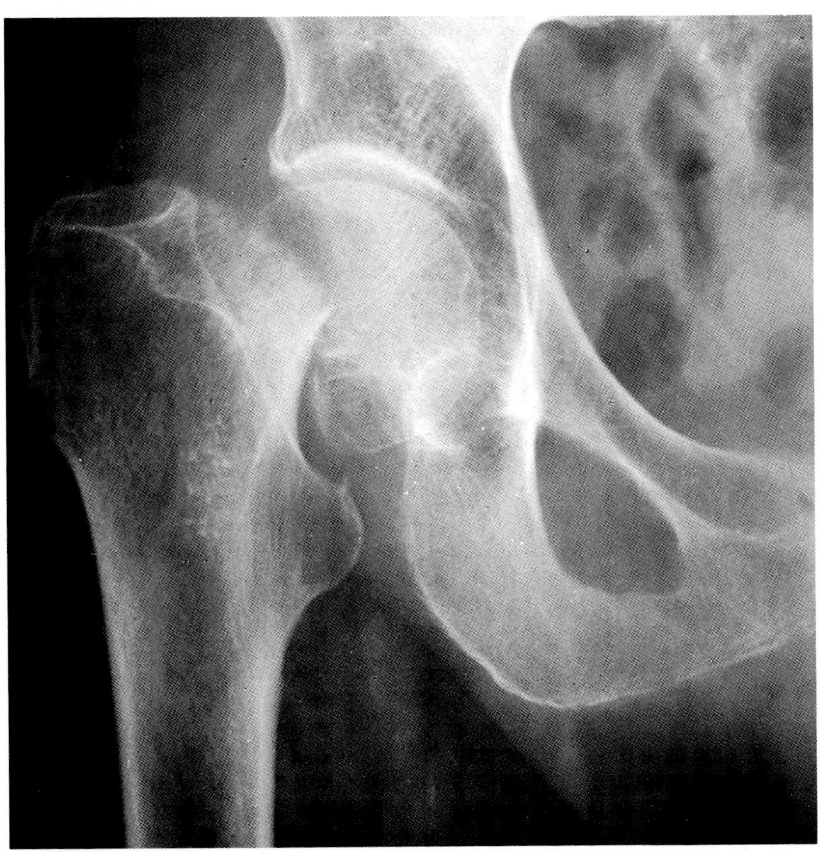

271 Fracture neck of femur. Xray showing a recent subcapital fracture through the neck of femur. This is a serious and disabling 'disease' of the elderly, especially women, and is associated with osteoporosis. Combined orthopaedic-geriatric units can do much in tackling this rapidly increasing disorder.

272 Bilateral fractures. This patient suffered from recurrent falls and sustained fractures of both necks of femurs, within months of each other. The right fracture is treated with Thompson's prosthesis and the left one with nail and plate.

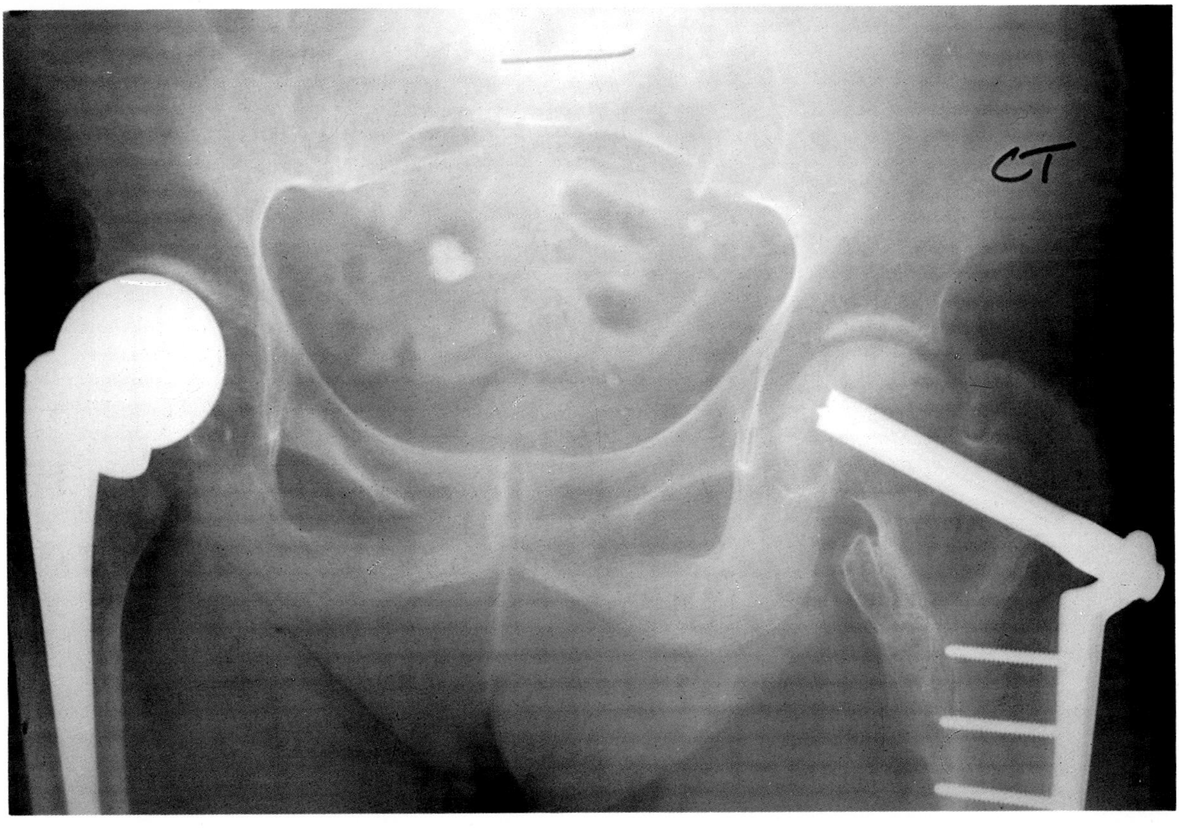

273
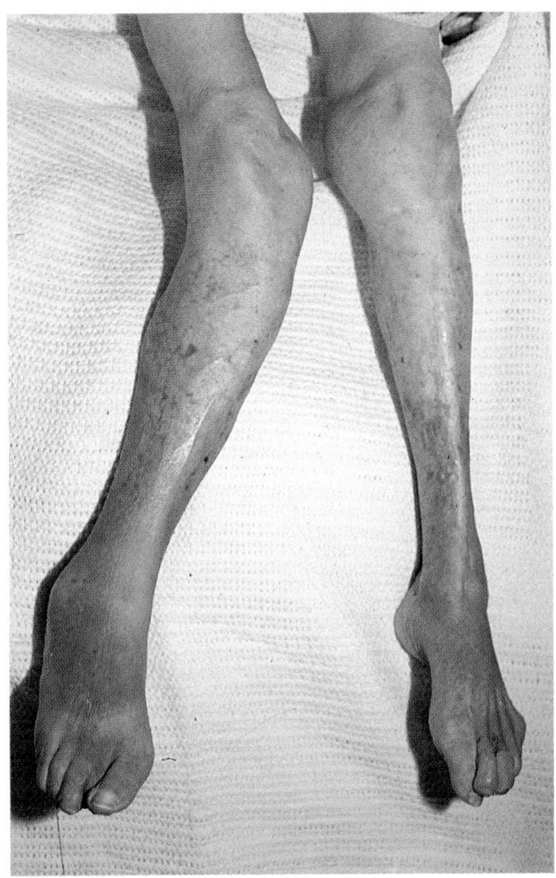

274
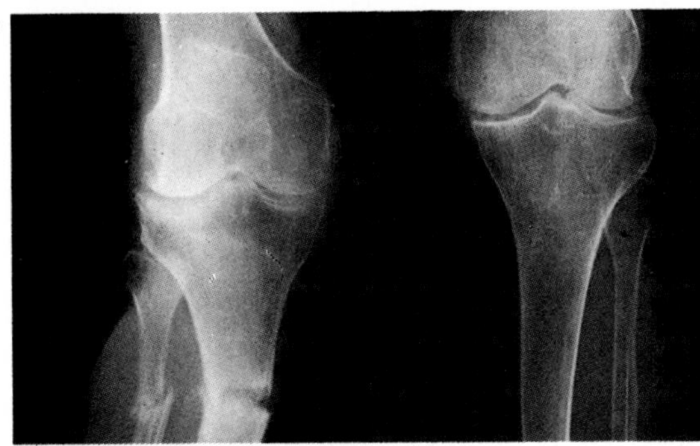

275
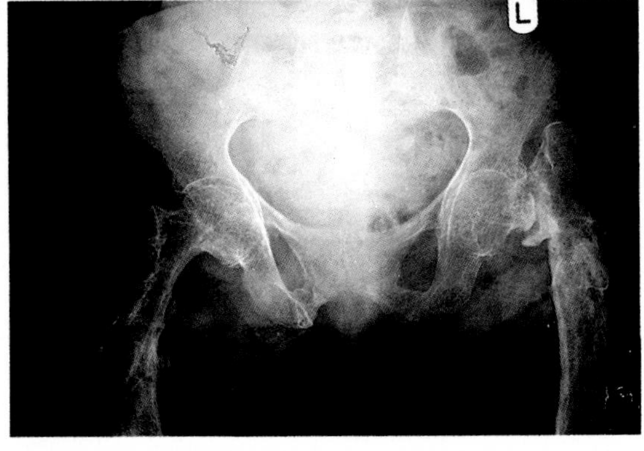

Osteomalacia
(softening of the bones)

Occurs in about 4 per cent of admissions to geriatric units. It is characterised by defective bone mineralisation with increase in osteoid tissue.

Aetiology

In the elderly the aetiology is multifactorial.

1 Vitamin-D deficiency
 Malnutrition – housebound, immobility, lack of sunlight, atmospheric pollution, inadequate diet.
 Malabsorption states and abnormal jugenal mucosa in some elderly.
 Post gastrectomy.

2 Abnormal Vitamin-D metabolism
 Liver disease
 Kidney disease
 Anticonvulsive drugs

3 Miscellaneous
 Malignant tumours
 Hypophosphatasia

Clinical features:

General deterioration in health
Anorexia and weakness
Non-specific aches and pains ('rheumatism')
Bone pains leading to bone tenderness
Proximal myopathy giving rise to waddling gait
Increased incidence of fractures, especially fractures of neck of femur
Depression
Immobility
Skeletal deformities

Diagnosis

Biochemistry –
 Low or normal serum calcium, low serum inorganic phosphate, raised serum alkaline phosphatase and low urinary calcium excretion.

Radiography –
 Reduced bone density with coexistant osteoporosis.
 Pseudo fractures (Looser's zones) in the cortex of bone are diagnostic.

Bone biopsy –
 Microscopic examination of bony tissue will show excess of unmineralised osteoid tissue greater than 40 per cent.

Isotope bone scan –
 Increased uptake by the bones with focal hot areas.

Therapeutic trial with Vitamin-D –
 A patient with osteomalacia will respond dramatically with rapid improvement of symptoms.

273 Osteomalacia. This elderly lady presented with painful bones, depression and immobility. Note the deformity of the right leg. Diagnosis of osteomalacia was confirmed by finding a raised serum alkaline phosphatase and low serum calcium and inorganic phosphate.

274 Osteomalacia. Xray of the same patient reveals a non-traumatic stress fracture of tibia and fibula. Response to Vitamin-D therapy was rapid and with physiotherapy she became mobile and independent.

275 Osteomalacia. Advanced osteomalacia in an elderly lady who was housebound for several years. Note marked bone translucency, old fracture neck of the left femur and Looser zone in the right femur.

276 Osteomalacia. Looser's zone seen near the lesser trochanter.

277 Osteomalacia. Looser's zone seen in the right superior pubic ramus.

278 Osteomalacia. Section of bone reveals the classic picture of osteomalacia. There are wide uncalcified seams of osteoid tissue with decrease in the staining intensity of calcification fronts.

276

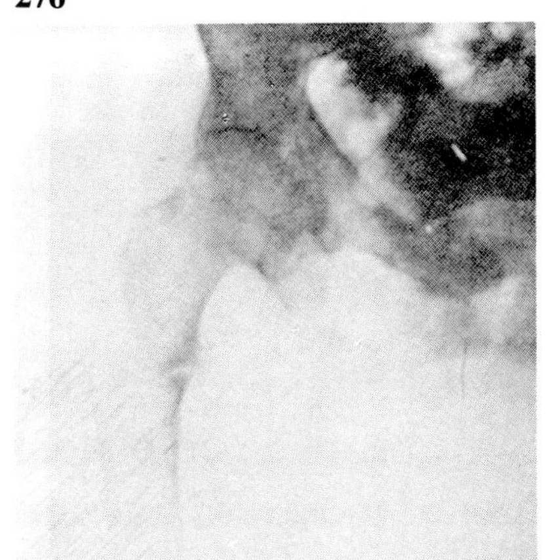

277

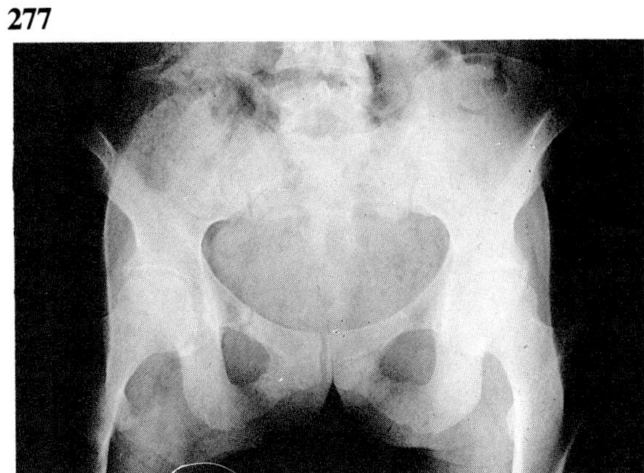

8

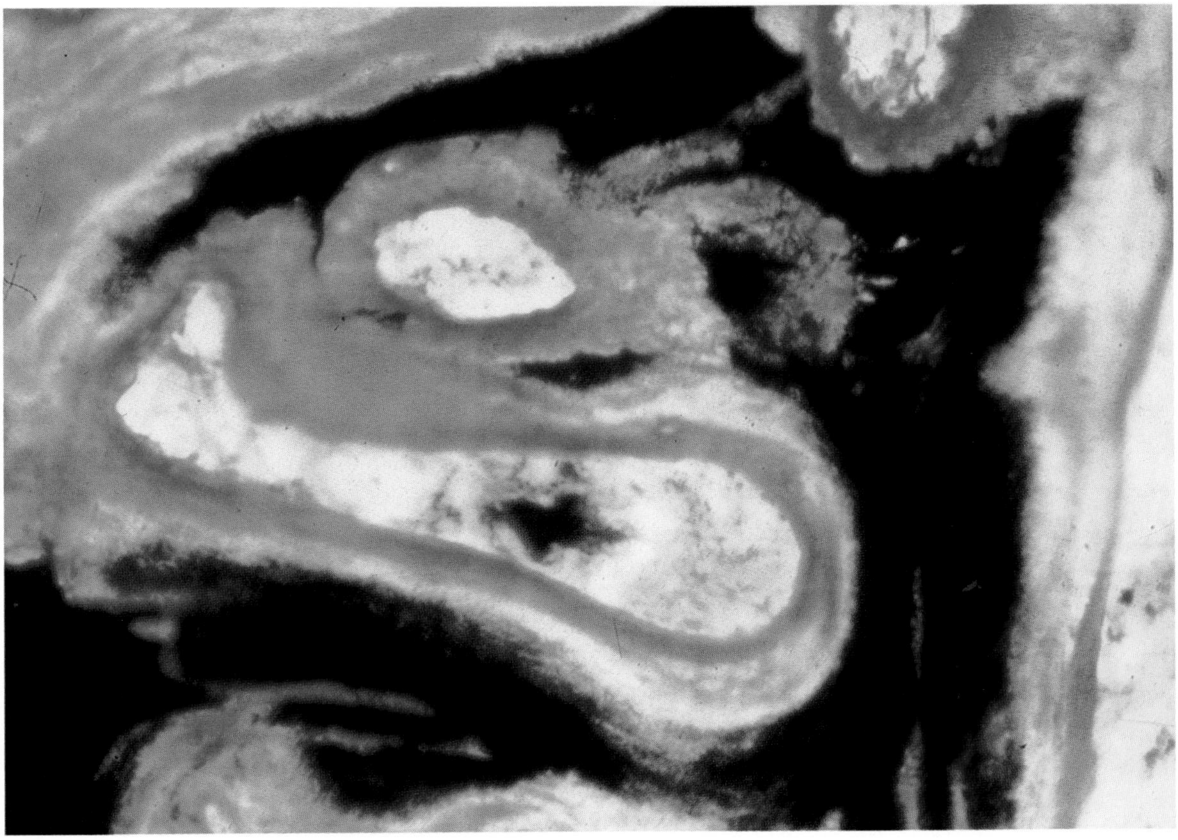

279

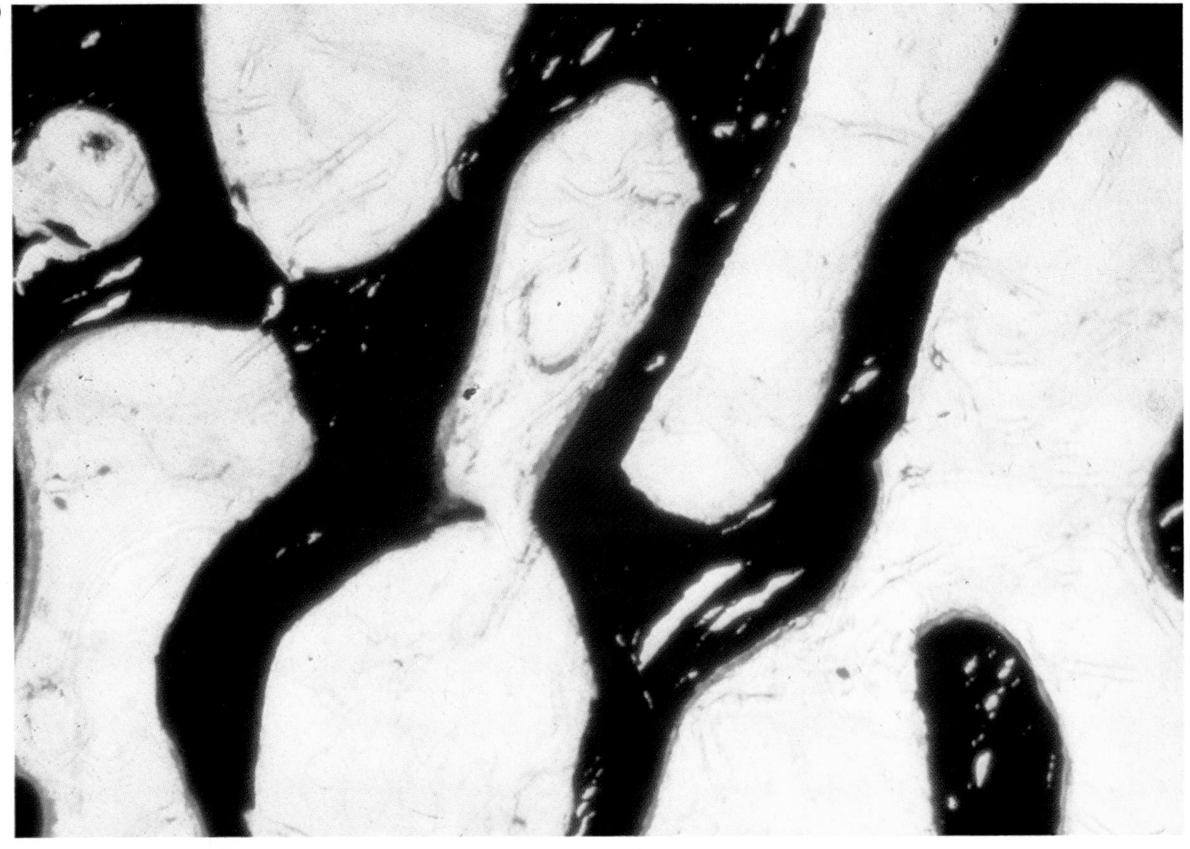

279 Normal bone. Section of normal bone shown for comparison. The calcified tissue stains black and the uncalcified matrix (osteoid) stains red (Von Kossa).

Paget's disease

Characterised by a combination of excessive bone breakdown and rapid bone replacement, resulting in deformity and increased fragility. Usually the condition is asymptomatic and is only revealed by routine xray or finding a raised alkaline phosphatase.

Clinical features

Bone aches and pain mainly in pelvis and legs
Bone deformities – bowing of tibia and enlargement of skull
High output cardiac failure
Deafness
Visual impairment
Rarely development of osteogenic sarcoma in the affected bone

Investigations

Serum calcium and phosphate normal
Serum alkaline phosphatase raised
Urinary hydroxyproline raised
Xrays – show lytic areas, zones of increased density, loss of trabecular patterns and deformity
Isotope scan – there is increased uptake by areas involved by the disease

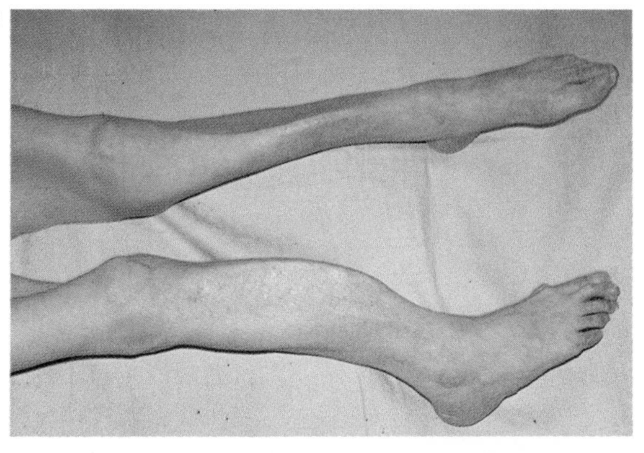

281

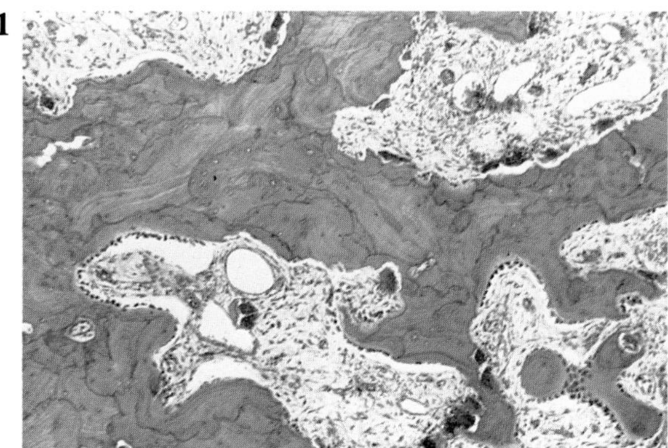

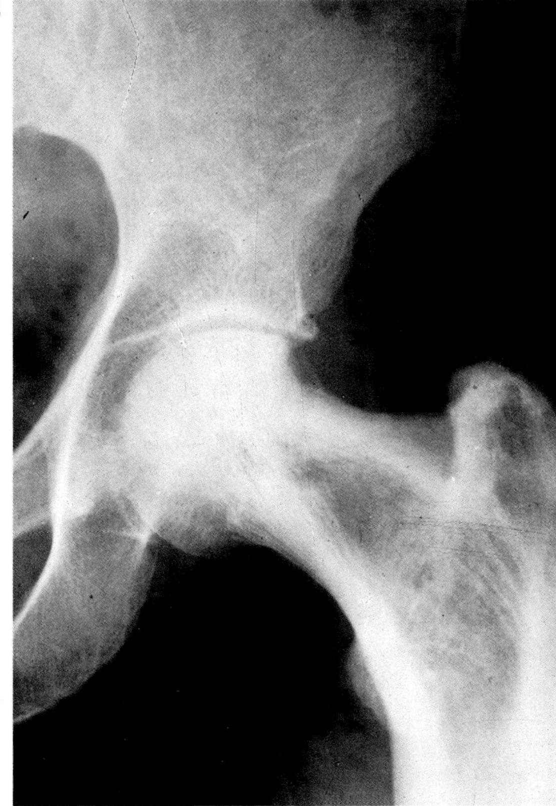

283

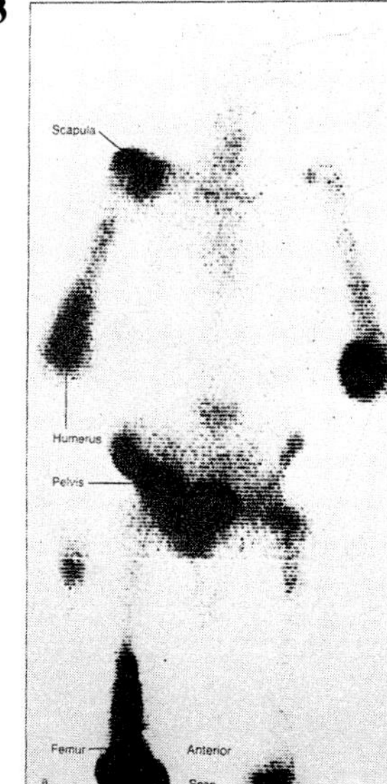

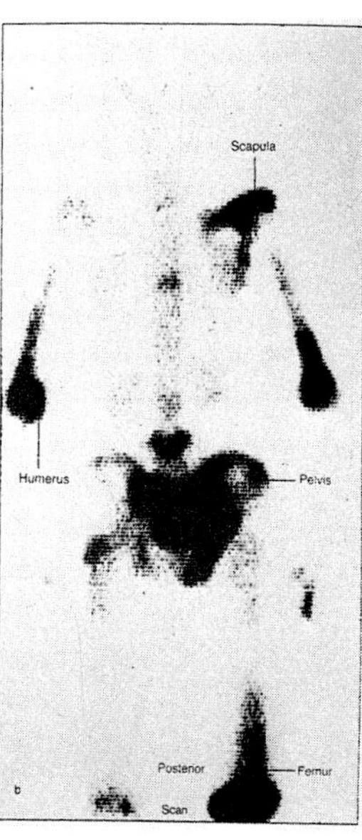

280 Paget's disease. Advanced Paget's disease of the bone showing deformity of the tibiae with bowing and thickening of the bones. This patient also complained of deafness and had cardiac failure.

281 Paget's disease. Histology of the bone showing grossly disorganised bony structure. There is rapid bone turnover with increased resorption and accelerated replacement. Note many osteoblasts along the trabeculae.

282 Paget's disease. Xray left hip showing Paget's disease of the head of femur.

283 Paget's disease. Isotope bone scan of skeleton showing the extent of active Paget's disease. The dark areas indicate the patches of Paget's bone.

284

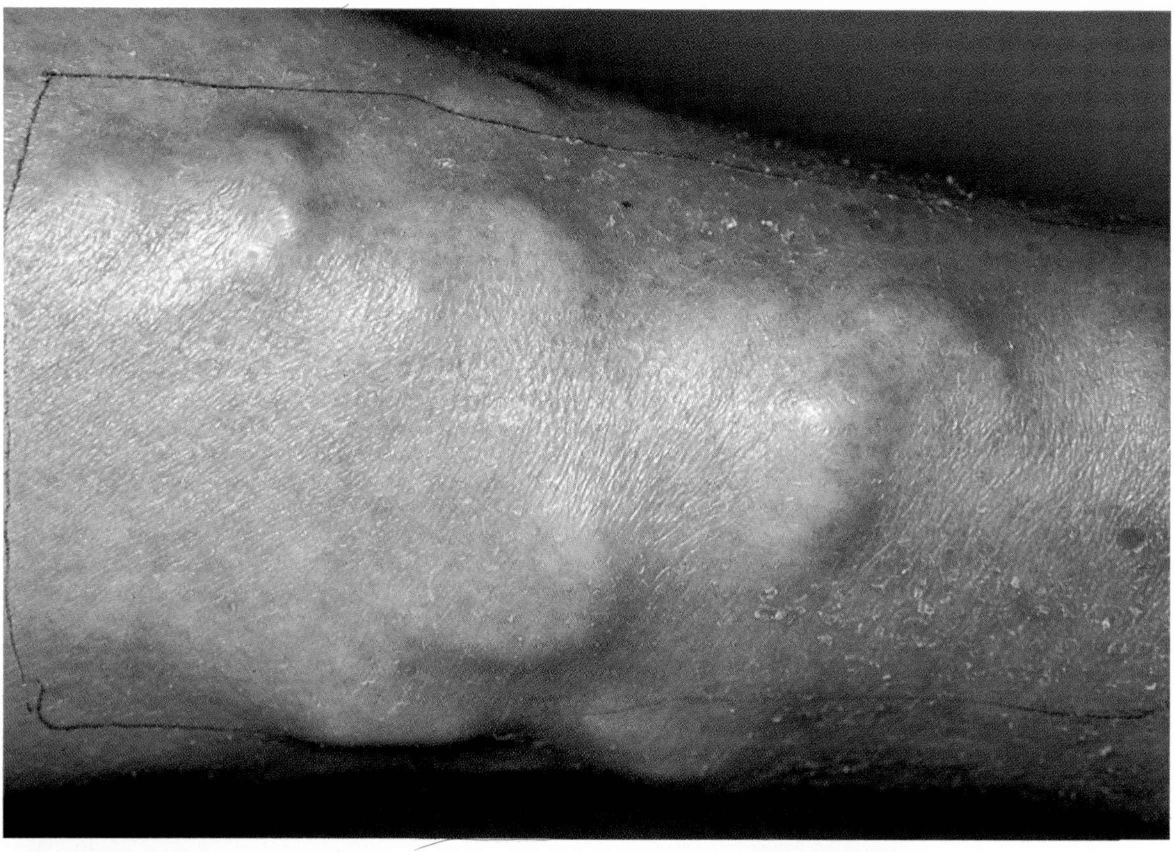

285

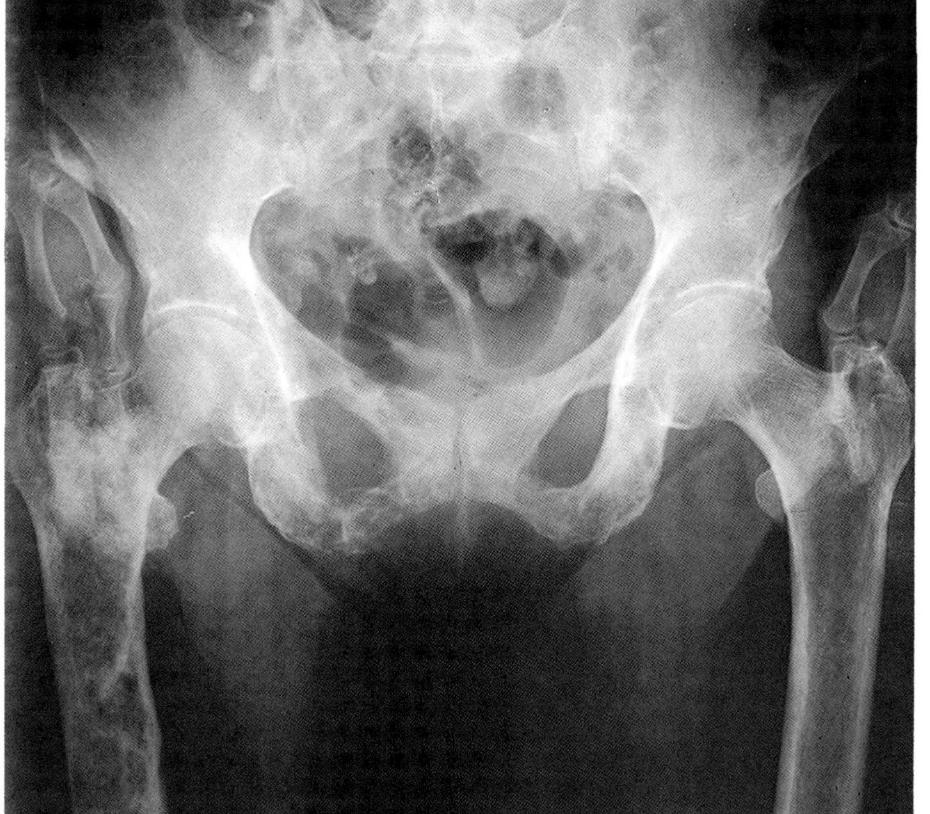

284 Varicose veins. Dilated, tortuous superficial veins with incompetent valves. The greater and lesser saphenous systems are most commonly involved. When varicose veins occur as a result of deep venous obstruction, the patient may go on to develop a postphlebitic syndrome.

285 Bony secondaries. Multiple osteolytic secondary deposits in the pelvis, and right femur, from a primary in the lung.

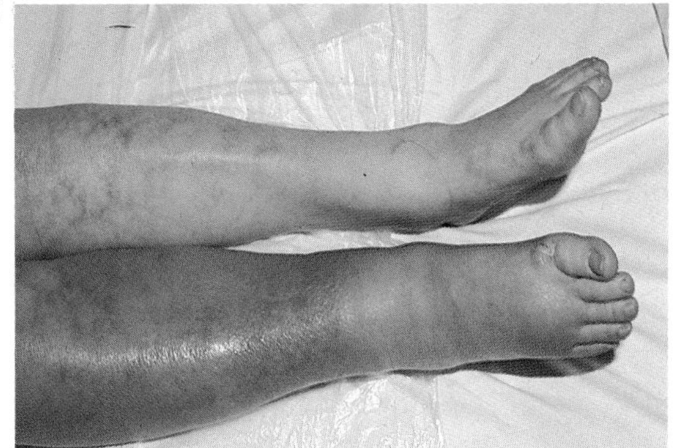

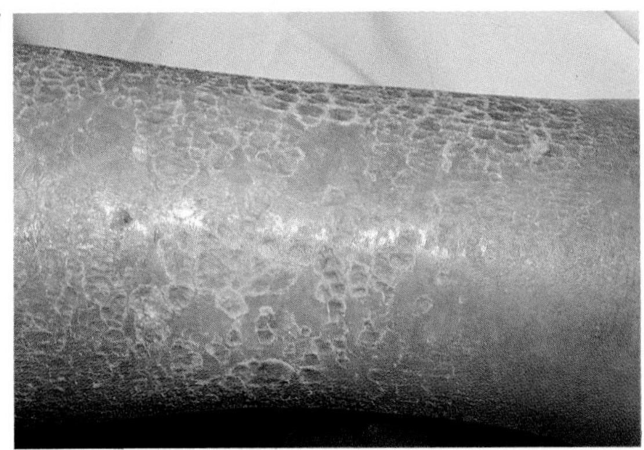

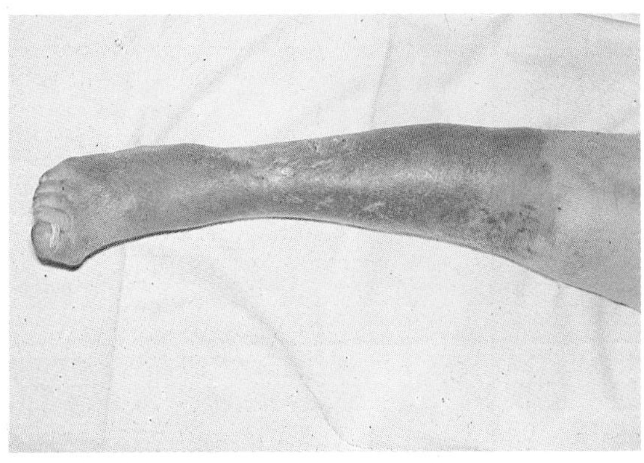

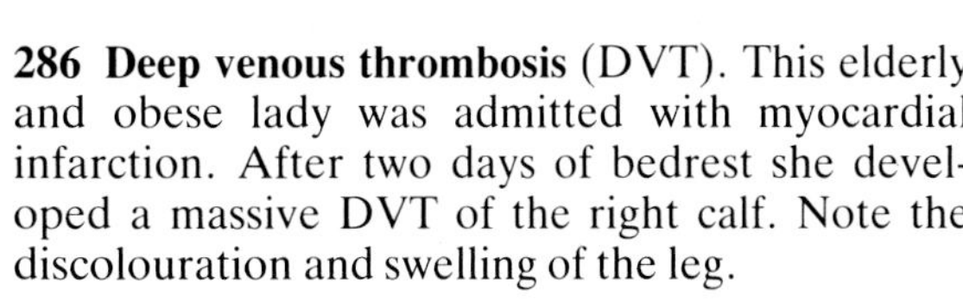

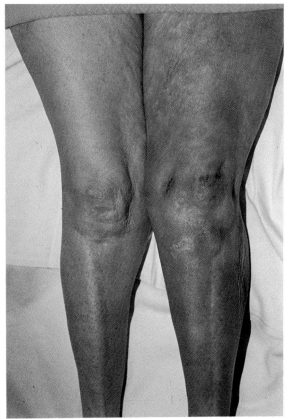

286 Deep venous thrombosis (DVT). This elderly and obese lady was admitted with myocardial infarction. After two days of bedrest she developed a massive DVT of the right calf. Note the discolouration and swelling of the leg.

287 Post-phlebitic leg. Dry, thin, scaly skin with oedema and pigmentation caused by haemosiderin deposit in subcutaneous tissues.

288 Cellulitis. Considerable soft-tissue inflammation with pain and fever as a result of a minor trauma to the foot.

289 Ischaemia of the left leg. Sudden arterial occlusion caused by femoral artery thrombosis. The leg may be saved with early vascular surgery.

Deep vein thrombosis

Important aetiological factors:
- Bedrest and immobility
- Postoperative
- Occult cancers, e.g. cancer of pancreas
- Thrombophlebitis migrans
- Paget-Schrotter's disease – in arms
- Phlegmasia caerulea dolens
- Obesity
- Lymphomas
- Dehydration
- Congestive cardiac failure

290

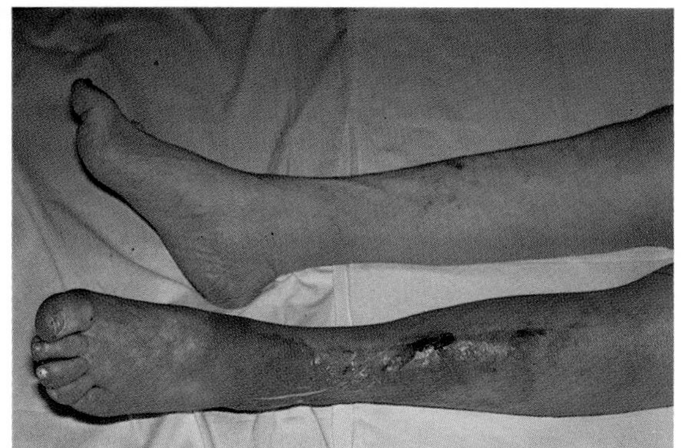

291

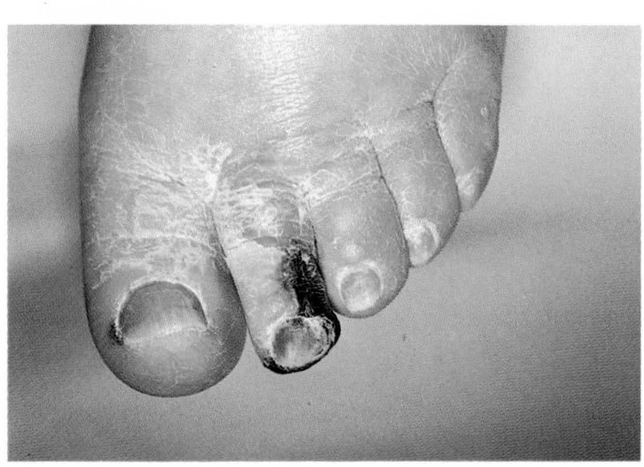

292

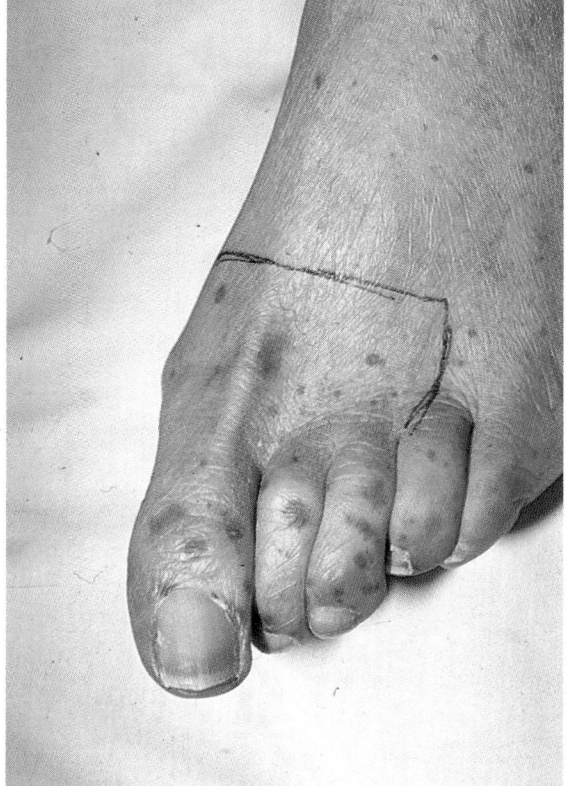

Peripheral vascular disease

Aetiology

Atherosclerosis, embolism, diabetic microangiopathy, giant-cell arteritis, vasculitis with collagen diseases, Buerger's disease, cold injury, increased blood viscosity, e.g. polycythemia, dysproteinaemias, Beta-blocking drugs

Clinical features

Asymptomatic in the early stages
Cold feet, feelings of numbness
Parasthaesia in feet
Intermittent claudication
Rest pain
Large blood vessel bruits
Loss of peripheral pulses
Cyanosis
Ischaemic ulcers
Gangrene

Some changes in bacterial endocarditis in the last 20 years in the UK

1 More common in elderly now. In 1945, 18 per cent of patients were over 60 years of age, but now 25 per cent are over 60 years of age. Prognosis is usually poor with mortality of 70 per cent and frequently occurs as a terminal illness.
2 Streptococcus viridians is still the commonest causative organism but relatively less than before – still over 50 per cent.
3 The underlying heart disease is now less often rheumatic mitral disease and is more frequently aortic valve disease of uncertain aetiology.

293

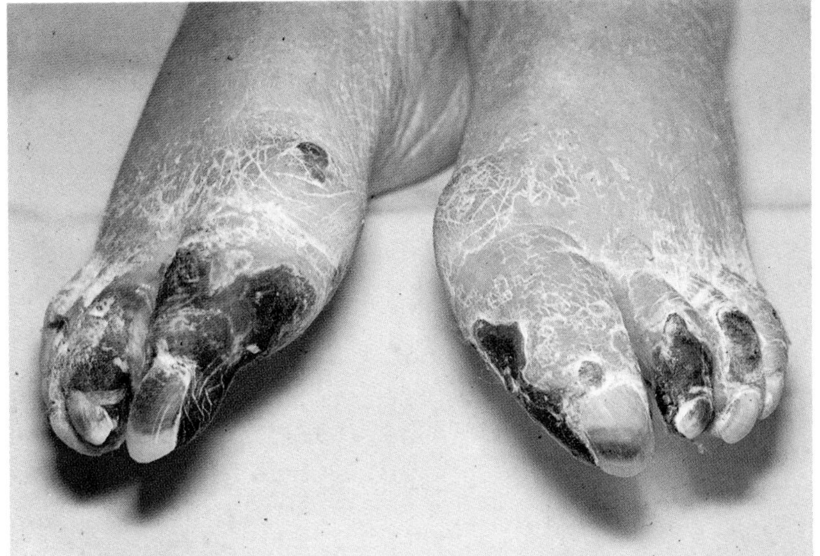

294

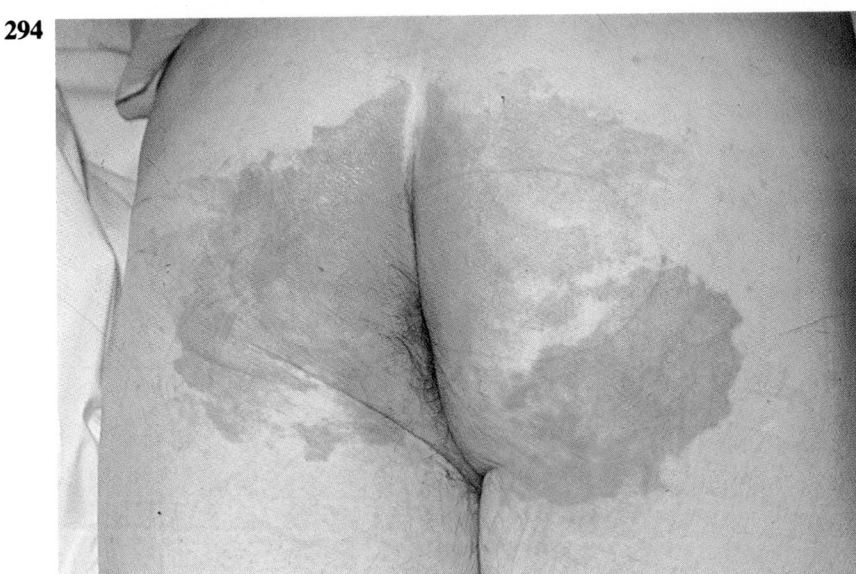

290 Acute arterial occlusion. Caused by atheroma in the femoral artery secondary to an abdominal aneurysm. The tissues of the leg are non-viable and early surgical intervention is required.

291 Peripheral vascular disease. There is ischaemic necrosis of the second toe, with dystrophy of the toenails and the skin is shiny and atrophic. The dorsalis pedis artery was not palpable.

292 Subacute bacterial endocarditis. Showing small embolic infarcts on the toes. The patient had low-grade fever, anaemia, and mild cardiac failure. The blood cultures were positive for streptococcus viridans.

293 Polyarteritis nodosa. Severe vasculitis resulting in ischaemic necrosis of the toes. The patient also had arthralgia, renal involvement, and hypertension. Several toes had to be amputated, but postoperatively the patient made a good recovery.

294 Urinary rash. Skin rash caused by urinary incontinence. Untreated, this can predispose to a pressure sore in an immobile patient.

295
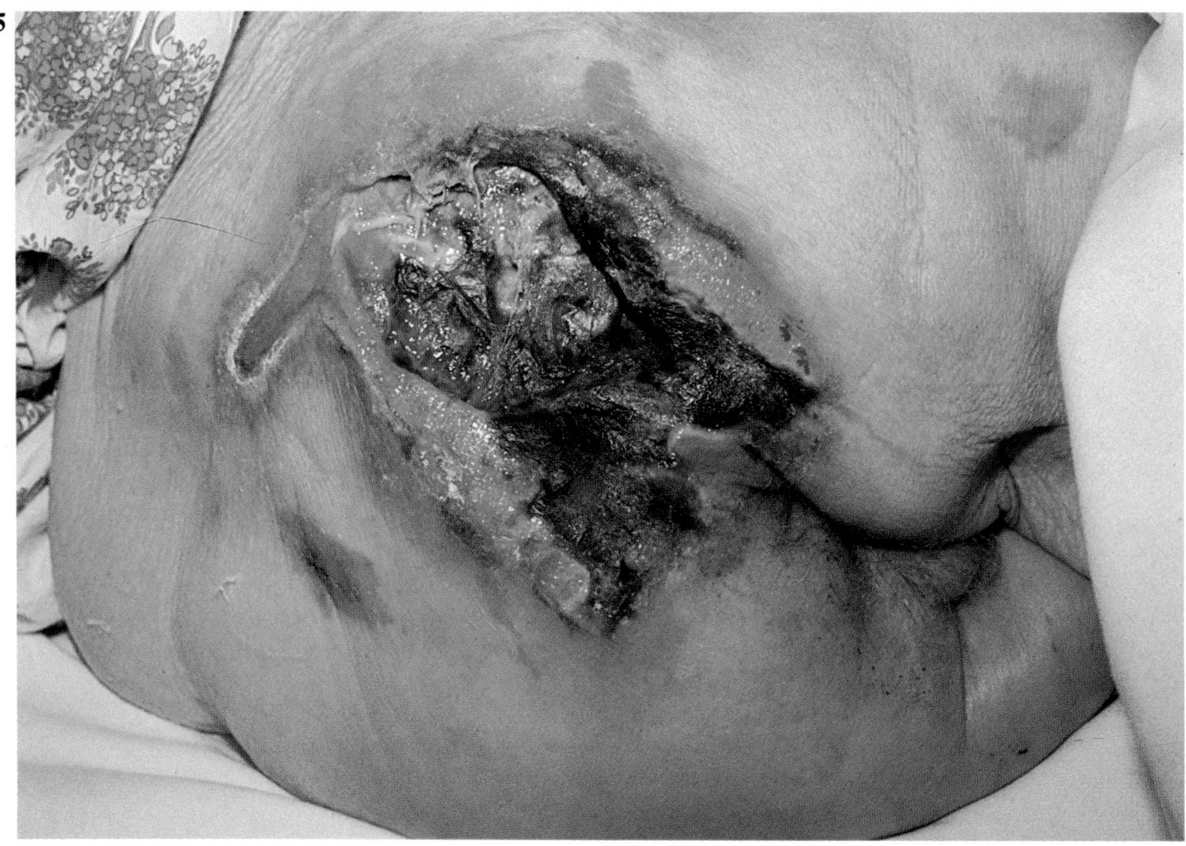

Pressure sores

Two main types:

A Superficial – good prognosis if actively treated
B Deep-tissue necrosis present

Predisposing factors

Mainly compression and shearing forces, plus:

1 Poor tissue perfusion
2 Immobility and paresis – CVAs, arthritis, fractures
3 Poor general health – malnutrition, anaemias, carcinomas
4 Hypoxaemia
5 Urinary incontinence causing skin maceration

Exton-Smith's clinical score for patients at risk

Patients scoring over 7 points are considered to be at risk.

General condition	*Mental state*	*Activity*	*Mobility*	*Incontinence*
0 Good	0 Alert	0 Ambulant	0 Full	0 None
1 Fair	1 Confused	1 Walks with help	1 Slightly decreased	1 Occasional
2 Poor	2 Apathetic	2 Chairfast	2 Very decreased	2 Incontinent urine
3 Bad	3 Stuporous	3 Bedfast	3 Immobile	3 Doubly incontinent

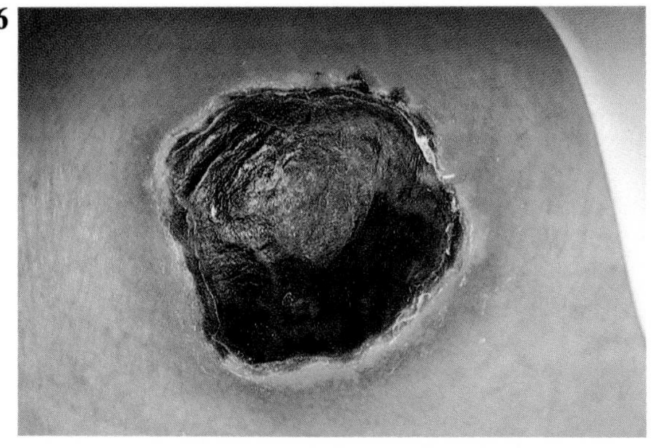

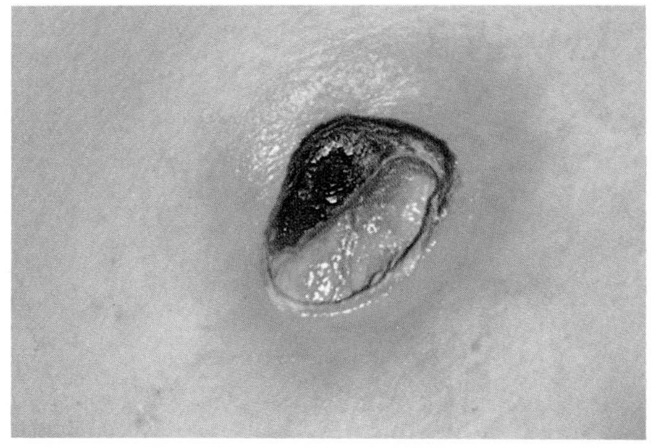

295 Pressure sore (decubitus ulcer). A large, deep, necrotic pressure sore over the sacral area. This resulted from immobility, urinary incontinence, dementia, poor nutrition, and general debility.

296 Pressure sore over the ischeal tuberosity with dry, black scab.

297 Pressure sore that is gradually healing. Note the appearance of new skin around the edges of the sore.

298 Oedema of the foot. Mild to moderate oedema of the feet is a common phenomenon in the elderly, especially in those who are immobile. Posture, gravitation, and poor venous return contribute to produce such dependant oedema.

299 Ill-fitting footwear. The sore areas on the toes are the result of wearing old, wornout shoes. Such lesions may become infected if there is poor foot hygiene. In the elderly, they may cause falls and immobility.

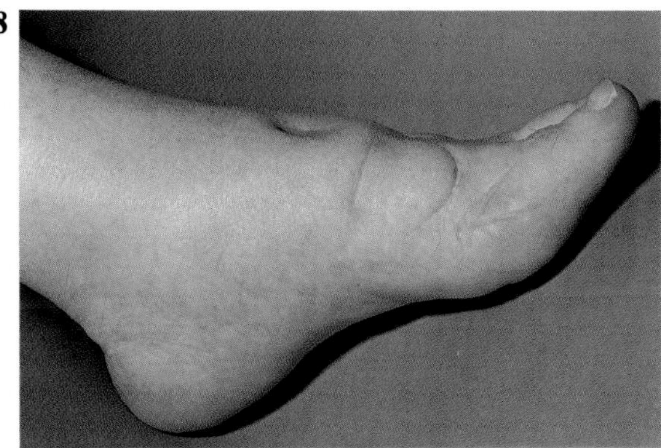

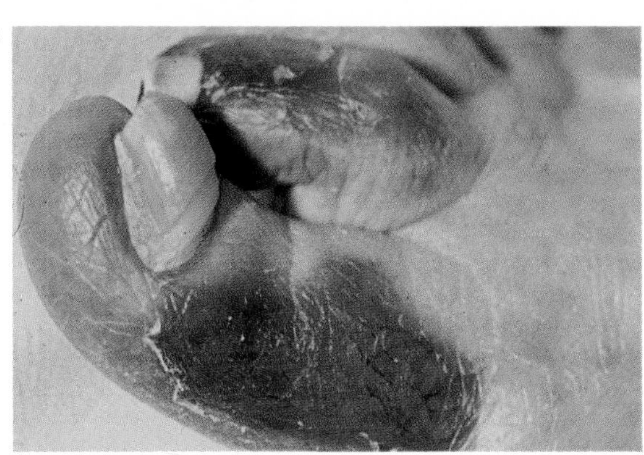

Peripheral oedema

1 Cardiovascular
- CCF
- Venous thrombosis
- Incompetent venous valves
- Cellulitis
- Immobility – gravitational

2 Lymphatic obstruction
- Neoplastic lymph nodes in groin
- Pelvic tumours
- Post-cellulitis

3 Hepatic failure

4 Renal – nephrotic syndrome

5 Hypoalbuminaemia

6 Drugs
- Steroids
- Carbenoxolone
- Indomethacin
- Phenylbutazone
- Oestrogens

300

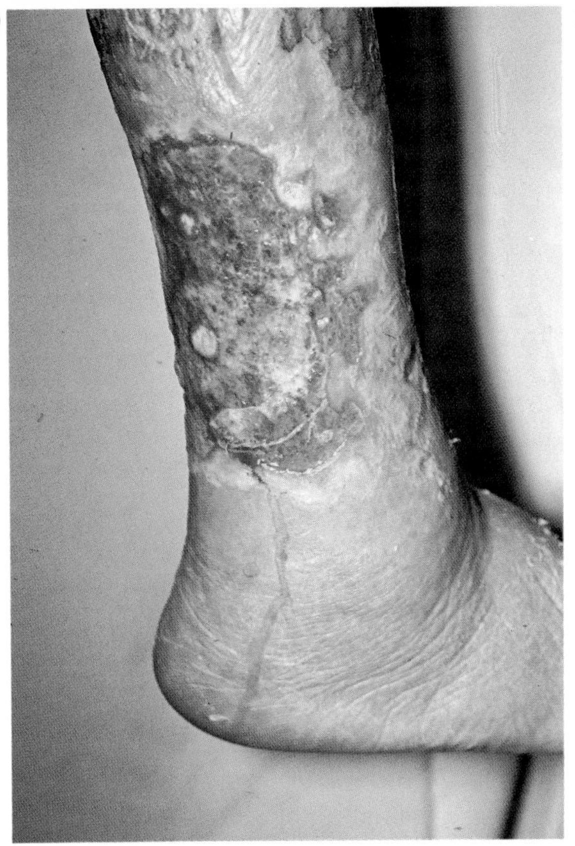

301

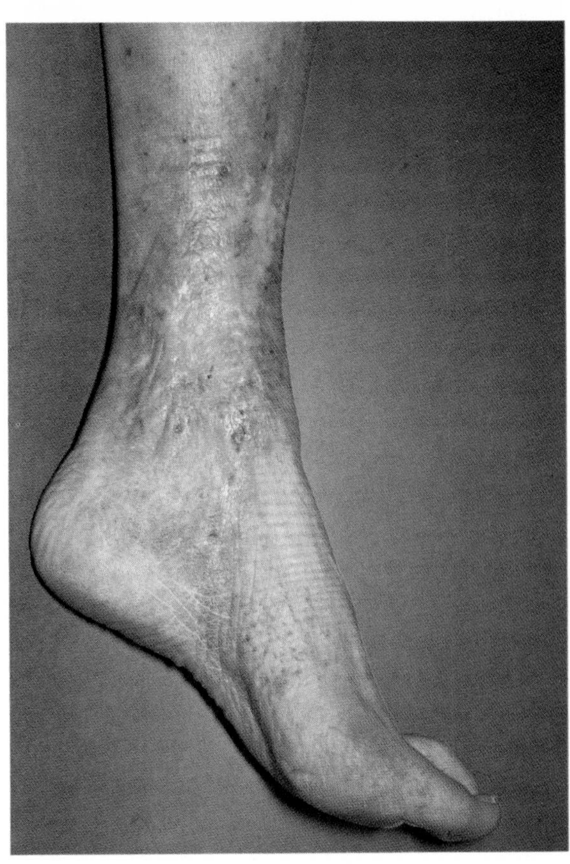

300 Varicose ulcer as a result of post-phlebitic syndrome. Such ulcers are slow to heal and require patient, meticulous nursing care.

301 Healed varicose ulcer. Note the clean healthy skin on the area where there was once a large varicose ulcer. Apart from prolonged nursing care and leg exercises, this patient also required treatment for anaemia.

Chronic leg ulcers in the elderly

Important aetiological factors:

- Varicose veins and impaired venous drainage
- Peripheral vascular disease plus poor foot hygiene, plus trauma
- Pressure sores, especially on heels
- Burns, e.g. erythema ab igne
- Neuropathy
- Ulcerating gouty tophi
- Pemphigus and pemphigoid
- Tumours, e.g. melanoma, basal-cell carcinoma
- Vasculitis, e.g. rheumatoid arthritis
- Dysproteinaemias
- Steroids
- Pyoderma gangrenosum

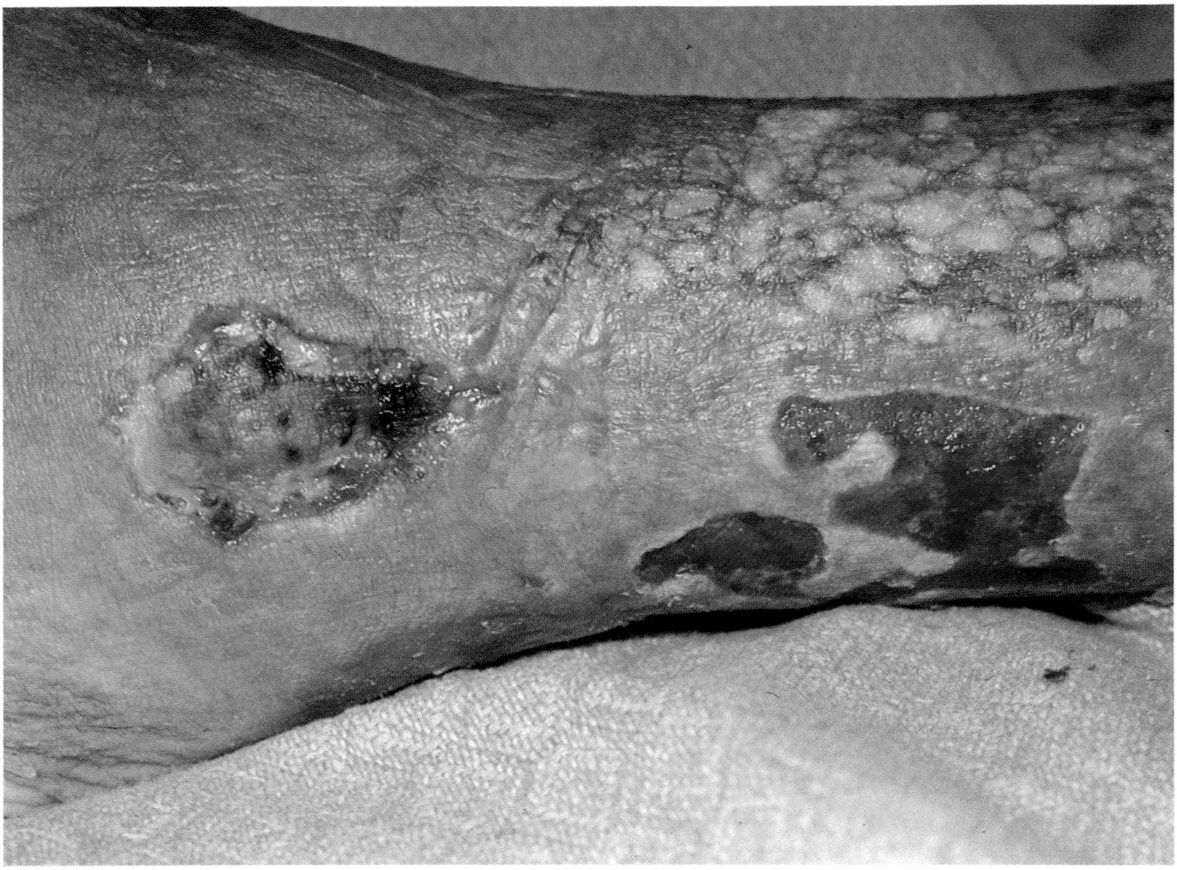

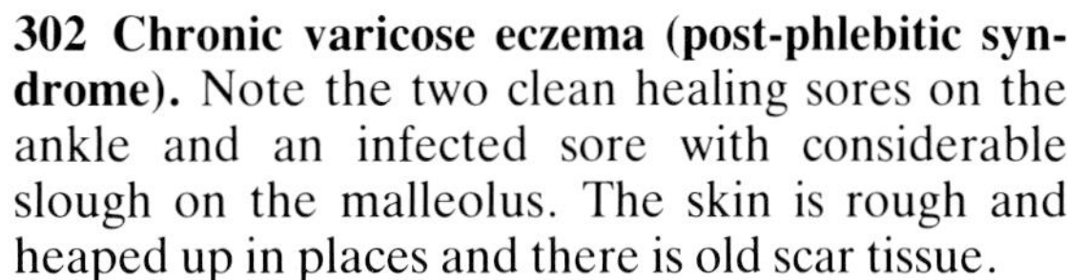

302 Chronic varicose eczema (post-phlebitic syndrome). Note the two clean healing sores on the ankle and an infected sore with considerable slough on the malleolus. The skin is rough and heaped up in places and there is old scar tissue.

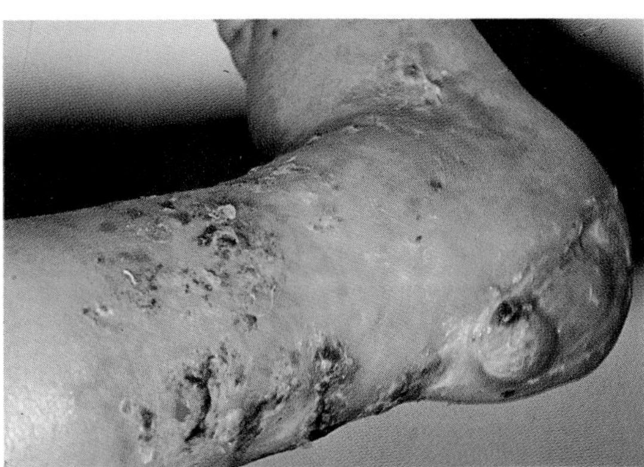

303 Chronic varicose eczema (post-phlebitic syndrome). The foot and ankle are affected. There are varicose ulcers surrounded by weeping, scaly, and sticky skin.

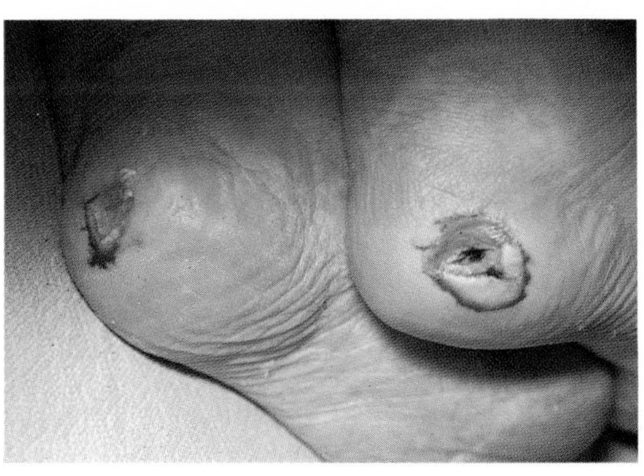

304 Heel sores. These ulcers are pressure sores. Contributory factors are stasis, arterial insufficiency, obesity, and general ill health.

305

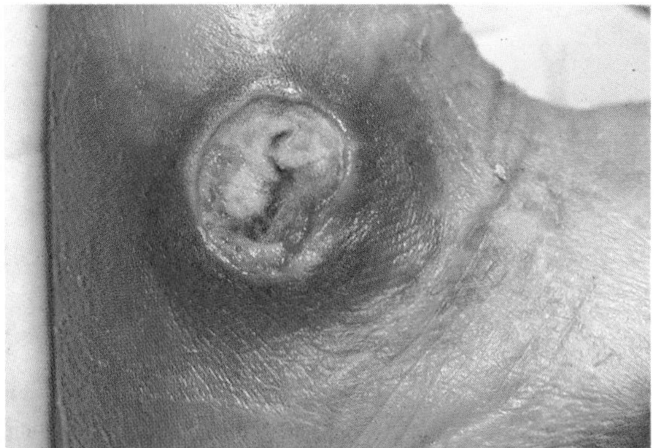

305 Diabetic ulcer on the lateral malleolus of an elderly diabetic. Note the clean edges of the sore. Such lesions are essentially arterial and occur with small-vessel disease.

306

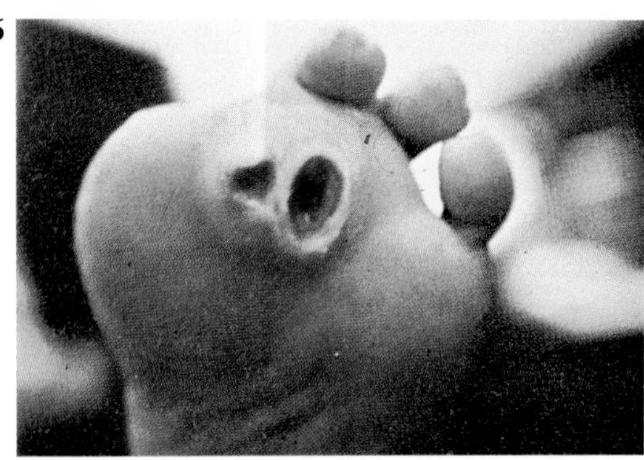

306 Diabetic ulcers on the sole of the foot. Note the two missing toes which had to be amputated.

307

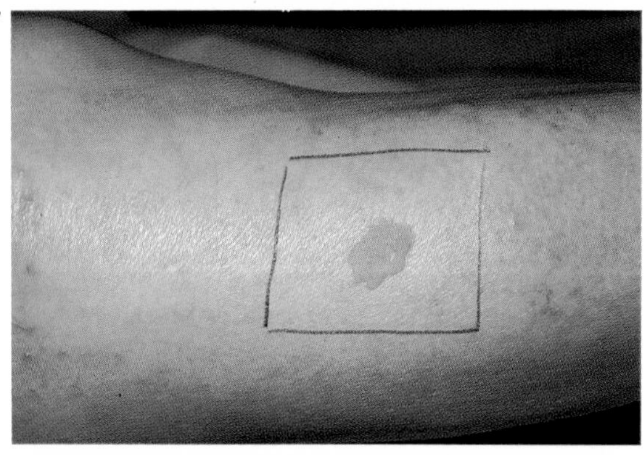

307 Xanthoma. Xanthomatous deposit below the knee joint. It consists of lipid accumulating in the tissues in association with large foam cells. This patient presented with a history of ischaemic heart disease.

308

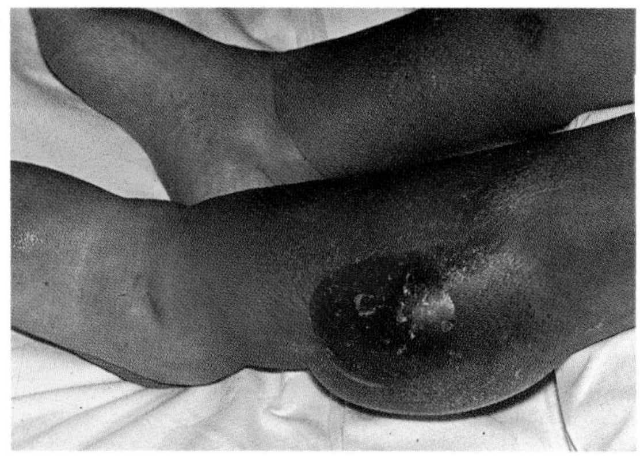

308 Traumatic bulla. A large blood blister caused by a fall in an elderly lady who was on longterm corticosteroid treatment for chronic asthma.

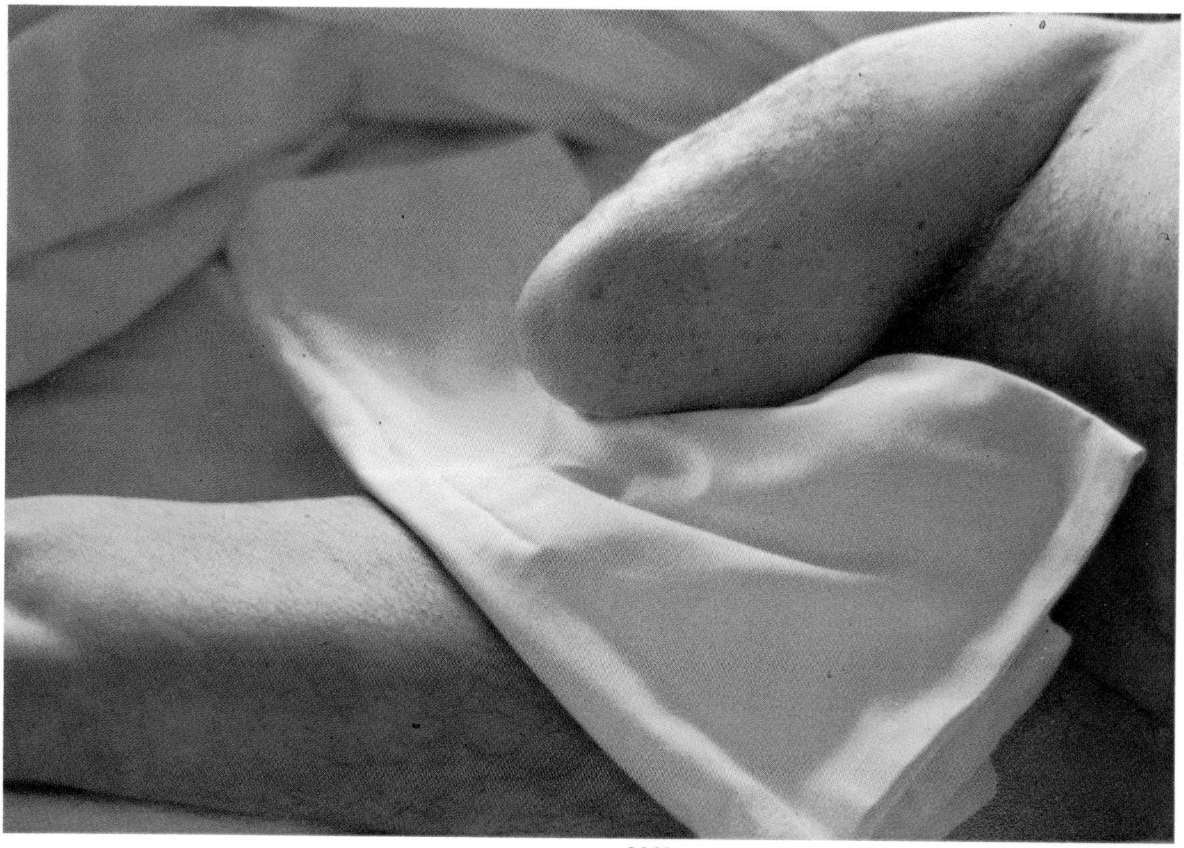

309a Above-knee amputation. This patient had ischaemic necrosis of the right foot. After amputation the patient required prolonged rehabilitation by a multidisciplinary team.

309b Ischaemic necrosis. Result of severe peripheral vascular disease caused by atherosclerosis. This patient required below-knee amputation.

309b

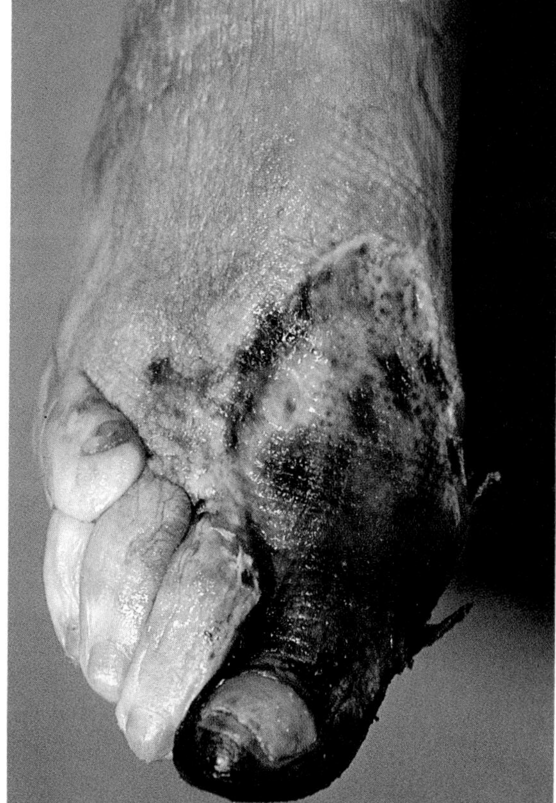

Problems after a limb amputation

1 Phantom limb sensations and pains
2 Grief and depression
3 Psychosocial problems and loss of occupation
4 Negative attitudes to the prosthesis

310

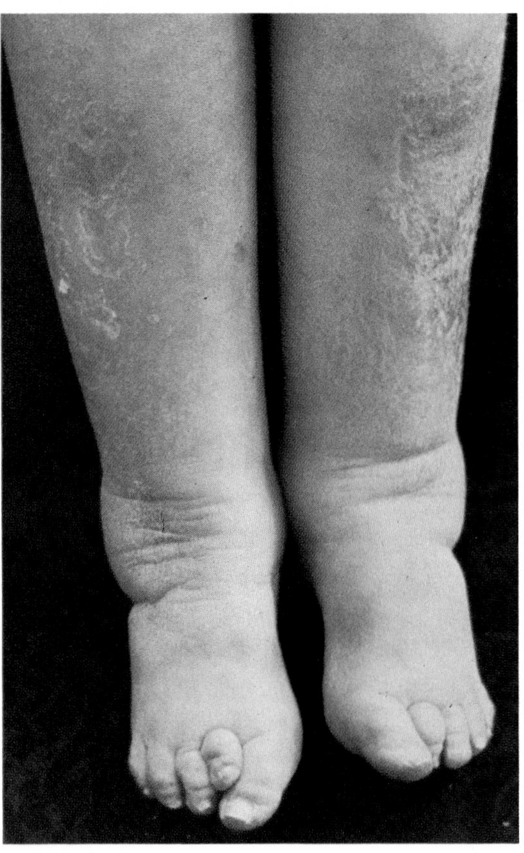

311

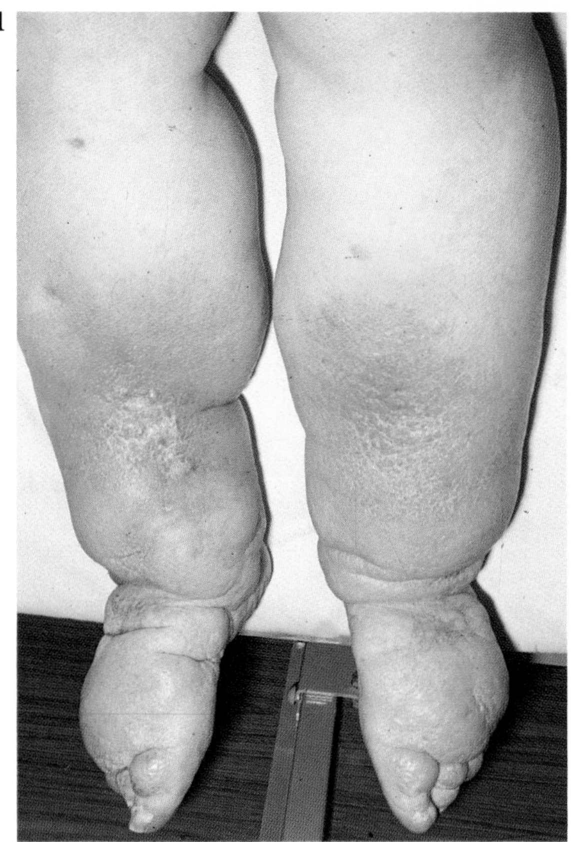

310 Lymphoedema of the legs. Post-thrombotic accumulation of lymph in the extremeties. The oedema is non-pitting and resistant to diuretic therapy.

311 Lymphoedema of the legs. An advanced case resulting from a combination of Milroy's disease, stasis, venous insufficiency, and chronic congestive cardiac failure.

312

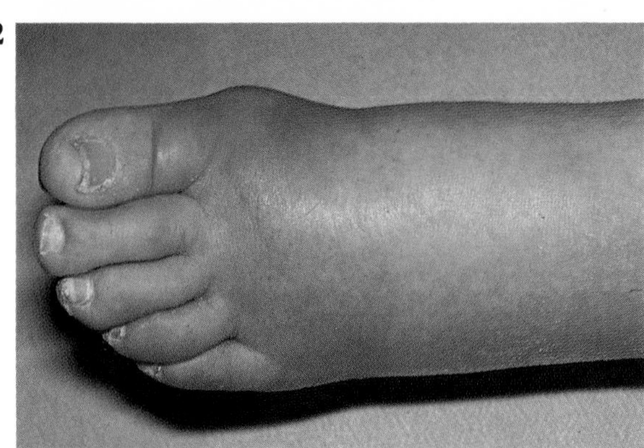

312 Gout. A classical attack of acute gout affecting the big toe and accompanied by fever and sickness. This elderly patient was obese and had a past history of renal stones.

313

313 Gout. Histology of tophus showing deposits of uric acid crystals surrounded by inflammatory infiltration.

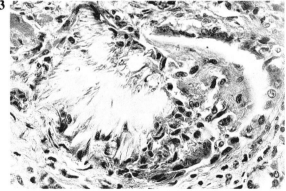

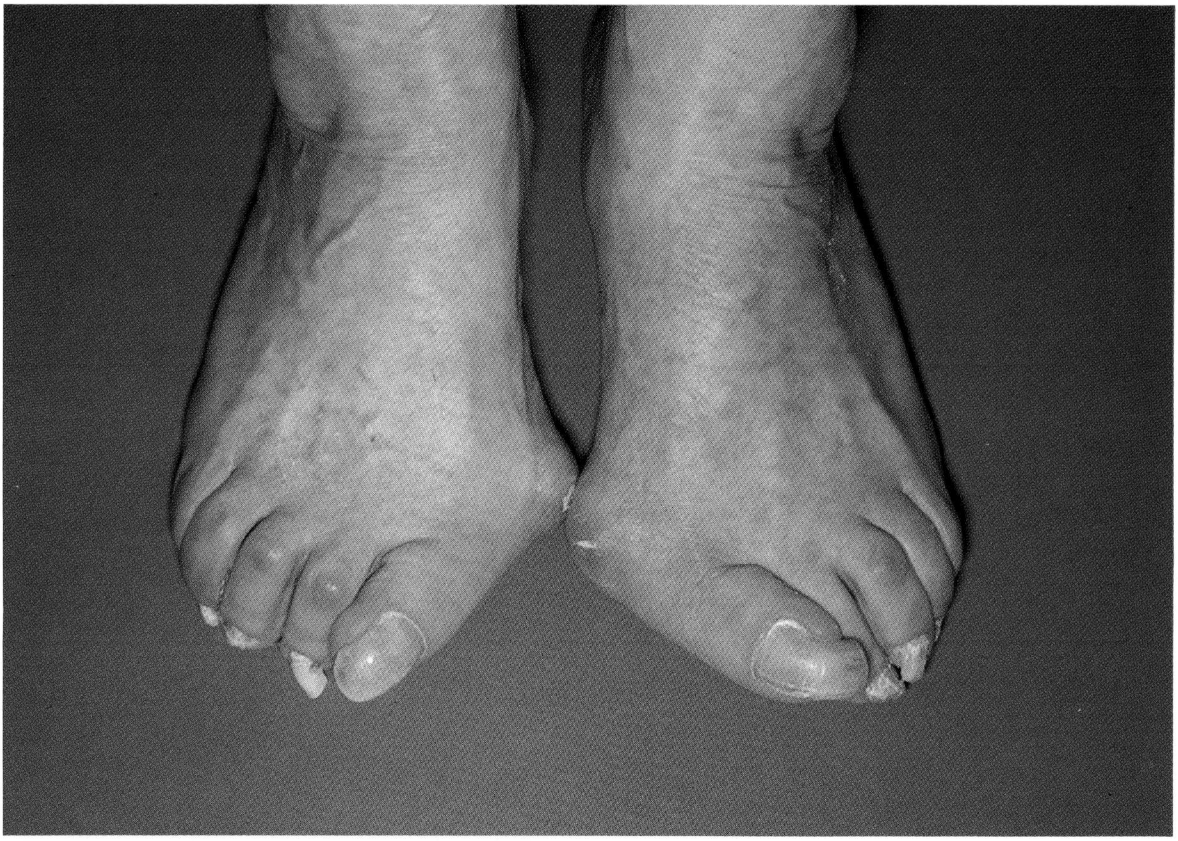

314 Multiple foot problems. Feet of an elderly lady showing onychogryphosis, hallux valgus, and bunions.

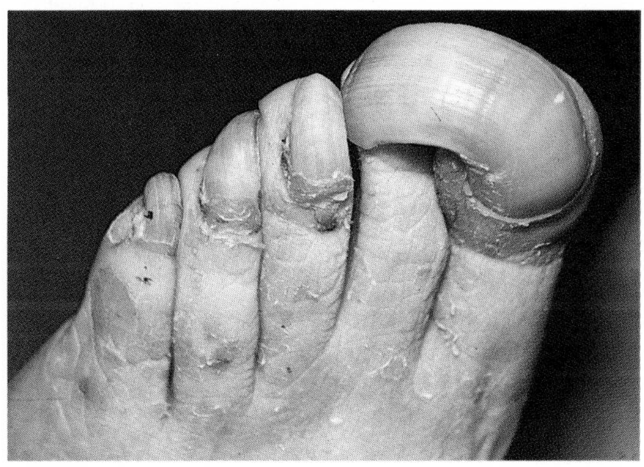

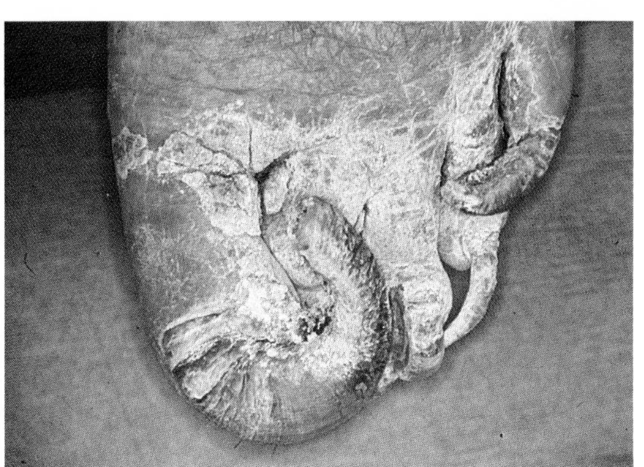

315 and 316 Onychogryphosis. Overgrown, claw-like toenails causing discomfort on walking, immobility, and falls. It is usually a sign of extreme neglect and deprivation.

Such patients require a thorough geriatric assessment with a full investigation of their social background and living conditions. Expert chiropody will be necessary in these cases.

317
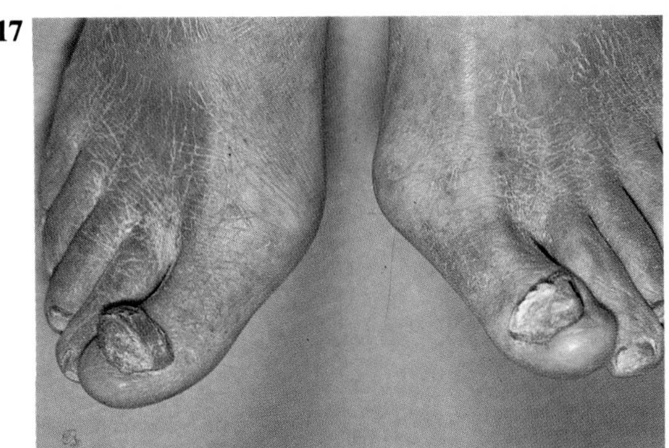

317 Nail dystrophy. Brittle, rough, and deformed toenails in a case of peripheral vascular disease and venous insufficiency. Note bilateral hallux valgus.

318
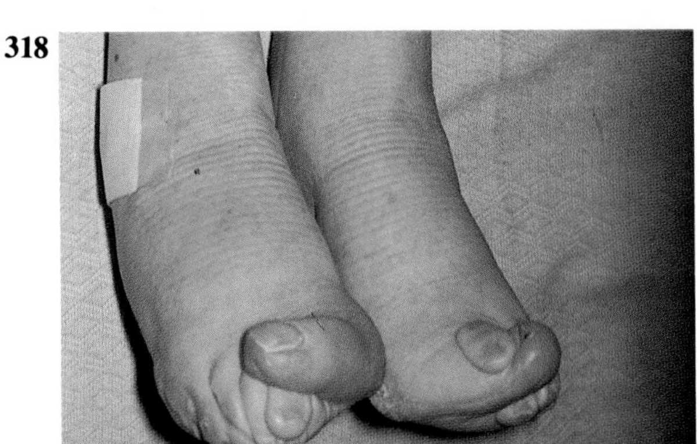

319

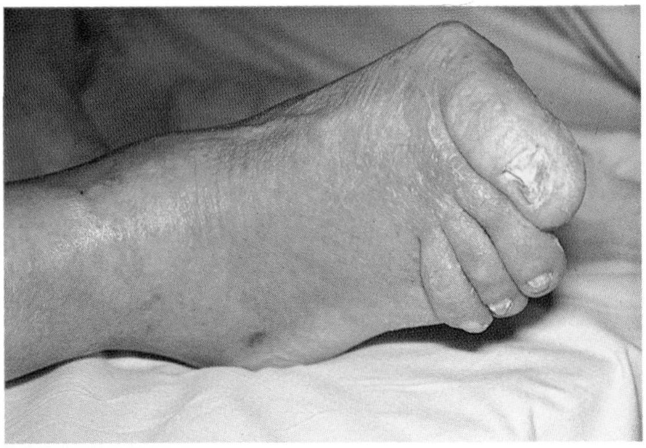

320
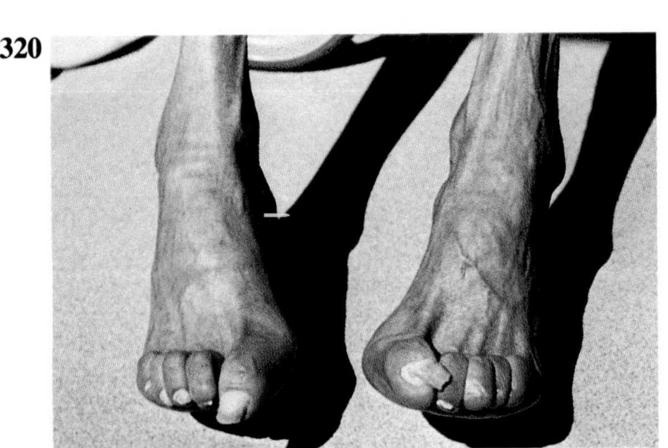

318 Bilateral hallux valgus. A common orthopaedic problem in the feet of the elderly. The big toe is abducted so that it lies on top of the other toes. Marked prominence of the first metatarsophalangeal joint occurs with the bony enlargement of the inner side of the first metatarsal head.

319 Hallux valgus. A bursa (bunion) has formed over the enlarged first metatarsal head. This is painful, interferes with mobility, and may ulcerate.

321
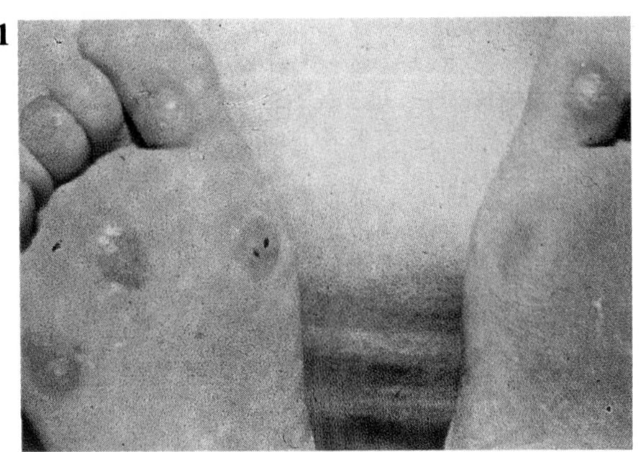

320 Hammer toes. A common problem in the elderly usually caused by prolonged use of ill-fitting footwear.

321 Corns on the sole of feet, causing pain on walking.

2

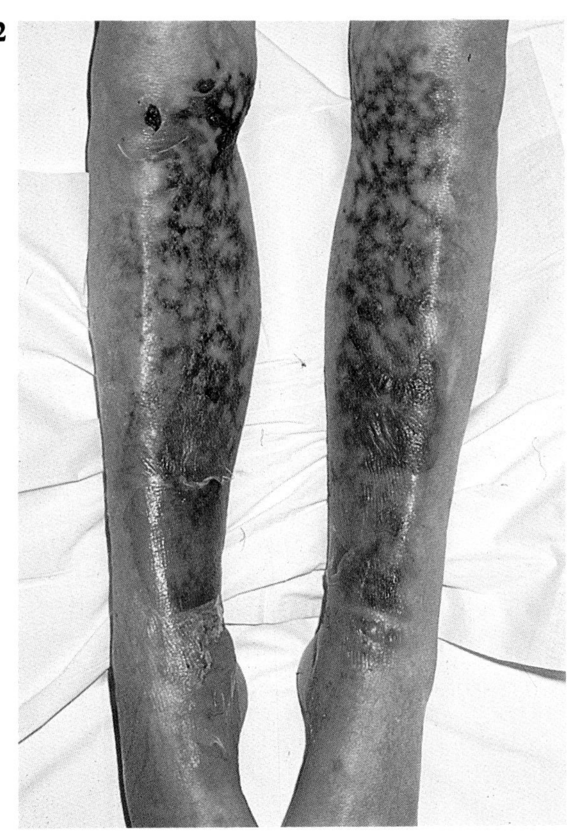

322 Erythema ab igne. The result of sitting too close to a fire. The condition is commonly seen in old people who live in cold houses and have a tendency to sit too near the fire for long periods. Such patients should be investigated for hypothyroidism.

323 Erythema ab igne showing an area of superficial burn.

3

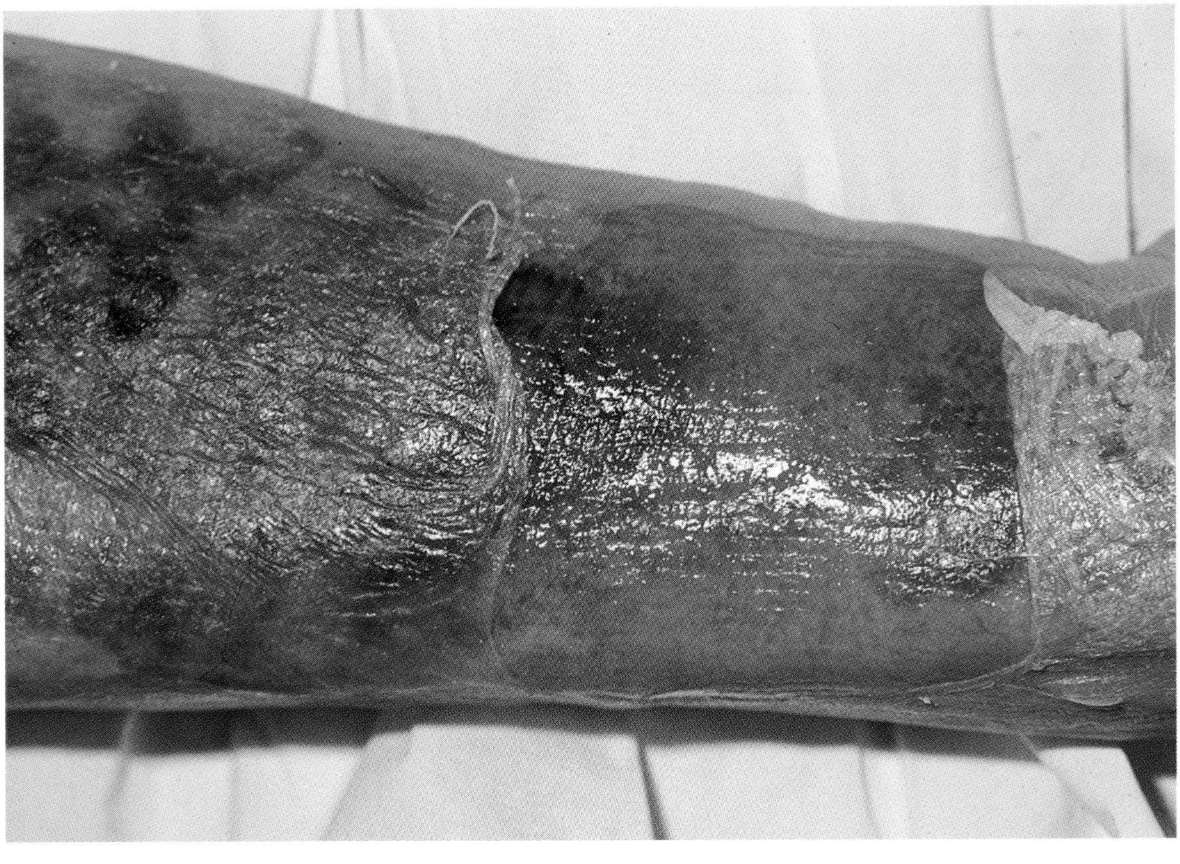

10 Disorders of the skin

324 Dry skin (asteatosis). Dry, tissue-like, atrophic skin caused by the loss of collagen and associated with advancing age.

325 Loose skin. A sign of ageing exaggerated by weightloss and dehydration.

326 Dry skin (ichthyosis). Dry skin with cracks in stratum corneum and rhomboidal scales with flaky edges. The histopathologic changes consist of epidermal atrophy and hyperkeratosis. This condition sometimes occurs in association with lymphoma, but in the elderly it is usually chronic and benign.

327 Prominent capillary network. Telangiectasia-like vascular pattern on the cheeks of an elderly man. This is a type of benign degenerative change seen more frequently in white-skinned people who are exposed to high-intensity ultraviolet radiation.

324

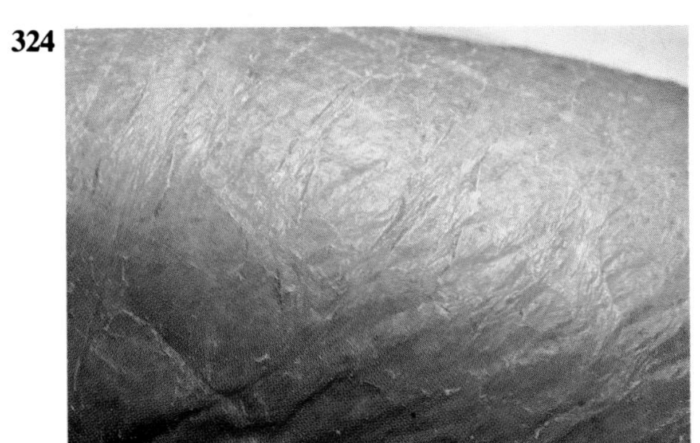

325

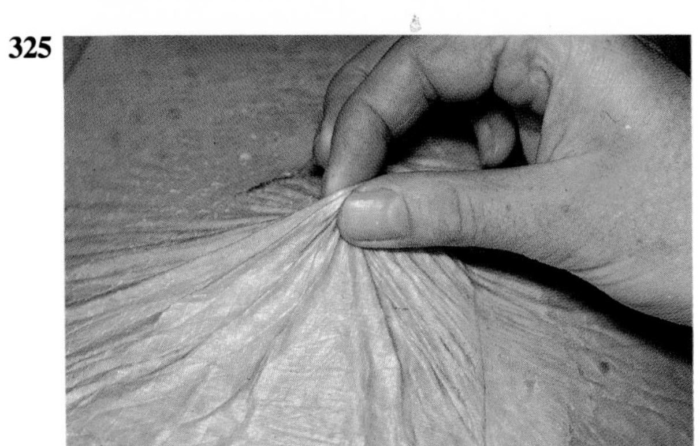

326

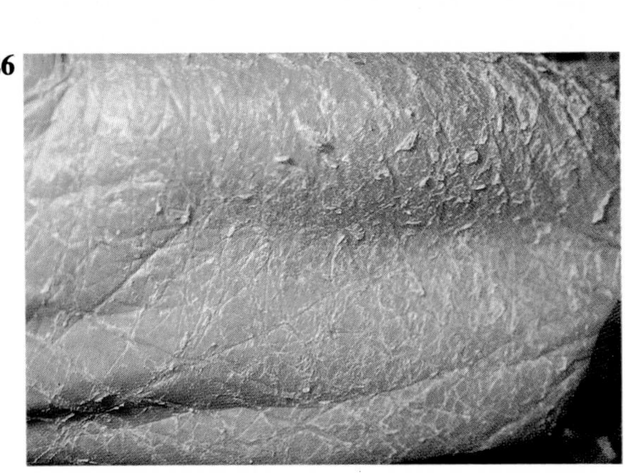

327

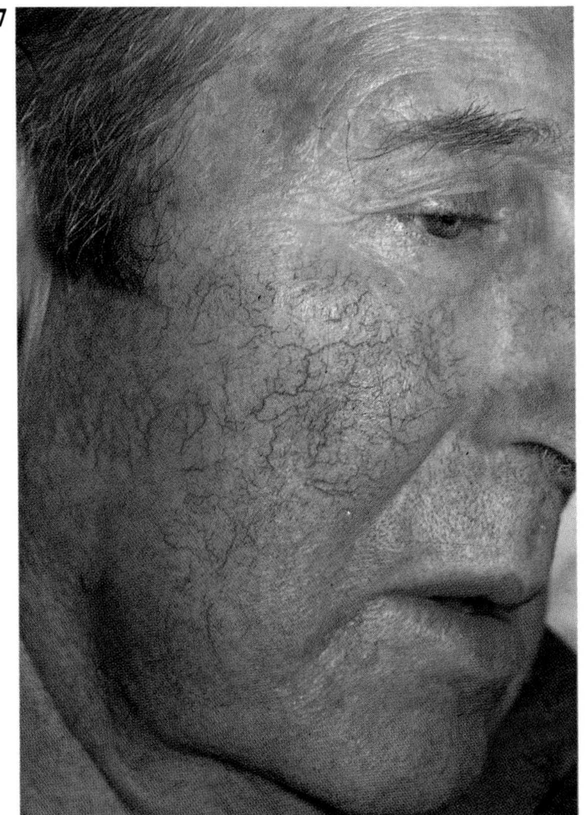

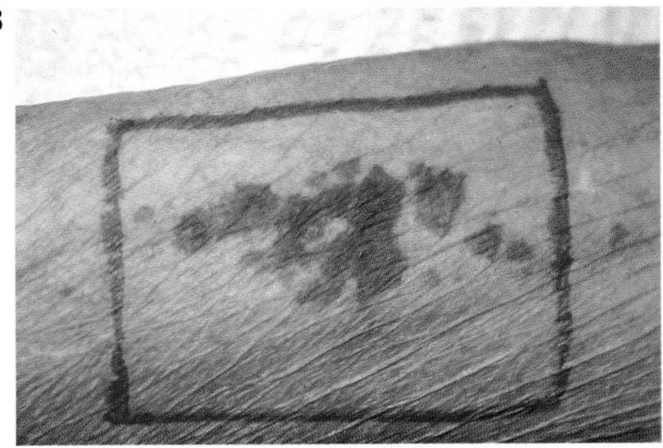

328 Senile purpura caused by a combination of increased capillary fragility, atrophic skin, and trauma. Typically skin on the dorsum of the hands and the extensor surfaces of arms. Tests for clotting mechanism are normal in such cases.

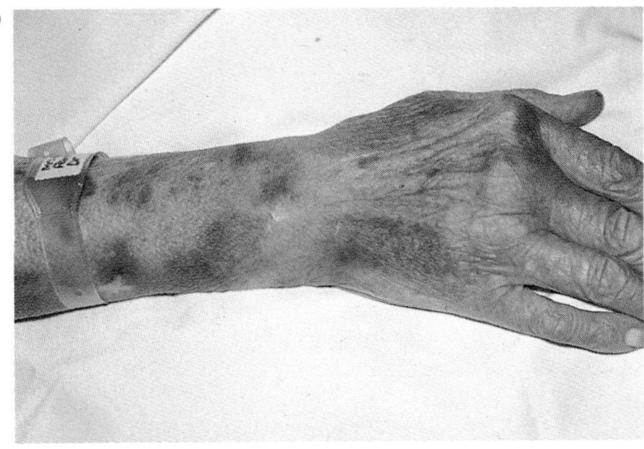

329 Steroid purpura. Large recurrent bruises on the forearm induced by long-term corticosteroid therapy.

330 Drug-induced purpura. Purpuric rash caused by damage to capillary endothelium induced by penicillin. The platelet count and bleeding time are usually normal.

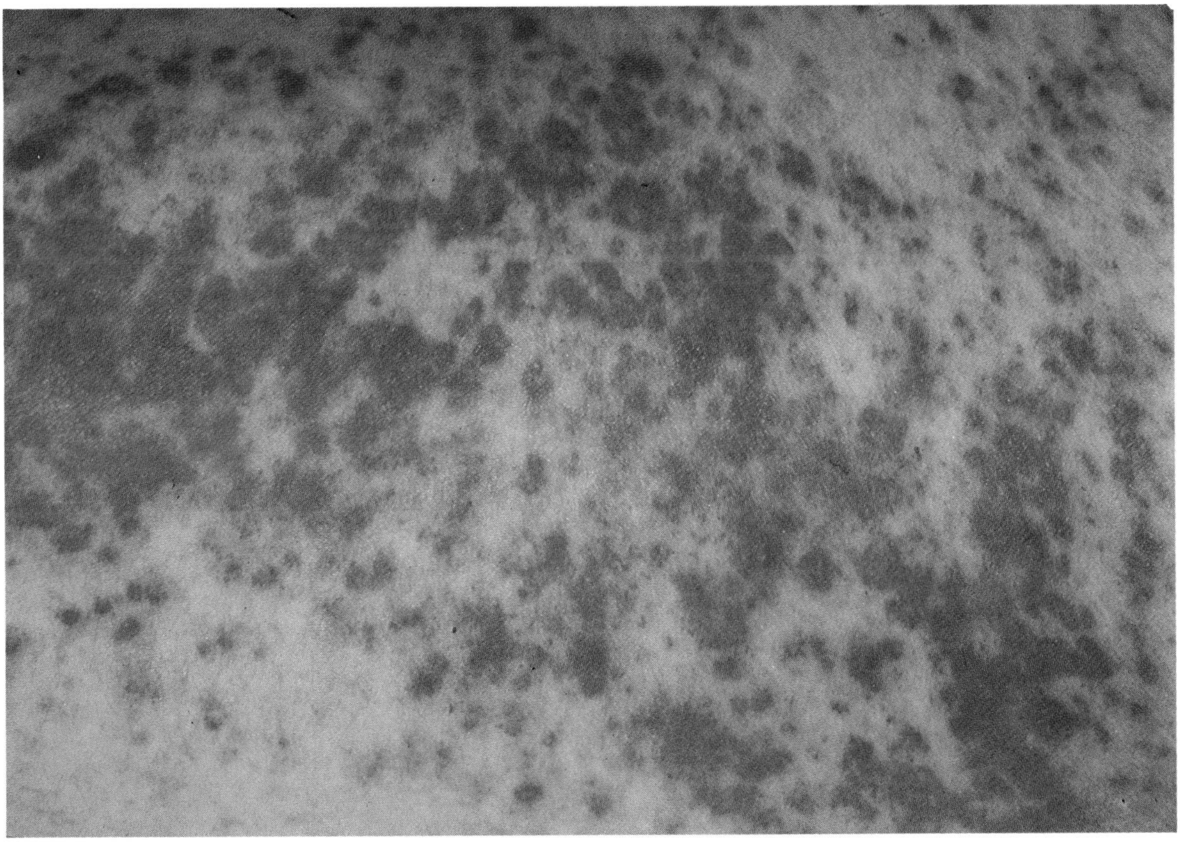

331a

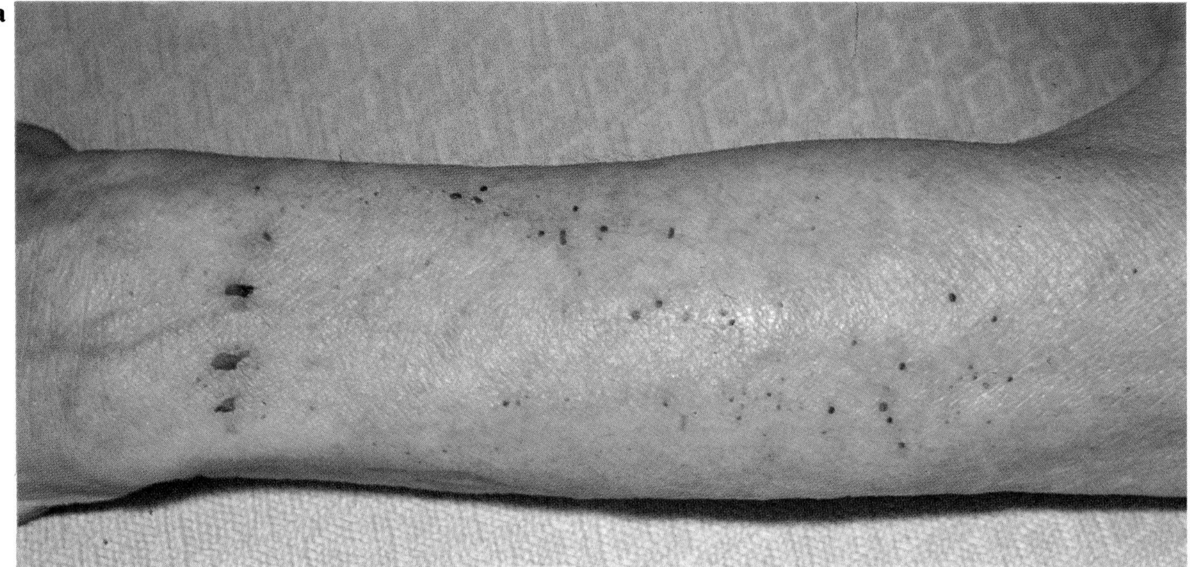

331b

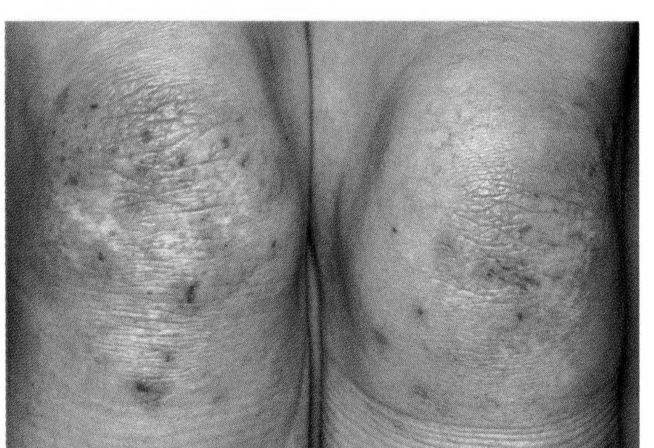

332

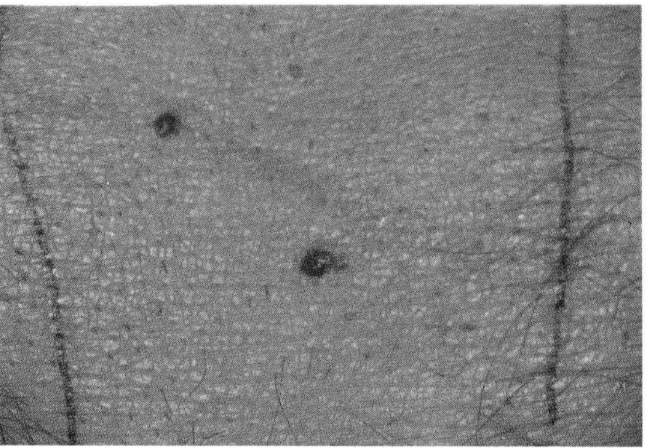

331a Pruritus caused by a combination of iron-deficiency anaemia and dry skin (asteatosis) in an elderly man.

331b Lichen simplex. A frequent cause of chronic pruritus with no obvious aetiology. Sometimes also called 'neurodermatitis'.

332 Senile angiomas (Campbell-de-Morgan spots). Small, bright red, raised spots on the skin of the trunk and shoulders. This condition is common in elderly male Caucasians and has no pathological significance.

Pruritus in the elderly

A *Skin diseases*
- Scabies, insect bites, pediculosis
- Eczema
- Lichen planus
- Dermatitis herpetiformis
- Lichen simplex

B *Systemic causes*
1. Hepatic, e.g. obstructive jaundice
2. Chronic renal failure
3. Endocrine, e.g. myxoedema, hyperthyroidism
4. Blood diseases, e.g. malignant lymphoma, myeloproliferative disorders, iron deficiency
5. Cancer, e.g. lung, stomach, colon
6. Drugs, e.g. allergic drug reactions, morphine
7. Psychogenic — 'senile pruritus'

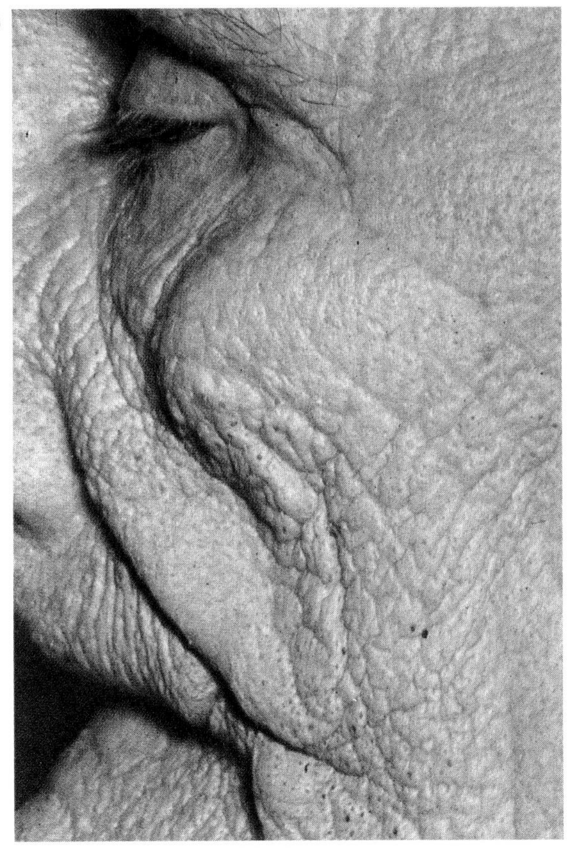

334

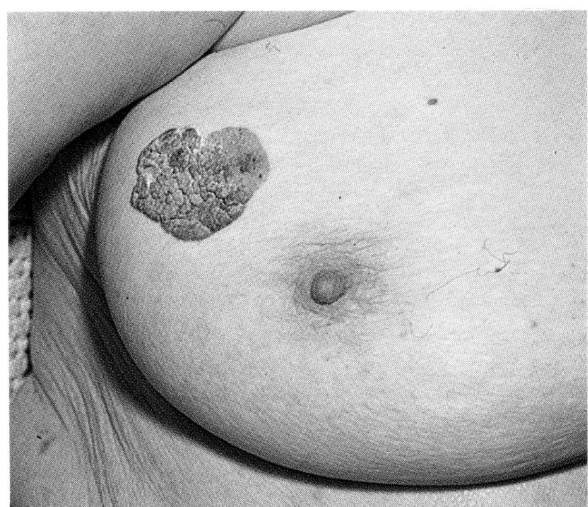

333 Solar elastotic degenerative change. Excessive wrinkling of the skin caused by changes in dermal collagen. It occurs after lifelong exposure to environmental factors, particularly sunlight.

334 Seborrhoeic wart (senile wart). Papillomatous, greasy, friable, and dark warty lesion. Increasingly common with ageing and appears predominantly on the unexposed Caucasian skin. The growth is benign.

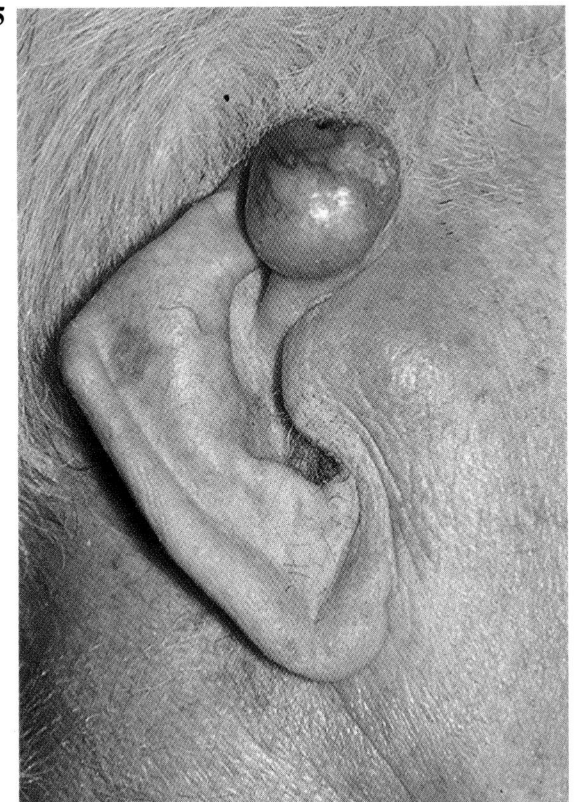

335 and 336 Basal-cell epithelioma. Commonest skin cancer in the white races. Arises from the epidermal or hair follicle cells of the face. The lesion is invasive but metastases are rare. Predisposing factors are mainly actinic radiation and rarely epidermal naevi and xeroderma pigmentosum.

336

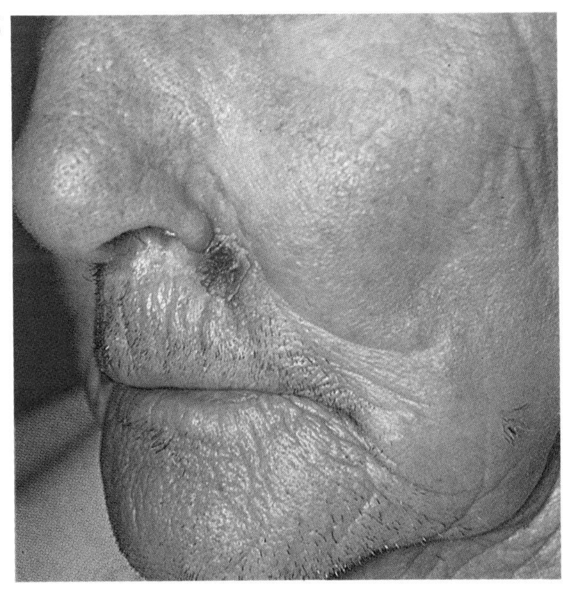

337

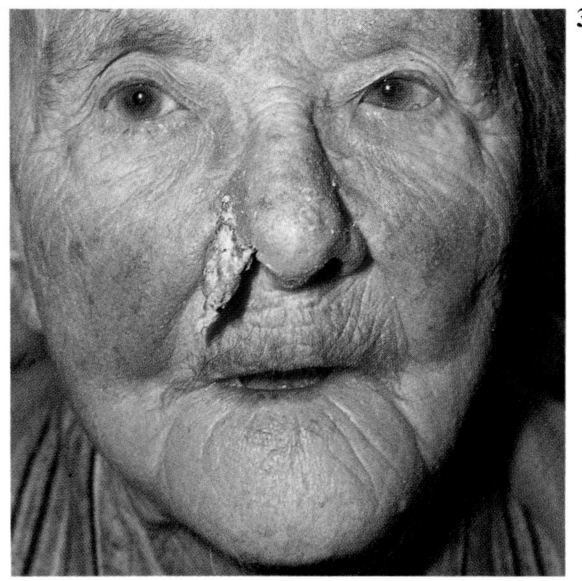

338

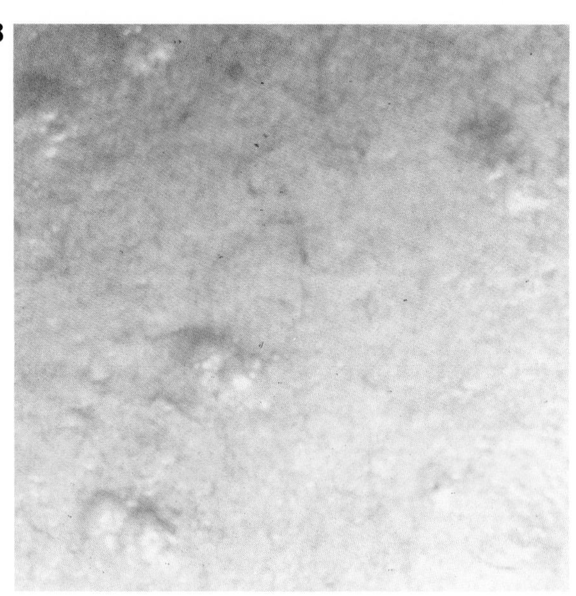

337 Squamous-cell epithelioma. This tumour of the epidermis and mucosae arises in premalignant sun-damaged skin. It is locally invasive and likely to metastasise. In this case there is a large mass arising from the nostril.

338 Senile sebaceous gland hyperplasia. A benign condition occurring in the elderly and sometimes confused with other skin diseases.

339a

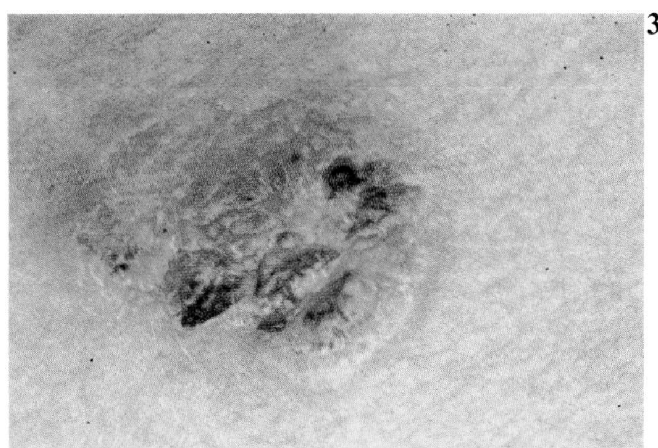

339b

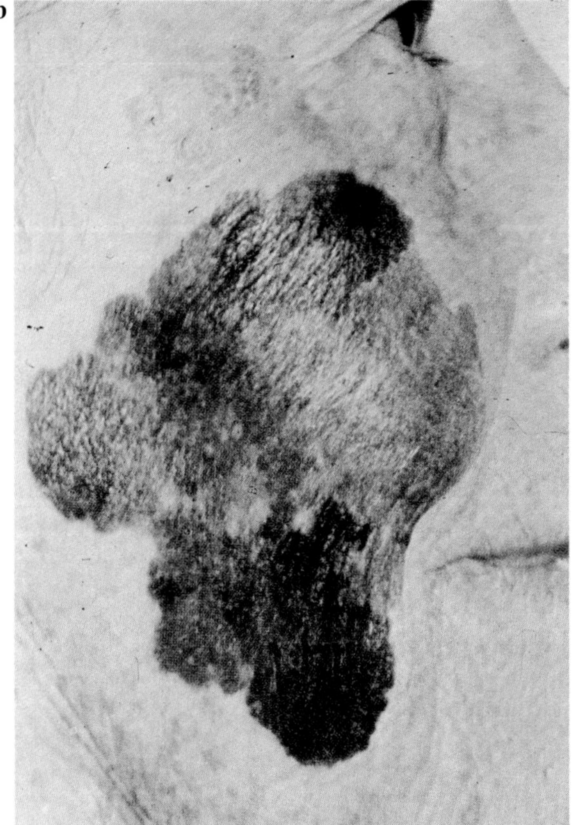

339a Actinic (solar) keratosis. These lesions occur after long exposure to sunlight and are potentially malignant, with a latent period of usually over 10 years. The commonest sites are forehead, cheeks, dorsum of hands and forearms, and in men ears and bald scalp.

339b Lentigo. Pigmented lesion on the face. Senile lentigo is benign, but lentigo maligna develops into an invasive melanoma in about one-third of cases.

0

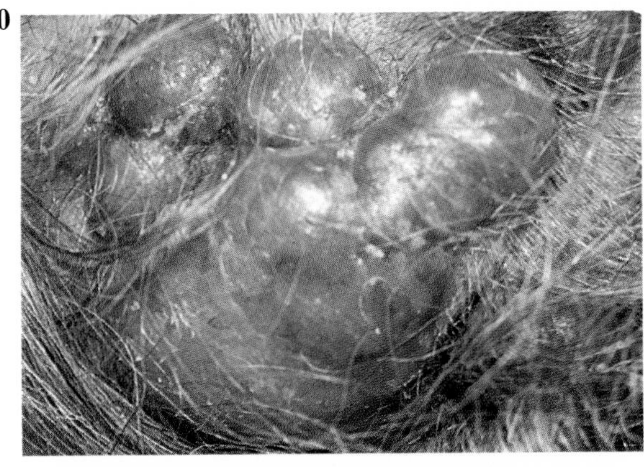

1

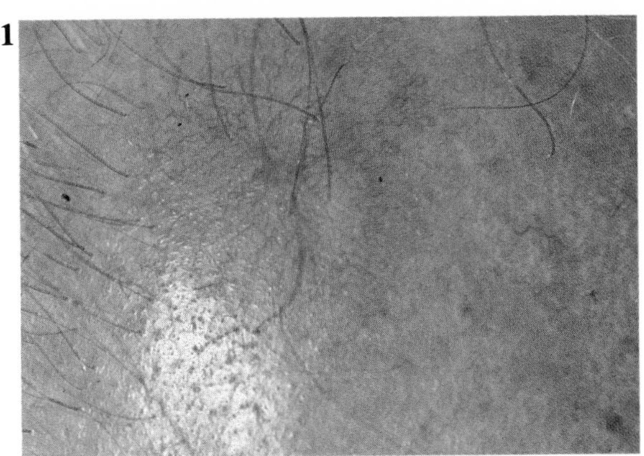

340 Skin secondaries. Cutaneous deposits from internal malignancies are seen occasionally in carcinomatosis. In this case there is a secondary deposit in the scalp from carcinoma of the lung.

341 and 342 Spider naevus on the forehead of an elderly man who had alcoholic liver cirrhosis.

343 Scabies. Producing areas of intense pruritus on the lower limbs. This infestation occurs in those elderly people who have poor personal hygiene with self-neglect.

344 Chronic varicose eczema showing hyperpigmentation around the ankle.

2

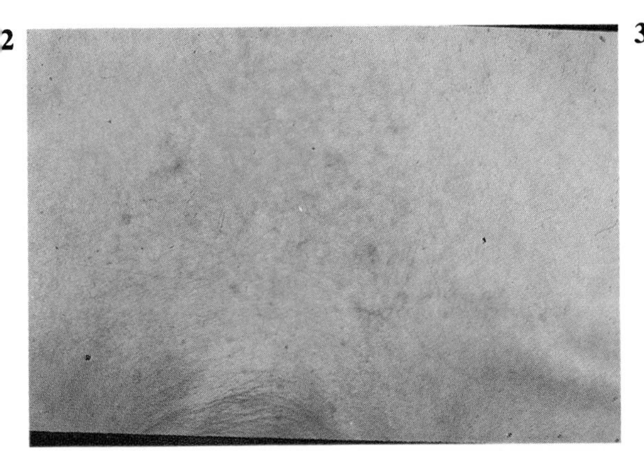

3

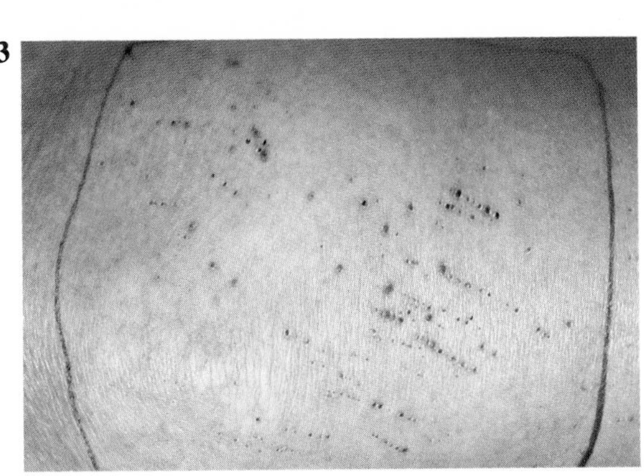

344

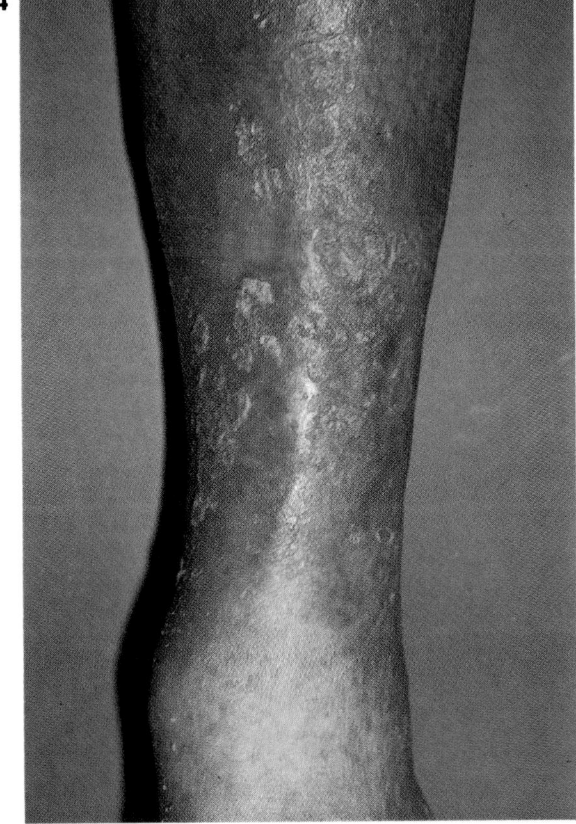

346

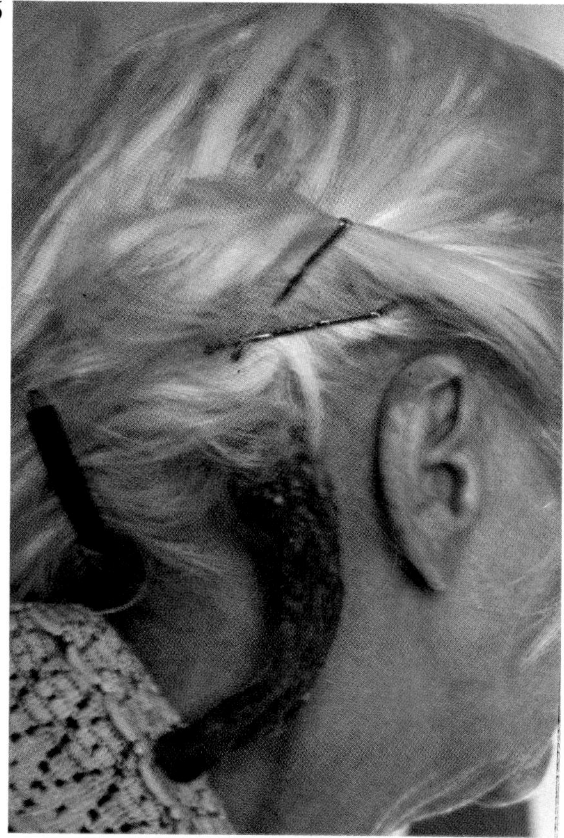

345

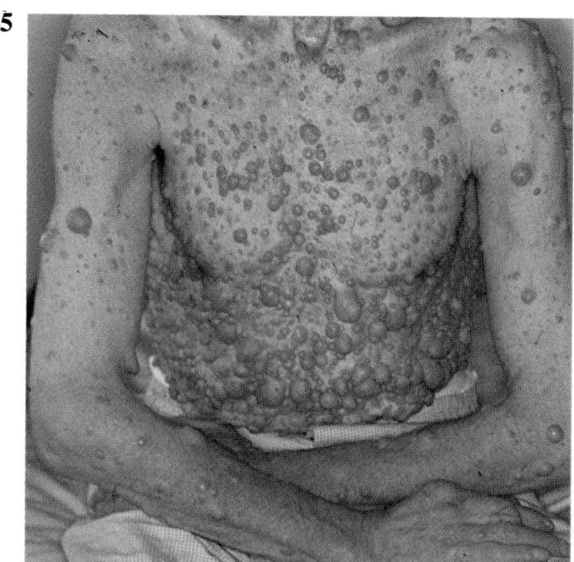

347

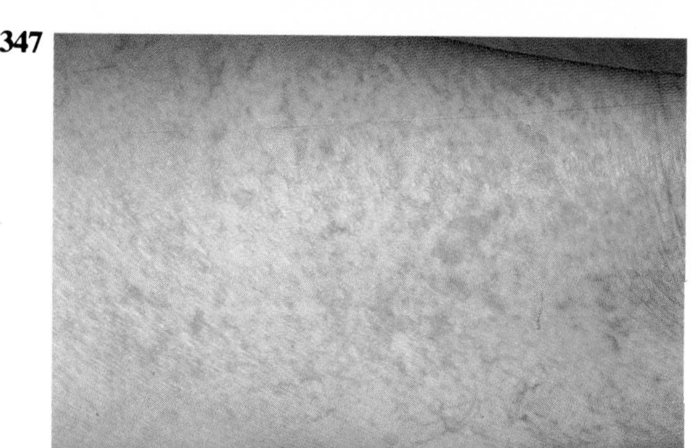

348a

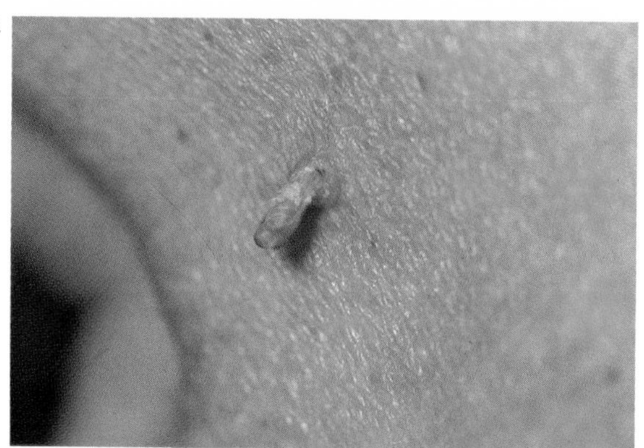

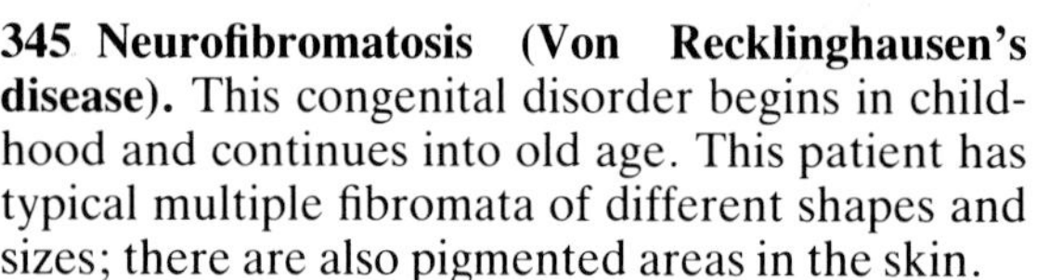

345 Neurofibromatosis (Von Recklinghausen's disease). This congenital disorder begins in childhood and continues into old age. This patient has typical multiple fibromata of different shapes and sizes; there are also pigmented areas in the skin.

346 Sebaceous horn (large). An oddity, sometimes seen in the elderly. It arises from the epidermis and grows slowly. Malignant change occurs rarely in the base of the horn.

347 Drug rash. Widespread macular rash as a result of taking an antibiotic, which also caused mild pruritis.

348a Sebaceous horn (small). A much smaller cutaneous horn. These lesions usually occur on the face or scalp in elderly persons who are seborrhoeic subjects or who have been exposed to strong sunlight.

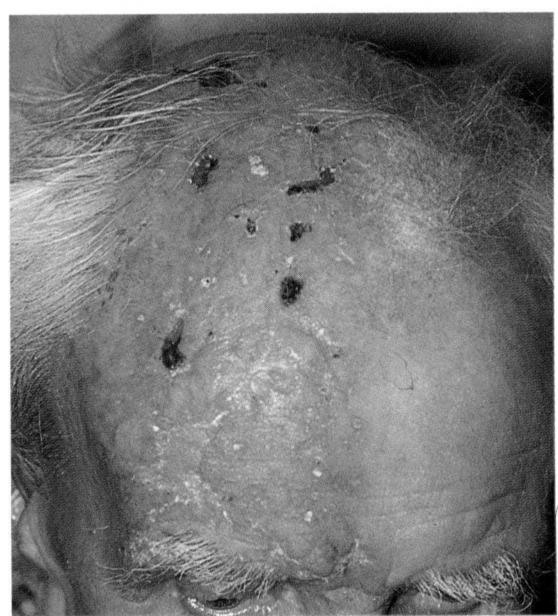

348b Herpes Zoster. Frequent cause of painful skin rash in the elderly. In this case, the rash is resolving, but the patient was left with post-herpetic neuralgia.

349

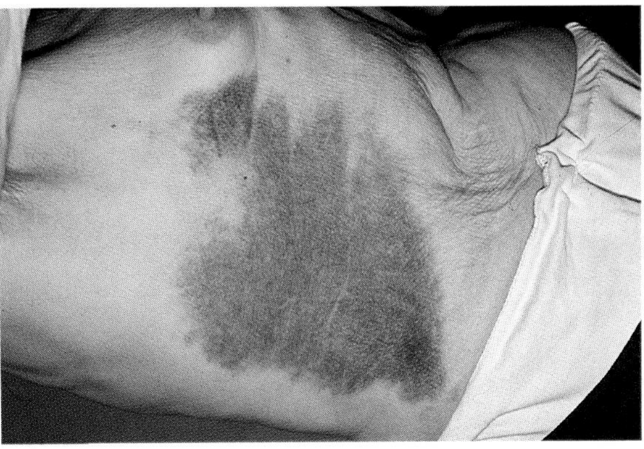

349 Traumatic bruise. A large bruise on the lateral aspect of the chest wall. This injury was caused by a fall and there is considerable pain due to suffering fractured ribs.

350 Erythema craquele (severe xerosis). Typical reticulation and rhomboidal scaling on the legs, commonly seen in the elderly.

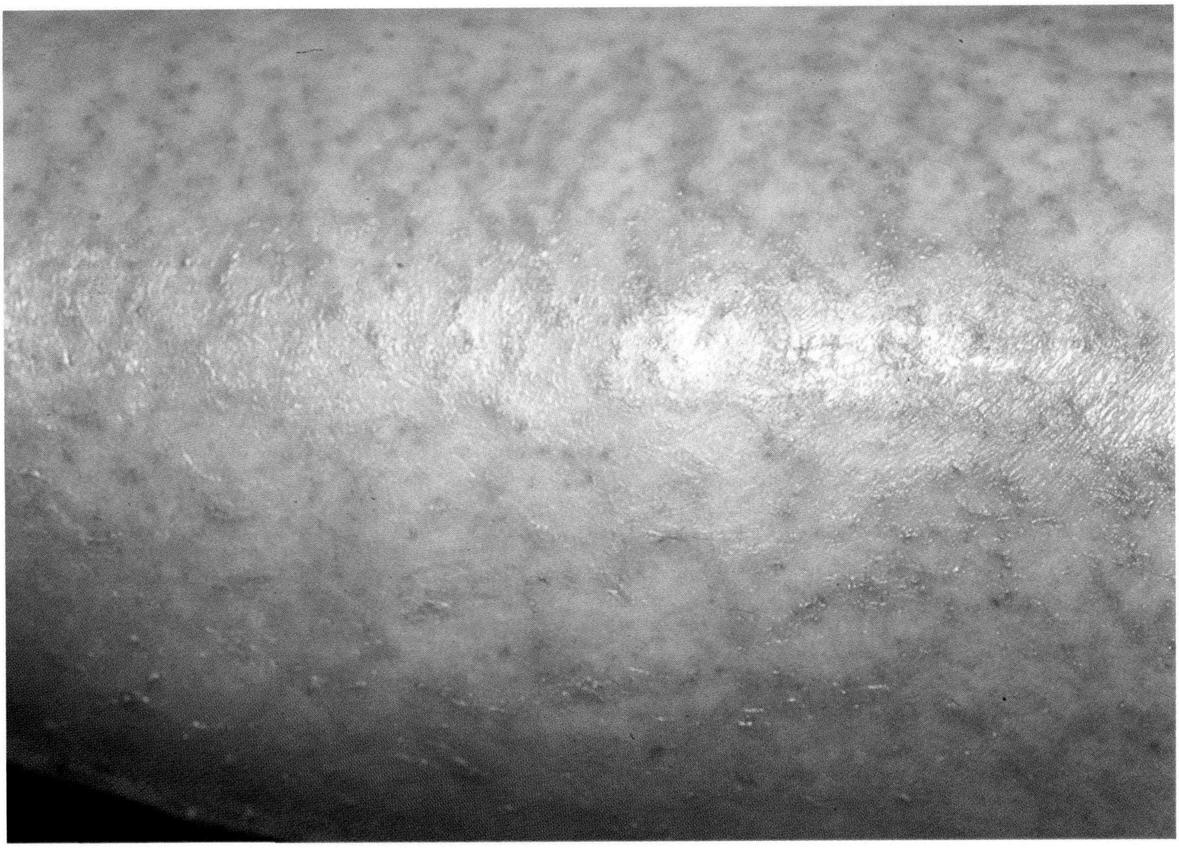

351

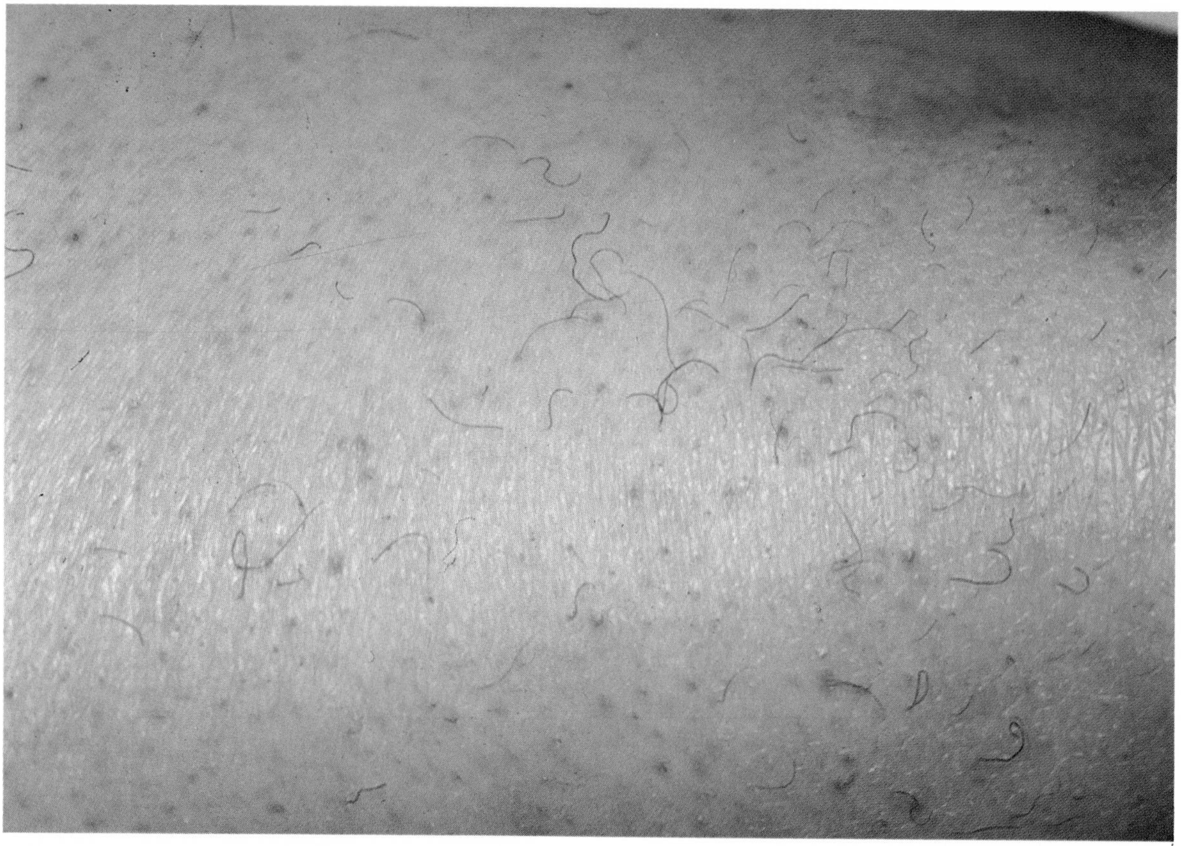

352

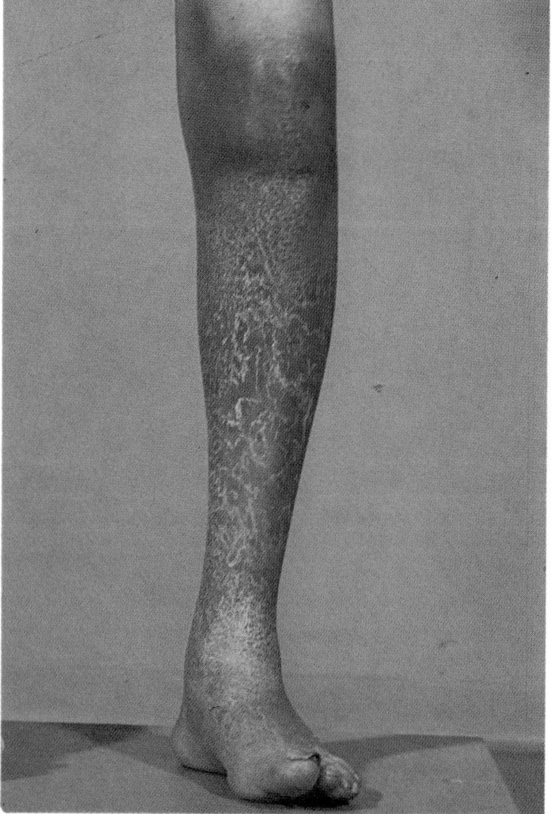

353

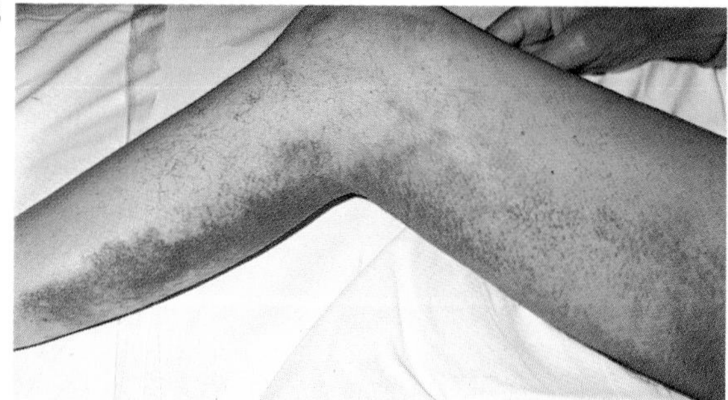

351 Scurvy. Typical 'cork-screw hairs' with perifollicular haemorrhages in an elderly bachelor who had hypovitaminosis-C caused by dietary deficiency.

352 and 353 Scurvy. Sheet haemorrhages in the legs of two other patients with Vitamin-C deficiency. The first patient was an elderly man who lived alone and had a past history of alcoholism.

Hypovitaminosis-C scurvy

'Bachelor scurvy'

Sometimes seen in elderly men, living alone in poor conditions

Clinical features:

Hyperkeratotic papules
Perifollicular haemorrhages
Gum lesions occur only in teeth-bearing jaws
Anaemia
GIT bleeding
Nasal haemorrhage

Bullous skin lesions

Some frequent causes in the elderly

Pemphigus vulgaris
Pemphigoid – 80 per cent of cases in over 60-year-olds
Stevens-Johnson syndrome
Drugs, e.g. bromides, iodides, barbiturates, penicillamine

354

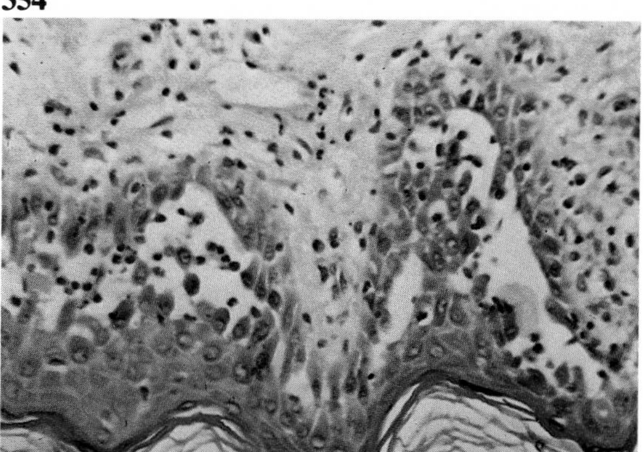

355

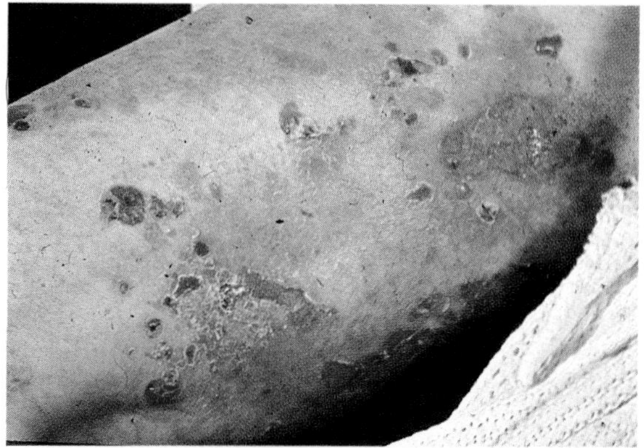

356

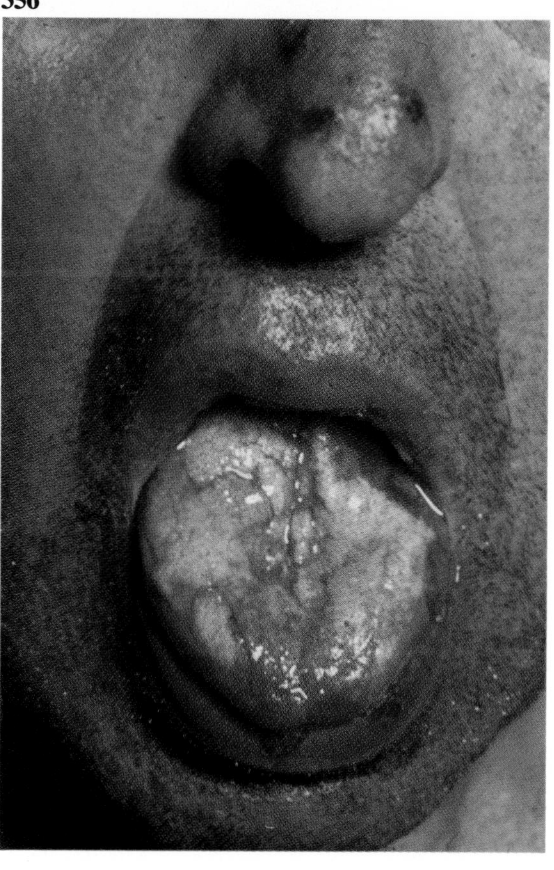

354 Pemphigus. Skin histology showing the characteristic of cell splitting within the epidermal layer called acantholysis.

355 Pemphigus vulgaris. Extensive involvement of the skin. Most of the bullae have burst and the patient is toxic. This is a disease of later life which may involve the mucous membranes as well as the skin.

356 Pemphigus vulgaris showing painful oral lesions. Such patients can be severely ill and may suffer from pain, dehydration, secondary infection, and toxaemia.

357

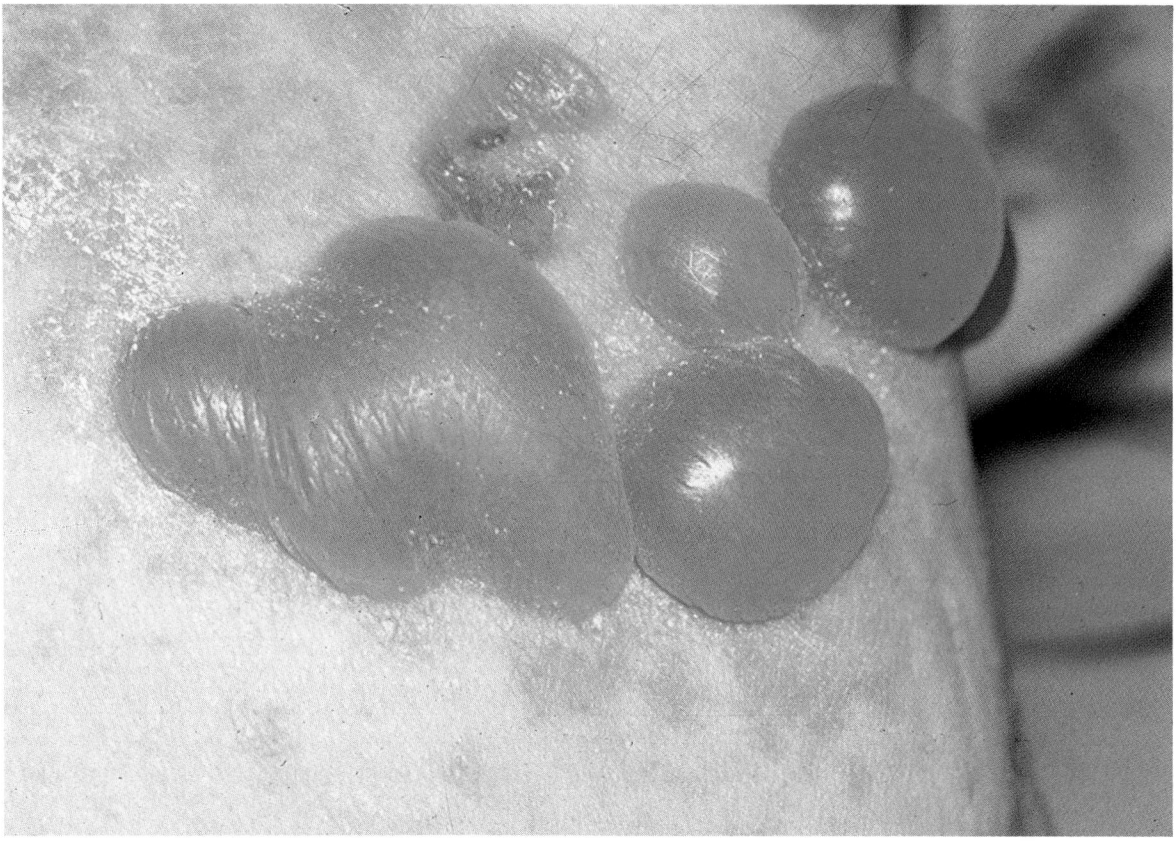

358

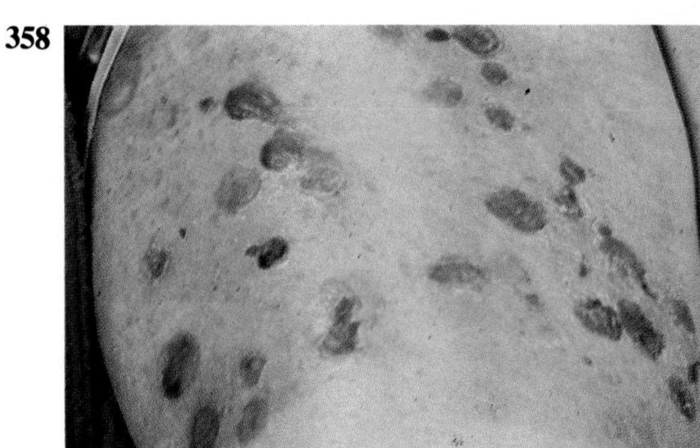

359

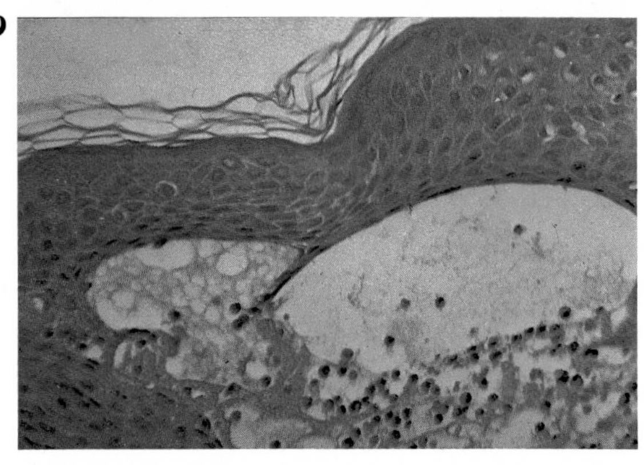

357 Pemphigoid blisters. Tense bullae caused by pemphigoid – disease of old age in which the mucous membrane is affected less commonly than in pemphigus.

358 Pemphigoid blisters. Here the disease is a few days old and some of the blisters have burst.

359 Pemphigoid. Histology showing that the blister is below the epidermis separating it from the dermis.

360

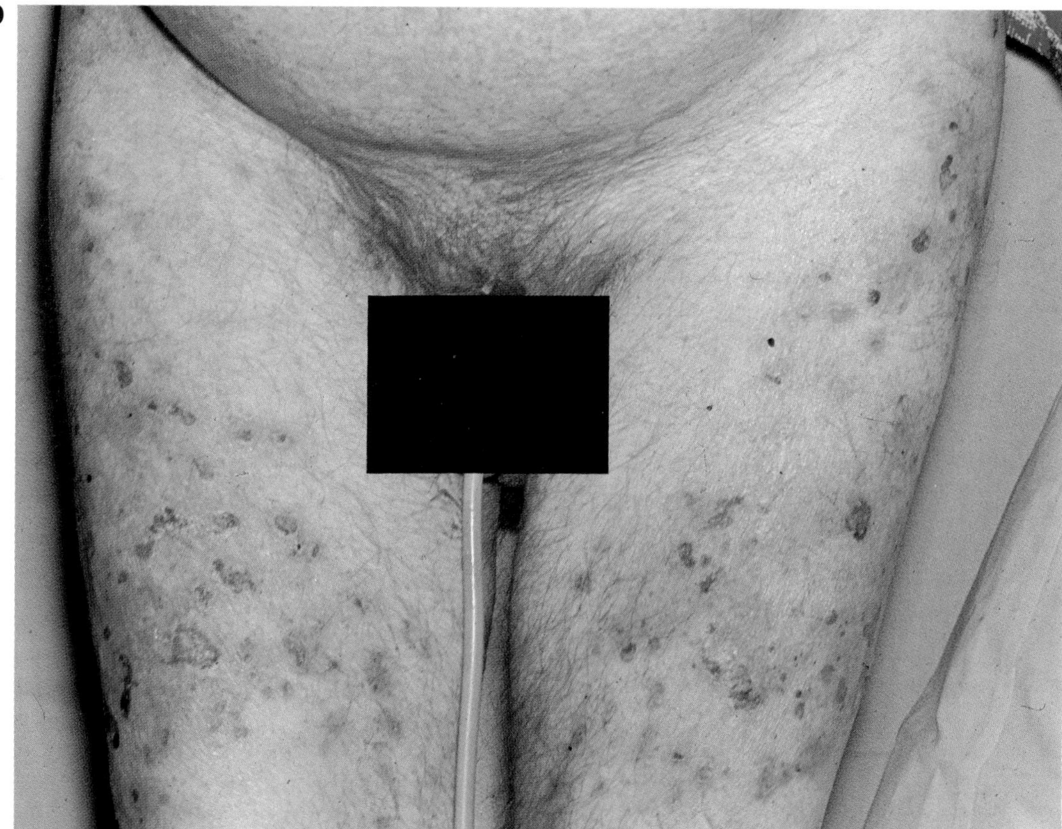

361

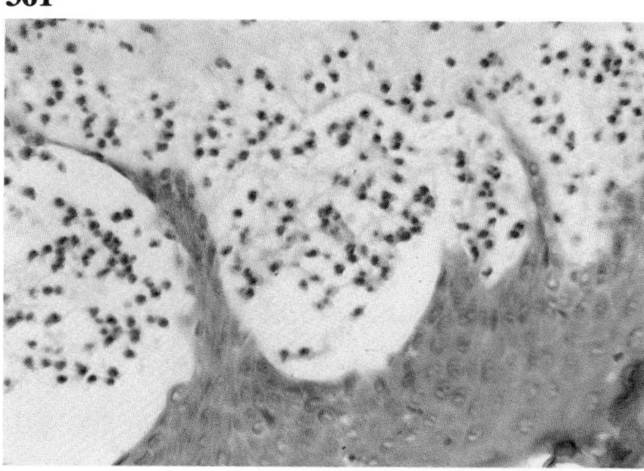

362

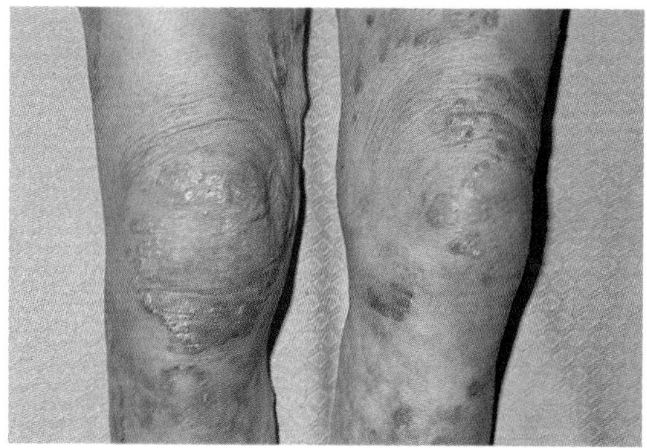

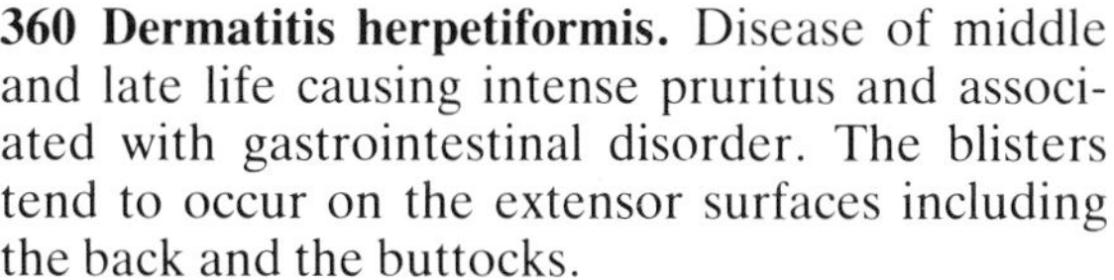

360 Dermatitis herpetiformis. Disease of middle and late life causing intense pruritus and associated with gastrointestinal disorder. The blisters tend to occur on the extensor surfaces including the back and the buttocks.

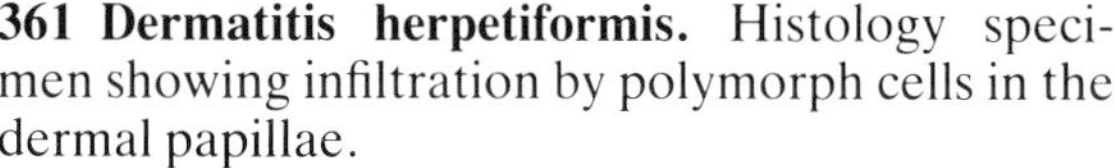

361 Dermatitis herpetiformis. Histology specimen showing infiltration by polymorph cells in the dermal papillae.

362 Psoriasis. A skin disorder seen frequently in the elderly. It is sometimes accompanied by arthropathy and nail changes.

11 Hypothermia in the elderly

A person is said to be hypothermic when his body temperature is below 35°C (95°F). It carries a high morbidity and mortality in the elderly.

A survey carried out by the Royal College of Physicians in 1965, involving ten British hospitals, revealed that over a period of three winter months 0.68 per cent of admissions were the result of accidental hypothermia: 42 per cent of these patients were over 65 years of age. Another study in 1977 revealed that in two London hospitals, over a period of three winter months, 3.6 per cent were elderly patients with hypothermia. A national survey done in 1973 showed that out of 1,020 elderly people living at home 0.52 per cent were hypothermic. The figures for hypothermia are almost always underestimated because:

1 The condition is not recognised
2 Rectal temperature is not checked
3 Patient is found dead in the house

Pathophysiology

There is an increasing gradient of body temperature from the skin outside to tissues deep within the body, the latter being called the central deep or core temperature; it is this core temperature which is important in terms of body metabolism. The easiest and the most reliable method of measuring core temperature is by a low-reading rectal thermometer.

When a person is exposed to cold, the peripheral blood vessels in the skin contract, directing blood away from the periphery and the cold, so preserving core temperature. The difference between central core and superficial skin temperatures can be thought of as a reflection of the body's thermoregulatory efficiency. There is strong evidence that the body's thermoregulatory efficiency declines with age.

The impairment of thermoregulatory efficiency in the elderly is usually multifactorial in origin.

The main aetiological factors are:

1 Physiological fall in body temperature with age
2 Old people are more likely to live in conditions of cold environment
3 Impaired mobility in the elderly
4 Cerebrovascular disease may damage the thermoregulatory centre in the brain
5 Autonomic disturbances in the elderly leading to decreased heat conservation
6 Drugs – for example, sedatives, hypnotics, tranquillisers, alcohol
7 Hypothermia is a frequent complication of myxoedema

There are **four** main reasons why the elderly are so vulnerable to hypothermia:

1 They often live in cold houses to which they have become accustomed
2 Reduced sensitivity to cold
3 They therefore respond poorly to cold temperature; that is by putting on extra clothes, lighting the fire, etc
4 Those who become hypothermic appear to be unable to increase heat production by shivering and are incapable of efficient heat conservation by cutaneous vasoconstriction

Clinical features

Between the temperatures of 35°C and 30°C the mortality is about 33 per cent. Below 30°C the mortality is about 70 per cent. Clinical features vary as the body temperature drops. In the early stages there is mild drowsiness, sluggishness of movement and thought, slurring of speech, mild mental confusion. The skin of the patient, including the abdomen and axillae, feels cold. The patient becomes apathetic, may develop restlessness, and suffer from falls. In the central nervous system, apart from slurring of speech and drowsiness, the patient may have ataxia, increased muscular rigidity, increased neck stiffness, and sluggish tendon jerks.

In the cardiovascular system there is bradycardia and the patient may develop various dysrhythmias. In moderate to severe cases the ECG shows typical features including prolonged PR interval, prolonged QT interval, inversion of T wave, and appearance of J wave.

In the respiratory system there may be hypopnoea, periodic respiration, and bronchopneumonia is usually the terminal feature.

Table 2 Main complications of hypothermia

Bronchopneumonia
Intravascular thrombosis causing – stroke
– myocardial occlusion
– mesenteric occlusion
– peripheral gangrene
Pancreatitis
Pressure sores
Hypoglycaemia may occur, particularly during rewarming

Prevention of hypothermia

Prevention remains the most important aspect of reducing the incidence of hypothermia in the elderly.

Old people should be educated and warned about the dangers of hypothermia. In the UK the Health Education Council publishes various booklets and leaflets which explain in simple language, the methods of preventing, detecting, and managing hypothermia; for example, 'The Winter Warmth Code', 'Looking After Yourself in Retirement', 'Keeping Warm in Winter'. Attention should be directed at housing – especially home insulation and draught-proofing, diet, clothing, supplementary pension, heating allowances, unnecessary drugs, and dangers of polypharmacy and detecting and treating disorders which are associated with hypothermia. Professionals such as the doctor, nurse or health visitor can help particularly if there is anxiety about an old person's health. Another source of help in the UK is the local Social Services Department.

Hypothermia in the elderly is a condition which can be prevented. All efforts should be made to reduce its incidence in old people.

Management

Hypothermia in the elderly is a medical emergency and requires urgent treatment. When confronted with a case of hypothermia, outside the hospital, then:

1 Warm the room up as much as possible
2 Give warm and nourishing drinks or soups
3 Wrap up the person well
4 Keep the patient in bed or sitting in a comfortable chair
5 Call a doctor or an ambulance

Do not do the following:

1 Load heavy blankets on to the person as they trap cold air
2 Use hotwater bottles or electric blankets
3 Encourage movement about the house
4 Give alcohol because this prompts further heatloss

In hospital the treatment is aimed at rewarming the patient at the rate of 0·50°C – 1°C per hour while carefully monitoring the blood pressure. This is best achieved by wrapping the patient in blankets. Nursing should be carried out in a room at a temperature of about 25°C. Other measures consist of rehydration, oxygen inhalation if required, antibiotics given prophylactically; occasionally intravenous hydrocortisone may be required, and if there is convincing evidence of hypothyroidism, then parenteral Tri-iodothyronine should be given.

363

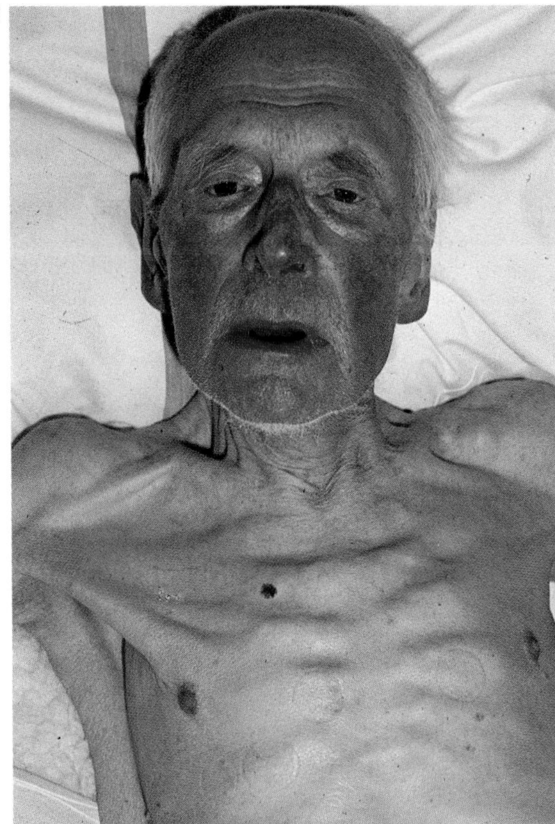

363 Hypothermia. This elderly man lived alone. In spite of being reasonably well-off, he neglected his diet and would not spend any money on domestic heating. He was admitted with bronchopneumonia and hypothermia.

364 Hypothermia. An elderly lady with accidental hypothermia. She had fallen at home and was unable to get up. She lay on the floor through the night and by next morning her rectal temperature was 29°C.

364

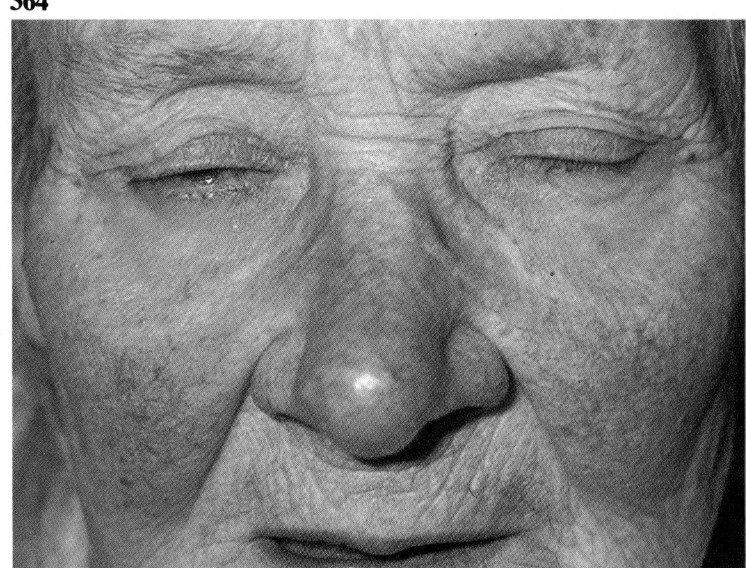

365 Anaemia and hypothermia. This lady was admitted twice with hypothermia over a period of six months. She suffered from chronic anaemia and was taking both diuretics and tranquillisers.

365

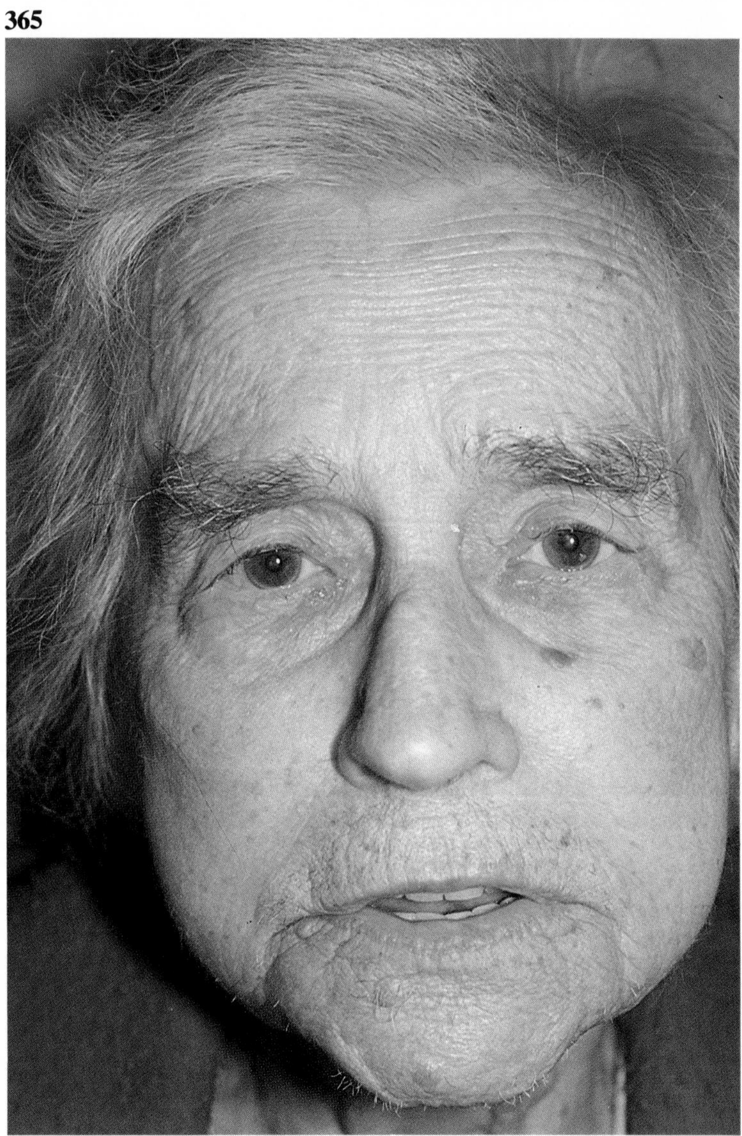

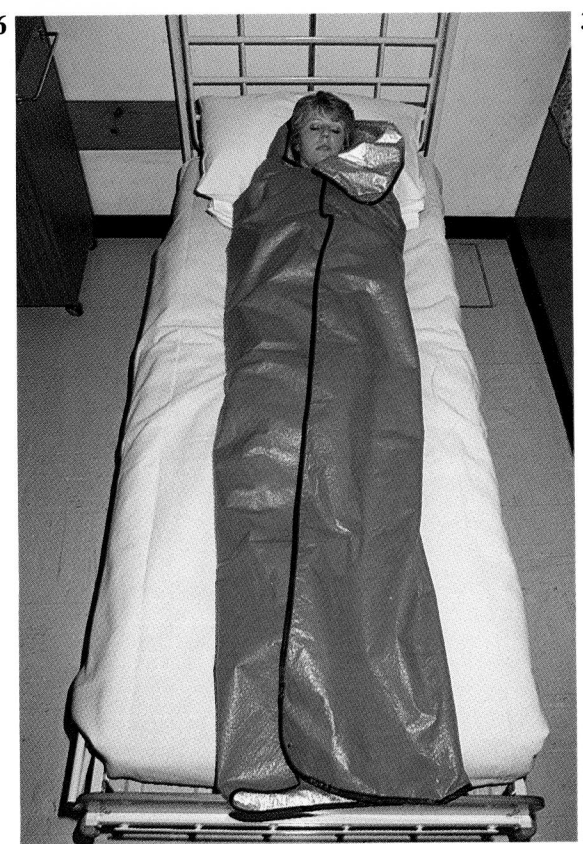

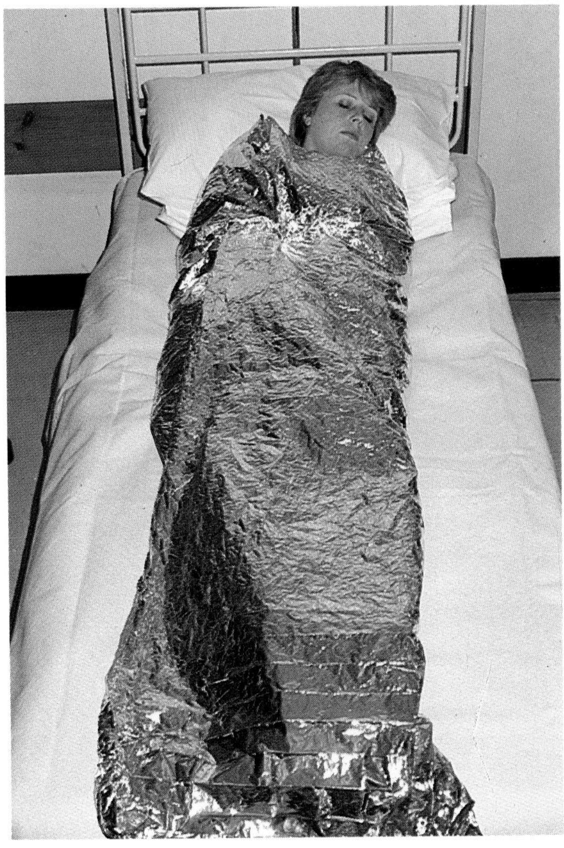

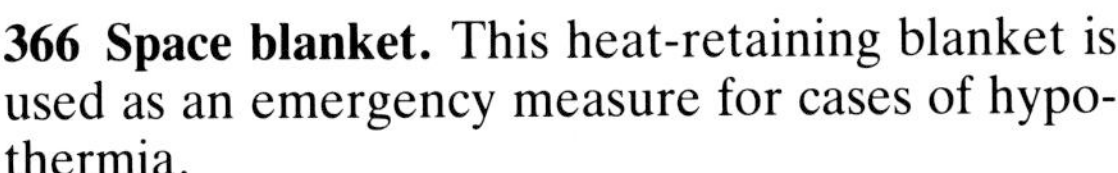

366 Space blanket. This heat-retaining blanket is used as an emergency measure for cases of hypothermia.

367 Foil blanket. Lightweight heat-preserving foil blanket is a good alternative to a space blanket.

368 Bottle of pills. This bottle of pills was found on an elderly lady who suffered with recurrent falls and came to hospital with hypothermia. She was taking about ten different drugs. She took these tablets in a most haphazard manner. She was a victim of 'polypharmacy', 'self medication' and iatrogenic illness.

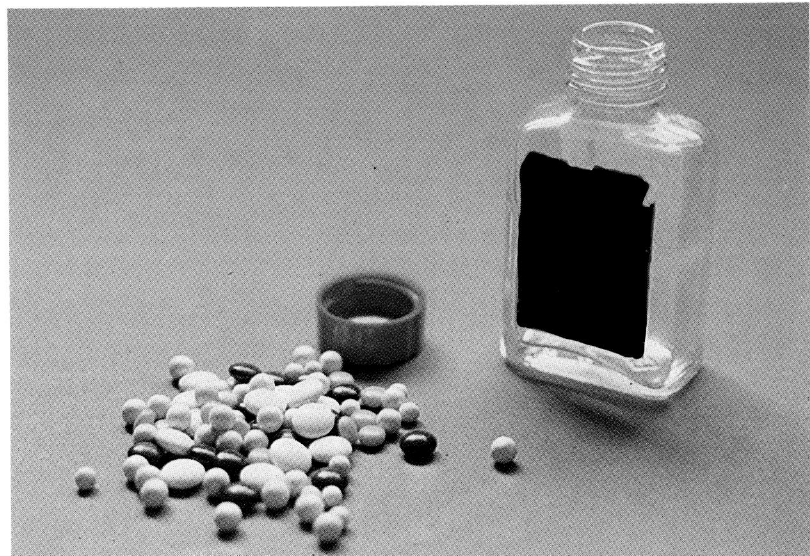

Reference

Bates, C.P., Whiteside, C.G., and Turner-Warwick, R., 'Synchronous cine/pressure/flow/ cystourethrography with special reference to stress in urge incontinence', *Brit. J. Urol.* **42,** 714–723, 1970.

Suggested reading

Anderson, W. F. and Judge, I. G. (editors), *Geriatric Medicine,* Academic Press: London and New York, 1974.

Brocklehurst, J. C. and Hanley, T., *Geriatric Medicine for Students,* Churchill Livingstone, London and New York, 1976.

Brocklehurst, J. C. *Textbook of Geriatric Medicine and Gerontology,* 2nd Edition, Churchill Livingstone, London and New York, 1978.

Coni, N., Davison, W. and Webster, S. *Lecture Notes on Geriatrics,* Blackwell Scientific Publications, London, 1977.

Hodkinson, H. M. *Common Symptoms of Disease in the Elderly,* Blackwell Scientific Publications, London, 1976.

Irvine, R. E., Bagnall, M. K. and Smith, B. J. *The Older Patient: A Textbook of Geriatrics,* 3rd Edition, Unibooks, Hodder and Stoughton, 1978.

Isaacs, B. *Recent Advances in Geriatric Medicine,* Churchill Livingstone, London and New York, 1981.

Pitt, B. *Psychogeriatrics: An introduction to psychiatry of old age,* Churchill Livingstone, London and New York, 1982.

Rai, G. S. and Pearce, V. *Databook on Geriatrics,* MTP Press Ltd., Lancaster, 1980.

Reichel, W. and Schochter, M. (editors), *The Geriatric Patient,* H.P. Publishing Co. Inc., New York, 1978.

Index

Numbers in medium type indicate page numbers; those in **bold** refer to figure and caption numbers.